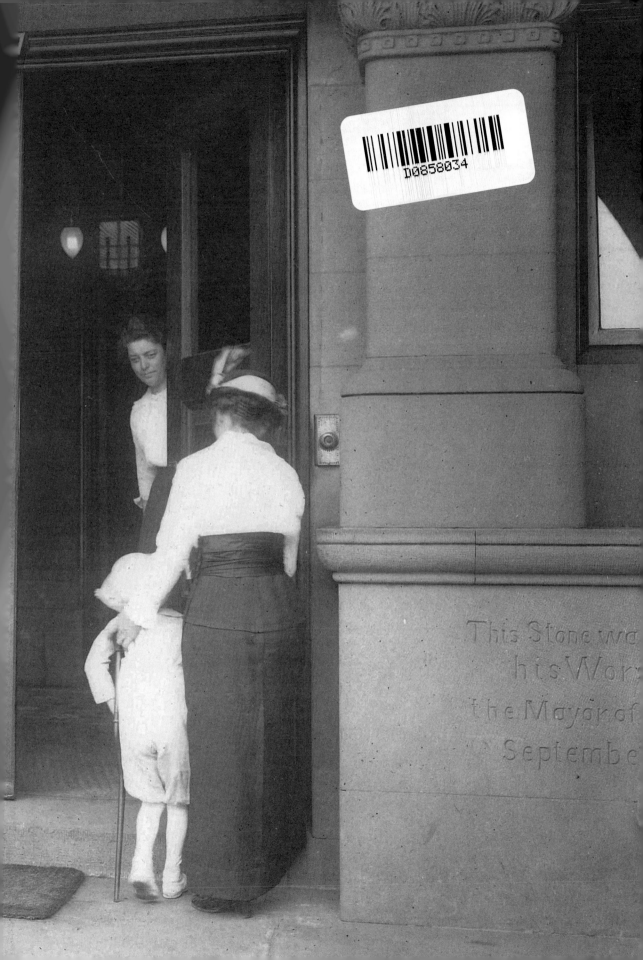

This Stone wa
hts Wor
the Mayor of
Septembe

SickKids

The History of The Hospital for Sick Children

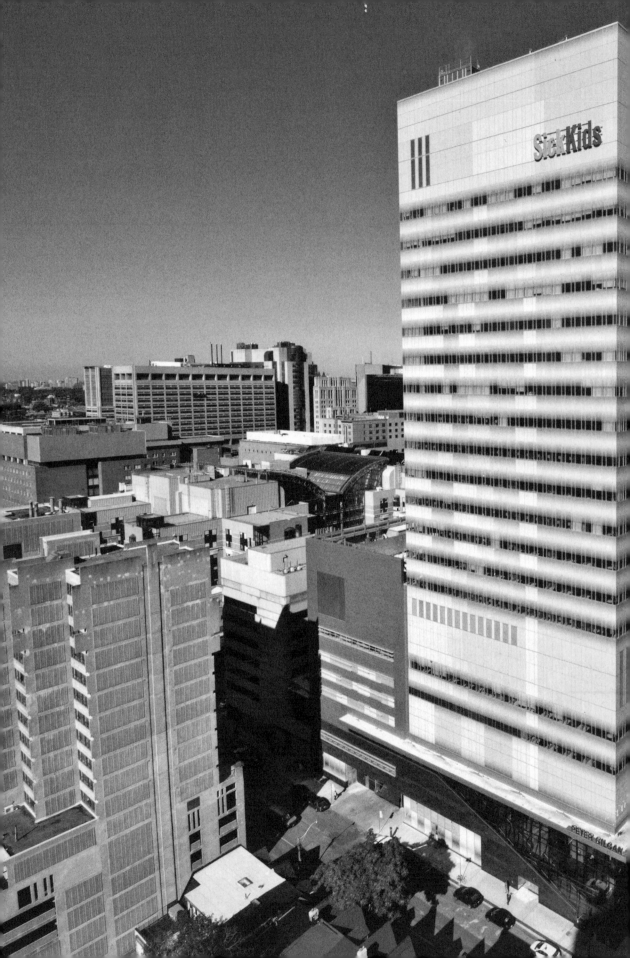

SickKids

The History of
The Hospital for Sick Children

David Wright

University of Toronto Press

Toronto Buffalo London

ISBN 978-1-4426-4723-7

∞ Printed on acid-free, 100% post-consumer recycled paper with
vegetable-based inks.

Library and Archives Canada Cataloguing in Publication

Wright, David, 1965–, author
SickKids : the history of The Hospital for Sick Children / David Wright.

Includes bibliographical references and index.
ISBN 978-1-4426-4723-7 (hardback)

1. Hospital for Sick Children – History. 2. Children – Hospitals –
Ontario – Toronto – History. I. Title.

RJ28.T6W75 2016   362.198920009713′541   C2016-905064-5

University of Toronto Press acknowledges the financial assistance to
its publishing program of the Canada Council for the Arts and the
Ontario Arts Council, an agency of the government of Ontario.

Canada Council   Conseil des Arts
for the Arts   du Canada

ONTARIO ARTS COUNCIL
CONSEIL DES ARTS DE L'ONTARIO
an Ontario government agency
un organisme du gouvernement de l'Ontario

Funded by the   Financé par le
Government   gouvernement
of Canada   du Canada

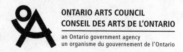

Canadä

SickKids®

Contents

List of Images, Tables, and Charts

Images

Tables

Charts

Foreword

I spent thirty years at The Hospital for Sick Children, known today as SickKids, including ten years during which I had the honour of serving as president and CEO. I experienced the extraordinary power of determination, great medicine, courage, and compassion. And I believed it was important that the rich history of this revered and remarkable hospital be written. The history of SickKids is anchored in Toronto's past, in Canadian history, and in an evolving health-care system. It's the story of an expanding city, waves of immigrants, changes in the way children (and families) have been treated, and the increasingly sophisticated medical interventions they have received. From its early beginnings in the 1870s, this institution proclaimed and maintained its deep and ambitious commitment to the well-being of children.

The story of SickKids needs to be shared, because it has touched the lives of hundreds of thousands of children and their families; it has launched the careers of clinical and scientific trainees who came here to learn and grow and become great contributors to child health around the world; it has garnered the support of philanthropists from all walks of life, who have enabled our mission; and it has galvanized dedicated staff who are the heart and soul of the hospital.

We are indebted to the thousands of people and organizations who have supported our vision for "Healthier Children: A Better World" through their generosity of time and resources. We are deeply grateful, in particular, to Patsy and Jamie Anderson, whose kind donation made this book possible.

I thank author David Wright, a talented Canadian historian whose tireless efforts in researching our past has inspired an optimism for our future. Finally, I am grateful to members of my Advisory Committee – Dr. Denis Daneman, David Estok, Jim Garner, Judith John, Jeff Mainland, Dr. Susan Tallett, and

Dr. Stanley Zlotkin – and to Len Husband and Lynn Fisher of University of Toronto Press for their advice, guidance, and commitment to this project.

It is my hope that, through understanding our early beginnings and the fullness of our past, SickKids leaders and staff will continue this profound commitment to children and families; will strive for excellence in care, research, and teaching; and will embrace the challenge to find answers to the most complex issues that affect the health and well-being of children and youth. Through exemplary care, scientific and medical advances, breakthroughs and setbacks, the SickKids team will be creating the next chapter of our history.

Mary Jo Haddad
Past President and CEO (2004–14)

Acknowledgments

I am deeply indebted to the many people who have implicated themselves in this book over the course of the last four years. First and foremost, I must thank Patsy and Jamie Anderson, who generously donated the money to fund this history project. The manuscript was nurtured by the tireless advocacy of Mary Jo Haddad, the former CEO and president of SickKids. Jim Garner, the former vice-president of the hospital, quarterbacked many of the administrative aspects of the project, with the able assistance of Mirella Andrade. The research enjoyed the enthusiastic support of Denis Danemen, the former chief of paediatrics, who was also co-applicant on internal Research Ethics Board approvals. Mary Jo, Jim, and Denis belonged to a hospital editorial advisory committee that also included Judith John, Jeff Mainland, Stanley Slotkin, Sue Tallett, and David Estok. I feel deeply humbled that they would provide me with unfettered access to hospital resources and also trust my instincts as a researcher to author a scholarly and balanced history of this remarkable hospital.

The Hospital for Sick Children boasts an impressive library in the University Avenue building. I am grateful to the staff, and in particular David Wencer, the hospital archivist, who supported the project through his unrivalled knowledge of SickKids history. Several scholars have already published directly or indirectly on some of the topics covered in the book: the full list of historians can be found in the Further Reading section at the end of this book. I would like to acknowledge, in particular, the scholarship of Judith Young, Annmarie Adams, Jim Connor, Chris Rutty, Edward Shorter, and Noah Schiff. It is clear that long-standing clinicians and administrators at the hospital have important historical perspectives of their own, among them Paul Swyer, the former chief of neonatology, who shared reflections and even family photos. Finally, several McGill undergraduate students assisted along the way, including Honor Lay and Peter Shyba, who inputted and coded hundreds of donations from the annual reports of the last two decades of the nineteenth century, and Martin Ciglenecki, who tracked down patients in the nineteenth-century decennial censuses.

The book profited from sixteen targeted oral interviews of former staff, volunteers, and donors to the hospital that were arranged as part of the project and subject to the hospital's research ethics board protocols. As a consequence, these participants must remain anonymous; however, their insights proved crucial in determining the "anchoring themes" of many chapters as well as providing some timely quotations. In addition to these interviews, the book borrowed generously from previous oral history projects that involved medical practitioners in Toronto and were conducted under the direction of Associated Medical Services (formerly the Hannah Institute for the History of Medicine). Six of these were physician-participants with involvement in The Hospital for Sick Children, and some transcripts included invaluable anecdotes and reflections on periods dating back as far as the 1930s and 1940s. These interviews, conducted in the 1970s, are publicly available at the University of Toronto and are therefore not anonymized. Finally, there have been a small number of internal histories – specifically of paediatrics and nursing – which themselves include transcripts or partial transcripts of the testimony of former medical staff at the hospital. These are also in the public domain and therefore not anonymized. Of course, there are literally hundreds of interviews and testimonials from patients, volunteers, donors, and staff that can be retrieved from newspapers, journals, reels of telethons, radio broadcasts, and television.

The manuscript covers a long time period – over 140 years – and a vertiginous array of medical and historical topics, some of which required a certain degree of technical and scholarly assistance. Historians seek to provide the most historically accurate evidence in their histories. But we are not perfect. Instead, we rely on colleagues to spot glaring, and potentially embarrassing, errors through the formal and informal process of peer review. I would therefore like to acknowledge individuals who donated their time to read chapters, or multiple chunks of chapters, for errors, inaccuracies, omissions, or lack of clarity: Annmarie Adams, John Court, Marlene Goldman, Geoffrey Hudson, Susan Lamb, David Martin, Shelley McKellar, James Moran, Sasha Mullally, Thomas Schlich, and Devon Stillwell. Of course, I would also like to acknowledge the comprehensive feedback of two (anonymous) peer reviewers. Noeline Bridge, who has now indexed many of my books, continues to impress with her organization and professionalism. It was a pleasure, as always, to work closely with Len Husband, Lisa Jemison, Lynn Fisher, and the wonderful team at the University of Toronto Press. Their support, patience, and guidance clearly demonstrate why historians in Canada return over and over again to their publishing house. My mother, Jean Wright, read the entire manuscript (yes, it is true, my mother still reads my written work) and acted as the ultimate arbiter of what would be in the public interest. My wife, Mona, didn't read the transcript at all, but performed the equally important role of psychological counsellor as I missed multiple self-imposed deadlines. Yes, I know, I promised the book would be completed by the end of 2013. But what are two years in the grand sweep of history?

I must say more than a few words about my research assistant, Renée Saucier. I first met Renée when she was a final-year undergraduate history student at McGill University in 2012. I required a summer research assistant, and she was recommended warmly by a colleague in the department of history. After nearly twenty years as an academic, one can spot those special students almost instantaneously. Renée was frighteningly intelligent, mature well beyond her years, and – most important to me – almost entirely without immediate employment prospects. It was, as they say in Québécois, *le bon timing*. We have worked together for almost four years on a variety of projects, but principally on this book. Just as I did not expect the book to take as long as it did, I was equally startled to have the support and insights of Renée for the entire project, from push-off to publication. For this, I must thank the Department of Immigration and Citizenship Canada, who proved incapable of processing her application for Landed Immigrant Status in anything resembling a timely manner. As a consequence, Renée was tied, serf-like, to Toronto, forced to see this book to completion, when one might have reasonably expected someone so highly skilled to have moved on to something far more appropriate for her enviable skill set. Her hard work, attention to detail, and critical insights are interwoven throughout the book. Renée, what can I say? People really don't need more Canada. Canada needs more people like you.

It is impossible to write a book on the history of children and not reflect upon one's own. Indeed, there have been no few times when I, like the interviewee who opens the introduction, had to pause to gather myself. Writing about children, some of whom die from horrible diseases or debilitating congenital conditions, is no easy thing for a parent. One could easily retreat from the social history of paediatric suffering – providing instead a dry catalogue of the hospital's physical growth and administration – or indeed, err in the opposite direction and risk indulging in a maudlin account of childhood suffering and triumph over adversity. It is a difficult balance to strike. Writing history is, at the end of the day, an imperfect and rather humbling exercise in crafting narratives of understanding from fragmentary and often ambiguous sources. But perhaps no more humbling than being a parent.

It is fitting, therefore, that I should dedicate this book to my own *enfants terribles*: Naomi, Neil, and Gopika. May the authoring of your own histories be filled with wonder, optimism, and good health.

David Wright
Montréal, Québec

SickKids

The History of The Hospital for Sick Children

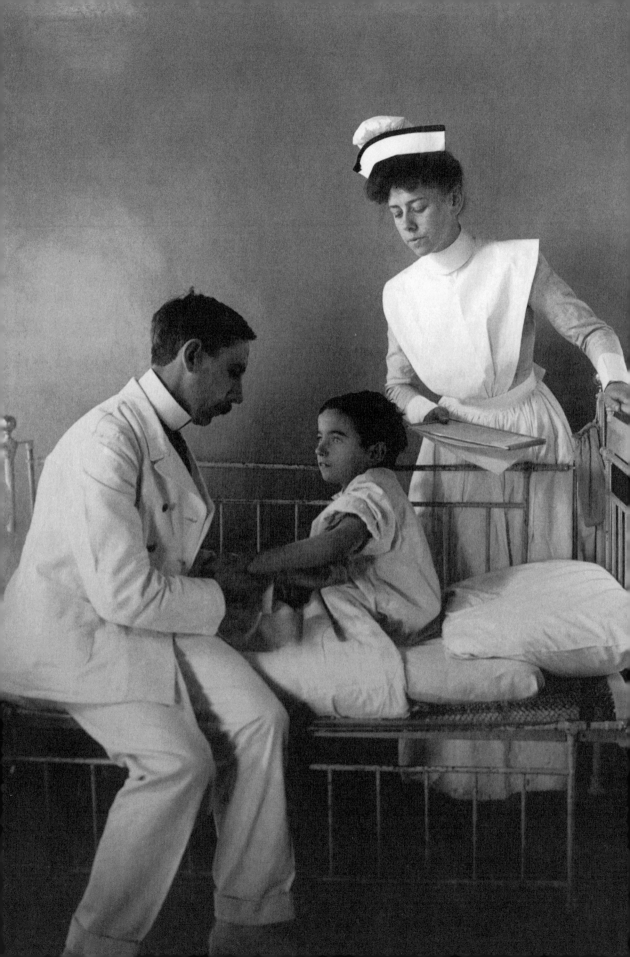

Introduction

The degree of confidence and affection on the part of the public is
sometimes frightening when one realizes that an institution is a collection of human beings who are subject to all of the frailties and
limitations of humans.[1]

> J.T. Law, Director of The Hospital for Sick Children, 1964

"So tell me ... what it was like on the wards with the patients when you began as
a staff member?" We were relaxing in a well-appointed condominium in North
Toronto, enjoying a latte. I was conducting one of over a dozen select interviews
that I completed on behalf of the project supporting this book. The retired
physician was amiable and generous with his time, recounting numerous
personal and professional anecdotes about why he had become a paediatrician, and how his field of clinical practice had been transformed immeasurably
over the decades. But suddenly his demeanour changed and his eyes swelled
with emotion. "Sure.... Well I think the first thing that happened, when I was
a resident in '65 or '66 ... there was this young girl, she was ten years old ... and
I stayed up with her and the parents all night to sit and watch her die ...
That was their only child." He paused to compose himself. "Sorry, getting a
little sentimental about this ..." He paused again. "Anyway, her mother ... I saw
her one day ... and I said, 'It just shows you what timing is in terms of medical
care. Here I am, four years later, and [with the evolution
of clinical techniques] I could have saved your child's
life.'" "Where did you meet her?" I inquired rather
awkwardly. "Oh ... she had become a volunteer for
the hospital and I ran into her on one of the wards."[2]

I.1 A doctor and nurse strike a
stylized pose with a patient,
symbolically representing the
modern medical encounter in a
formal institutional environment.

Hospitals occupy a prominent and complicated place in Western society. They encompass sites of death and birth, of cardinal discoveries and personal tragedies. The role they now fulfil in the complex of healing and suffering has never been constant: it has changed dramatically and, at times, unexpectedly over the course of history. Before the last decades of the nineteenth century, hospitals were predominantly religious and charitable institutions for the destitute of society, dubbed "gateways to death," with sanitary provisions scarcely better than those in the slums from whence their indigent patients came. Respectable members of society would never set foot in these institutions, tainted, as they were, by pauperism and despair. But slowly over the course of the last 150 years, hospitals emerged at the centre of a new, modern, and scientific infrastructure, where technology and laboratory science reshaped the architecture, patient population, and clinical practice of health care. By the mid-twentieth century, the hospital, for better or worse, became the defining element of medicine, the living laboratory in which scientific discovery would occur, the transformative site of birth and death, and the institutional locus around which universal health insurance would be constructed.

It should surprise few that, along with famous epidemics and biographies of medical pioneers, hospital histories have long been a mainstay of scholarship in the history of medicine. They are the most popular and accessible types of publication; they are also, at times, the most controversial and criticized. Unlike more abstract concepts such as "medical professionalization" and the "great epidemiological transition," people *know* hospitals; they see them, work for them, donate to them, and are treated in them. Hospitals attract lifelong attachments, deep loyalties and, from time to time, antipathies. They embody urban cultures and reflect civic pride. In a manner of speaking, they take on personalities in and of themselves. The more important they are, the more passions they engender, and the more public are their shortcomings.

Most hospital histories have been labours of love, initiated by long-serving and dedicated staff of a particular institution. These internal histories have garnered, perhaps unfairly, a poor reputation within academic scholarship. For critics, too much time was devoted to claiming firsts, enumerating heads of departments, and omitting uncomfortable truths. Patients' perspectives, and the social context of the institutions, were often left in the background, as were the subtle relations between disparate non-medical groups who found their way into the institutions. Hospital histories that coincided with landmark anniversaries hinted at an intention that a particular publication was more an exercise in institutional self-congratulation than reflective scholarship. Indeed, so ubiquitous were histories written by insiders that it became frowned upon for academic historians to even contemplate doing so. The medical historian Jim Connor, who would later go on to author an impressive history of the Toronto General Hospital, lamented a generation ago that his colleagues had abandoned serious scholarship in the history of hospitals in this country.[3]

The tendency of professional historians to steer clear of hospital histories was not from a lack of dedicated scholars in the history of medicine. Quite the contrary. Canadians outside of the academy may not necessarily appreciate – being the Canadians that we are – the remarkable depth and breadth of scholarship in medical history that has arisen over the last generation in this country. Foundations such as Associated Medical Services in Toronto, which established the Hannah Chairs in medical schools in Ontario and elsewhere; federal government initiatives such as the Canada Research Chairs program (of which there are at least ten in the history of medicine); as well as taxpayer-supported research through federal granting agencies have enabled significant programs of research in this exciting field (see Further Reading, at the end of this book). We now have an impressive scholarship in the history of health and medicine in Canada. Notwithstanding the history of lunatic asylums (which have always been popular), hospitals have tended to fulfil the role of mere supporting cast in some of the most famous discoveries in Canada – such as the discovery of insulin – as captured in the magnificent work of Michael Bliss.[4]

Such holds true for the most famous hospital in the entire country – The Hospital for Sick Children in Toronto – which still has no comprehensive history attached to it. This despite the fact that "SickKids," as it is popularly known, has been the site of some of the most important paediatric advances in the world, including the iron lung for polio victims, pioneering paediatric surgery on congenital heart malformations (the Mustard procedure), as well as the discovery of the genetic basis for certain diseases (such as the gene for cystic fibrosis), to name only a few among many. In the 1890s, through the generosity of newspaper magnate John Ross Robertson, the hospital's early proponents built an impressive hospital that powered it to the top of the paediatric world by the dawn of the twentieth century, with state-of-the-art surgical theatres, an X-ray department, and a convalescent home on the Toronto Islands. Scientific breakthroughs – such as the royalties

derived from its bestselling (if awful-tasting) nutritional cereal, Pablum —
would bankroll the hospital's research program for a good part of the
twentieth century.

By 1951, the citizens of Toronto responded to the physical decline of the
College Street hospital by supporting the largest-ever fundraising drive in
Canadian history, enabling a new hospital on University Avenue that was
the envy of the paediatric world. It drew leading researchers from all over
the globe. It was the "United Nations in the staff room," as one retired and
foreign-trained doctor recalls, as well as, for a while, reputedly the largest
children's hospital in the world. The positioning of the hospital as the only
paediatric hospital in a city that was, by the middle of the twentieth century,
fast becoming one of the largest urban centres in North America, gave it an
unparalleled monopoly on patients and public influence. Its affiliation to the
University of Toronto involved it in some of the most important discoveries
of medicine, including the Nobel Prize–winning researcher, Frederick Banting,
who would head the diabetes unit at the children's hospital in the 1930s. By
contrast, The Hospital for Sick Children was also the dramatic backdrop for
two of the most controversial events in late twentieth-century Canadian
medicine — the death of an indeterminate number of babies from apparent
digoxin poisoning in the early 1980s, and, almost two decades later, the controversy over hospital researcher Nancy Olivieri's whistle-blowing. Both events
shook it to its core, leading to a questioning of its management, its institutional
priorities, and the future of the hospital as it entered the twenty-first century.

I approach this subject with great familiarity with the field of medical
history but little prior knowledge of the hospital itself. My own research has
explored the history of childhood mental disability within the history of
Britain and Canada.[5] As for SickKids, I had no association with the hospital
itself before I began writing this book. I was never treated there, and lived
in Toronto for only three years of my life. My only personal connection to
SickKids was that my brother-in-law, now a paediatric neurosurgeon in the
United States, completed his residency (post-graduate training) at SickKids
over twenty years ago. It seems, however, that one cannot escape connection
to the institution. I found out, only during the latter stages of research for
this book and entirely by chance, that my great-uncle was treated as a polio
outpatient at the College Street hospital sometime in the 1910s.

During my own training as a social historian of medicine, the new scholarship in the field emphasized the importance of understanding medical
history from the perspectives of both patients *and* practitioners. Health care,

I was told repeatedly, must be understood historically as a dynamic encounter between these two parties, neither of whom was all-powerful. This warning to understand the interplay and bidirectionality of health care was certainly helpful in rebalancing a field (medical history) which had been, up to that point, too focused on "dead white men." In retrospect, however, the admonition was also far too binary; it omitted the fact that there were *multiple* parties who influenced the medical encounter – families, volunteers, donors, nurses, non-medical staff, and administrators. Hospitals were the point of intersection of many diverse communities whose interests and visions often coincided, and sometimes clashed. As a consequence, the history of clinical care of children is, indeed, central to this history of Toronto's Hospital for Sick Children, but it is only one of many interwoven stories and themes that animate the pages that follow.

This book, then, understands the history of The Hospital for Sick Children in accordance with professional standards of historical scholarship; it seeks to be intellectually honest, forthright, and balanced, accessible to an audience well beyond academic historians. No single history, of course, can do full justice to the complexity of any institution that has been in constant flux and that has treated, literally, hundreds of thousands of patients. All historical narratives involve a delicate and painstaking process of selection, ordering, and analysis. To be blunt: a lot of really interesting stuff had to be left out, and I suspect if there are any disappointments with the book, they will arise more from omission than analysis. I have tried, in the end, to emphasize failures as well as triumphs, and to embrace the ambiguities of historical action – the sacrifice as well as self-interest that came to play in many cardinal events. The hospital was, and is, a *public* institution, full of individuals, with their own hopes, dreams, ambitions, and frailties.

Over the course of my writing during the last three years, there remains little doubt that patients and practitioners, volunteers and donors, feel deeply passionate about SickKids. Despite its setbacks and public controversies, the hospital retains a profound affection in the hearts and minds of its former (and current) patients, their family members, and the medical and non-medical staff who have served in the institution. It is very difficult to find anyone living in Toronto who has not been treated in, volunteered on behalf of, or worked for The Hospital for Sick Children. To write a history of this famous institution, then, to borrow John Law's frank admission, is somewhat frightening. But, then again, the most fascinating research projects probably always are.

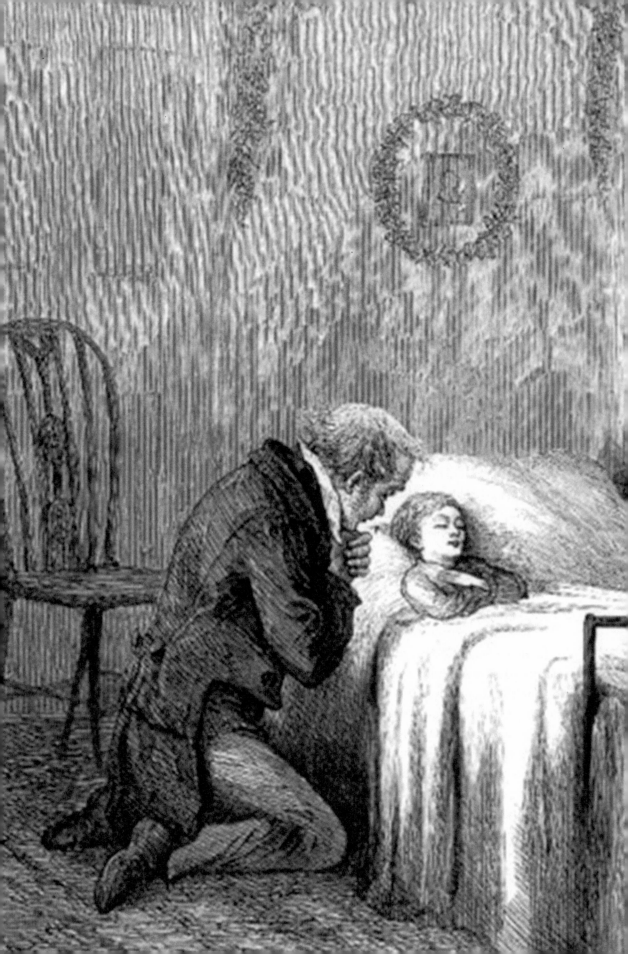

ONE

Between the Cradle and the Grave

"We want to move Johnny to a place where there are none but children; a place set up on purpose for sick children; where the good doctors and nurses pass their lives with children, talk to none but children, touch none but children, comfort and cure none but children." "Is there really such a place?" asked the old woman, with a gaze of wonder. "Yes, Betty, on my word, and you shall see it."[1]

Charles Dickens, *Our Mutual Friend* (1864–5)

The Invention of Childhood

Children haunted the landscape of industrial society. As poor families streamed in from the countryside to chaotic urban centres, communities struggled to maintain and reinvent family relations in unforgiving metropolitan environments. Abandoned infants, penniless orphans, petty juvenile criminals – they were all part of the social reality and literary imagination of industrial Britain and North America. Threadbare welfare systems, like the English Poor Laws and their much-caricatured workhouses, strained to sustain a mobile population for which they were ill-equipped and unintended. Unsupervised children wandering the streets and engaging in the informal and as yet

1.1 "Poor Tiny Tim!," from Charles Dickens's *A Christmas Carol* (1869). Such depictions not only captured childhood suffering but also served as an allegory for the crippling effects of industrialization.

unregulated market in child labour occasioned a mixture of disdain, resignation, and anxiety. The frightening levels of infant and childhood mortality have led some historians to conclude that children, in the early industrial world, were an "expendable commodity" in whom few affective relations could, or should, be invested. The life stage of *childhood*, with all our contemporary cultural assumptions and expectations, simply did not exist at the time.[2]

From the human drama of the industrial city, however, a new understanding of children began to emerge, one that challenged the more traditional view of them as "little adults" produced en masse for the transmission of property, for cheap labour, or as a hedge against infirmity when parents aged and became dependent themselves. In the English-speaking world, we associate this new, contested view of children's place in the world with the writings and social reform of Charles Dickens. Dickens's novels contain dramatic portrayals of the suffering, neglect, mistreatment, ill health, and disability of children. As Robert Newsom suggests, "Not just a reverence for the child, but an often intense fear for the child's welfare and a sometime morbid sentimentality hover about Dickensian children, many of whom die young."[3] Some scholars have speculated that Dickens's youthful experiences on the brink of poverty and later personal tragedies inspired his interest in the plight of children.[4] Regardless of the psychological origins of his fiction, Dickens played a vital role in the popularization of a new view of childhood, one that emphasized sentimentality, physical separation from adult pursuits, and a life stage — deserving protection, rights, and considerations — that differed fundamentally from adulthood.

In his voluminous writings, Dickens paid particular interest to "crippled children," representing them as blameless victims suffering from infirmities that were closely linked with poverty and deprivation. Disability, for this towering literary figure, was both a physical condition and a metaphor for the social ills of unrestrained capitalism. In *Nicholas Nickleby*, for example, Dickens presents the physical impairments of the inhabitants of Dotheboys Hall (a school for boys with physical disabilities) as inextricably linked to their social suffering. The moral vacuum created by industrial capitalism, according to the author, had injured physically, as well as emotionally, the youth of urban Britain. Children needed to be rescued from cruel circumstances in which they found themselves and over which they had no control. Amidst the depressing circumstances of the Industrial Revolution there was also a growing optimism that a new "age of improvement" was dawning. It was possible to ameliorate the plight of sick and impoverished children. What was lacking, Dickens implied, was the moral imperative to do so.[5]

Premature death was as much the focus of social reformers as permanent disability and disfigurement were. In early Victorian England of the 1840s and 1850s, the time during which Dickens began to write his early fiction, the estimated rate of infant mortality hovered around 200 per 1,000 live births. In less abstract terms, two children out of ten died before their first birthday; four in ten perished before reaching the age of five. Childhood death was thus an ever-present tragedy of all classes, even if it was a tragedy concentrated, unsurprisingly, among the poorest and most migrant groups of the cities. The reasons were multiple and are widely debated among medical historians. Certainly, outbreaks of infectious diseases played an important role. Cholera epidemics in 1832, 1848, 1854, and 1866 devastated the urban environments of Britain and North America, demonstrating the impact of "shock diseases" that destabilized communities as they travelled inexorably westward with migrant groups and trade. Typhoid, diphtheria, and measles all arrived and left in terrifying waves, accelerated by infected drinking water, crowded living conditions, poor sanitation, and inadequate nutrition. Even if governments were winning the war against smallpox – due, in part, to the controversial imposition of compulsory vaccination – there were many other childhood killers to replace this ancient plague. Less dramatic but no less lethal endemic scourges also left their mark, physically and socially, on the children of industrial Britain, including consumption (the Victorian term for tuberculosis) and its sister condition, scrofula.[6] Other childhood killers, such as scarlet fever (scarlatina), have now faded from memory, but were among the hordes of viral and bacterial infections that erupted from time to time in different urban locations and carried away the most vulnerable.

The emergence of government surveys in the nineteenth century, such as the decennial censuses and the civil registration of births and deaths, commenced with the beginning of Victoria's reign in the late 1830s.[7] These imperfect exercises in social surveillance generated the raw data that would lead to a new epidemiological concept during the early Victorian era – the belief in "excess" mortality. The comparative study of individual neighbourhoods in London in the 1840s, in particular, demonstrated fairly conclusively to contemporaries that where one lived had a direct impact on one's likelihood of dying. The logical extension was that the deaths of thousands of children (and adults) living in poorer districts were unnecessary and preventable. Such findings shook the centuries-old fatalism that high infant and childhood mortality was somehow a natural state of affairs about which nothing much could be done. It also promoted the view that poor sanitation, malnutrition, and poverty – rather than luck or Divine Providence – accounted for premature death. Dickens, who was on friendly terms with some of the prominent social scientists and medical reformers of the time, attempted to represent, in dramatic literary form, the physical toll of childhood deaths:

> In London alone, there die in a year young children enough to make an unbroken line of corpses, lying head to foot, along the kerb-stone on each side of the way, from Bow Church down the Bow-road, through Mile-end, and down the Mile-end-road, Whitechapel-road, Whitechapel, Aldgate, and on through Leadenhall-street, the Poultry, Cheapside, and on still through Newgate-street and Skinner-street, to line with dead children both sides of the whole length of Holborn and Oxford-street, to beyond Kensington-gardens.[8]

Although Dickens's "line of corpses," guiding visitors through the squalid and infested streets of Victorian London, might strike some as morbid and melodramatic, there was something raw and moving in his observations. As the returns of the new system of civil registration demonstrated, half of all deaths reported in any given year in the 1850s and 1860s were attributed to children under the age of five. Childhood death lurked everywhere and became a recurring theme in Victorian popular culture. To borrow just one illustrative statistic from hundreds, during each year of Victoria's reign – from 1837 to 1901 – no fewer than 7,000 people in Great Britain, mostly children, died every single year from measles alone.[9] Given the ever-present fear of their imminent demise, it is not surprising, then, that Dickens characterized children as occupying a precarious existence, somewhere "between the cradle and the grave."

Great Ormond Street

Charles Dickens contributed to a new, and – as some might consider – highly sentimentalized, view of childhood. He also helped promote one of the most important medical initiatives of the era – the founding of The Hospital for Sick Children on Great Ormond Street, London. Great Ormond Street began its life in 1852 as a small rented house with ten beds, under the stewardship of the influential physician Charles West and patronage of other men of eminence, such as the great Victorian peer and reformer, Lord Shaftesbury.[10] Plagued by financial issues during its early years, the new hospital was often at risk of failing for lack of support. As was the case for many medical charities, funding was a serious challenge during the early years; the hospital was established just before the outbreak of the Crimean War, and charities devoted to the orphans and widows of the over 20,000 fallen soldiers of that war siphoned off potential donations. With the help of Dickens, who wrote "Drooping Buds" in support of the fledgling hospital just six weeks after it was opened, the institution slowly gained a foothold in the crowded market of medical philanthropy in Victorian England. The growing appeal of children's charities, as well as innovative fundraising techniques, such as the annual "purchase" – meaning sponsorship – of individual cots (children's beds), helped consolidate the hospital's finances.[11] After years of financial turbulence, Charles Dickens agreed to preside at the hospital's first public dinner in February 1858, a feast that historians of that hospital have seen as a turning point in its fortunes. The dinner raised £2,850, and the author's reading of *A Christmas Carol* raised an additional £165.[12] The funds enabled the hospital to purchase a neighbouring property, stabilize its finances, and increase its inpatient capacity. In return, Dickens became an honorary governor of the hospital for life. Dickens wrote of the children's hospital in "Between the Cradle and the Grave" (1862) and featured it again in *Our Mutual Friend*, into which he incorporated much of his 1858 speech. Indeed, so close was Dickens to the fledgling medical institution that one literary scholar contends that "the sick and disabled characters in Dickens's writings came to be inextricably linked with the new hospital in the public imagination."[13]

The actual founder of the Great Ormond Street, the physician Charles West, envisioned an institution with three principal goals. First, he hoped the hospital would provide inpatient treatment and care dedicated to children of the metropolis aged two to twelve. The age range was suggestive of the contested boundaries of Victorian childhood. The decision to exclude infants and children under the age of two was likely a self-conscious act to suppress an association of the fledgling institution with the frighteningly high infant mortality rates of foundling hospitals (see below). The maximum limit of twelve years of age reflected a vague dividing line between the end of childhood and the beginning of young adulthood. By way of comparison, contemporary debates over mandatory elementary education

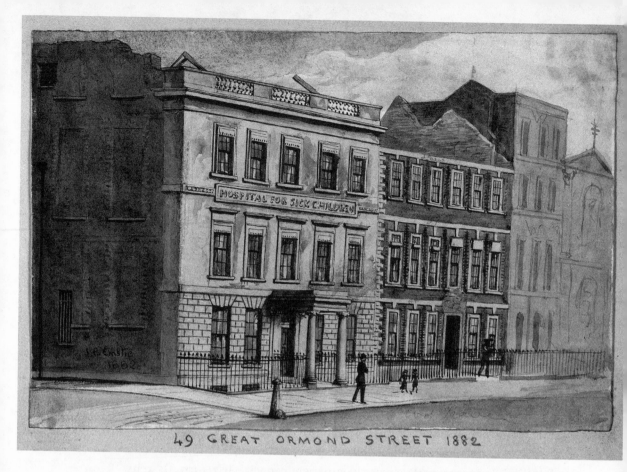

49 GREAT ORMOND STREET 1882

1.2 The Hospital for Sick Children on Great Ormond Street in London, England, in one of its earlier iterations. The famous Victorian hospital served as a reflection of the specialization of medical institutions in the nineteenth century and an inspiration for similar projects throughout the British Empire.

in England often proposed that all children, regardless of background, be schooled to the age of twelve or fourteen. This was also the age at which young boys were often sent out for apprenticeship, signalling the beginning of the adult phase of life. Second, West hoped to legitimize those medical practitioners who were particularly interested in childhood diseases. Paediatrics, of course, did not become formalized as a medical specialty until the twentieth century, but there were clusters of physicians and surgeons who were already being drawn to ailments and infirmities that disproportionately affected children. Thus, hospitals with inpatients provided a much-needed locus for medical professionalization and specialization, as will be discussed below.[14]

Like all children's hospitals of the nineteenth century, Great Ormond Street began with a very modest number of inpatients. During the first decades of the hospital, there were fewer than three dozen beds at the hospital. Medical staff and nurses most commonly treated children for tubercular diseases, respiratory ailments, and complaints of the heart. Before the 1870s, surgical interventions were uncommon, despite the advent and popularization of anesthesia in the 1840s and 1850s. Indeed, the board of the hospital did not open the first surgical wards until 1871, nor did it have sufficient funds to construct an operating theatre until 1875.[15] Rather, the children's hospital focused on shelter, Christian values, and nutrition. "Insufficient food and unwholesome living are the main causes of disease among these small patients," asserted Dickens, "so nourishment, cleanliness, and ventilation, are the main remedies."[16] Like many children's hospitals modelled on it, Great Ormond Street initially excluded those children visibly afflicted by contagious diseases.[17]

The British tradition of medical charity is central to our understanding of the founding of the children's hospital in Toronto. Great Ormond Street was first and foremost a medical *charity*, established primarily for the benefit of the poor, and in particular for the "deserving" poor. The provision of free services for those deemed deserving – and modest fee-based services for those considered able to contribute something to their care – necessitated the use of various mechanisms to ascertain patients' degree of need and "worthiness." At Great Ormond Street, medical and nursing staff questioned mothers and children at length about their personal background; after 1875, parents were interrogated by specially appointed hospital clerks who determined whether they were appropriate recipients of aid. In some provincial children's hospitals, such as the one in Birmingham, several successive approaches were attempted to formalize this determination of worthiness, including requiring a certificate signed by two householders and investigating on site the particular family circumstances of prospective patients. A letter of support from a contributor to the hospital often greatly assisted admission. Such a social determination of who would be treated, however, was far from a Victorian invention. Rather, the cultural importance of ascertaining who was (and was not) the proper object of charitable giving – of who actually constituted the deserving poor – had emerged a century earlier and would inform all medical charity before the advent of universal health insurance in the twentieth century.[18]

The Gift Relation

The English tradition of medical charity can best be understood as arising in the eighteenth century, which witnessed a remarkable expansion of general infirmaries from the 1740s. Over thirty provincial infirmaries, from Bristol to Glasgow, from Manchester to Bath, were founded in England, Scotland, and Wales by the end the eighteenth century.[19] These general hospitals, if one can use that modern term, operated through a complicated system of local patronage, whereby the middle class and local gentry subscribed – that is, gave annual donations of prescribed amounts – to the hospital in return for influence over who was admitted. Annual lists of subscribers (and the amounts they gave) were published in municipal papers, thus conferring a hierarchy of philanthropic giving (and social standing) to the local elite. As the medical historian Roy Porter memorably framed it, this "gift relation" – between landed gentry and tenant farmers, between municipal commercial elites and their domestic servants, between factory owners and waged labourers – endowed the act of giving to hospitals with mutual dependence and engendered reciprocal duties of donors and recipients.[20] However, such a system of so-called *voluntary* financing was often precarious; annual donations fluctuated considerably, and hospitals constantly teetered on the brink of financial collapse. Most survived, however, and adapted to changing social circumstances, whilst attracting honorary (that is, non-remunerated) medical practitioners who were eager to donate an afternoon of gratis medical care to the poor in order to mix with the major patrons of the hospital (potential paying private patients, who would, of course, be treated in the privacy and relative comfort of their own homes). These large provincial infirmaries, however, were not really *general hospitals* in the modern sense, since the rules excluded large groups of potential patients. They tended to bar children from admission as inpatients, as well as lunatics and other "incurables," "women big with child," and fever cases. Due, in part, to the exclusion criteria of the general infirmaries, specialist hospitals emerged in England by the dawn of the nineteenth century, including a small network of charitable asylums for the "insane," lying-in (maternity) hospitals, and lock hospitals (for venereal diseases).

As institutional charity and welfare began to take shape over the one hundred years before the establishment of children's hospitals in the nineteenth century, various models for responding to the medical and welfare needs of children coexisted. One early institutional possibility was the foundling hospital, a residential institution for orphaned and abandoned children. London's Foundling Hospital, for example, was created in 1741, but was controversial, not least due to allegations of high mortality rates and suspicions of neglect towards those under its care. For those not convinced of the need, or the utility, of residential institutions, there was also a small number of formal dispensaries – the first of which operated for two decades in London, from 1769.[21] Another London institution, the Universal Dispensary for Children (which would evolve into the Royal Waterloo Hospital for Children and Women) opened in 1816, just two years after the creation of another charity, the East London Orphan Asylum in 1814. The latter, renamed the London Orphan Asylum, excluded "sick, deformed or infirm" children from admission.[22] In addition, some of the provincial infirmaries, discussed above, compensated for the exclusion of paediatric inpatient treatment by providing some limited outpatient dispensary services for mothers and children. Others made exceptions for emergent cases of children injured in accidents.[23] Seen in this broader context, Great Ormond Street and the Toronto Hospital for Sick Children did not emerge from a vacuum. Rather, they built upon a long, complicated, and fluid institutional context of medical services for different strata of society.

It should be remembered that the experience of children in welfare institutions was generally viewed as one of neglect, death, and despair. Thomas Malthus, in his *Essay on the Principle of Population* (1803), was one of many to rip into the legacy of residential solutions to the problems of children cast off by industrial society. As he caustically observed, "The greatest part of this premature mortality [of children] is clearly to be attributed to these institutions, miscalled philanthropic … If a person wished to check population, and were not solicitous about the means, he could not propose a more effectual measure than the establishment of a sufficient number of foundling hospitals."[24] Although Malthus was pointing to a combination of parsimony and prejudice, he might as well have been voicing the growing belief that

1.3 An early English-language medical treatise on the treatment of childhood ailments. Although paediatrics did not exist as a formal medical specialty before the twentieth century, a handful of medical practitioners gravitated to the diseases of childhood and used medical treatises such as this to disseminate knowledge and reinforce their claim to expertise.

closed institutions – prisons, workhouses, and hospitals – merely permitted the diseases of the few to multiply into the maladies of the many. Thus, he was giving voice to a widely held prejudice among the lay public that hospitals in the eighteenth and nineteenth centuries often did more harm than good, that they were often little more than "gateways to death."

In an era before effective medical interventions, and when the source of infectious diseases was still widely debated, much of the rhetoric in favour of children's hospitals conflated the therapeutic with the moral, and the moral with the economic. Some opponents expressed the concern that hospitals for sick children would encourage illegitimacy, exacerbating the underlying demographic tensions of a society that a vocal minority characterized as overrun by unsupervised offspring of the poor. Others, more compassionately, wondered about the extent to which institutional options, even charitable ones, would undermine the affective relations between mother and child. Advocates of charitable institutions for children countered these arguments by suggesting that the existence of children's hospitals would actually *strengthen* the labouring classes and make them more economically productive. Indeed, part of the push and pull of welfare in the nineteenth century was the contention that charitable institutions actually *lessened* dependency on state welfare by freeing up destitute fathers and mothers to enter the labour market. A particularly unkind vein of advocacy involved upbraiding poor families as the principal cause of their children's disability and infirmity. Some observers marshalled mid-century mortality statistics that rendered visible the elevated death rate of poor urban children as indictments of the habits and conduct of the poor themselves, rather than their environments or socio-economic circumstances. In this way, social and medical statistics challenged the prevailing predisposition to view the household as the safest and most "natural" place for a sick child, eroding one cultural opposition to the hospitalization of children.[25] Indeed, an enduring current of the justification of paediatric hospitals (at least by middle-class commentators speaking to middle-class patrons) was that these children needed to be rescued, in effect, from the home environments that had either caused or contributed to their sickness and disability in the first place.

The intentional separation of children from their parents was thus a source of tension in the nineteenth century, but the conflict was wider than that of the admission of children to specialized hospitals. Indeed, the status and rightful place of children was being contested and negotiated in many different spheres of life. The ongoing debate over child labour and the obligation of parents to send their children to elementary schools also elicited conflicting attitudes over the ideal locus of children and, equally importantly, who had the right to decide. Elementary schools, like children's hospitals, represented a separate space for children, distinct from their households, where new ideals of an educated, cultivated citizen could be forged in a location apart from adult life and the degrading environment of the streets. Charitable bodies like the National Society for Promoting the Education of the Poor pursued this agenda of compulsory education, one which was often resisted by poor families who were economically dependent upon the labour of their offspring. Advocates of hospitals emphasized that in addition to providing the nursing, treatment, and diet that children required, specialist hospitals could offer moral and spiritual instruction in a healthy environment for poor children whose physical and spiritual lives were endangered by a menacing industrial environment.[26]

Resistance to children's hospitals also came from within the medical profession itself. The founders of children's hospitals often had to face the opposition of existing medical institutions and general practitioners, who feared losing their patients to new institutions. The general infirmary in Glasgow, for example, opposed the establishment of a hospital for children for fear that the new institution would "siphon off" charitable donations.[27] In Boston, the Massachusetts General Hospital argued that a new hospital for sick children was not needed, as existing area hospitals already admitted children. Indeed, during the 1860s, one-seventh of all their admissions were children. The managers of the proposed children's hospital emphasized, in turn, the moral setting and nurturing that a children's hospital, staffed by charitable Christian women, would offer to its patients.[28] These tensions within the medical profession, reflecting competing professional interests, would continue throughout the last decades of the nineteenth century. At stake was not simply the viability of one medical institution versus another, but rather a broader question about the desirability of specialization.

The Medical Interest in Childhood Diseases

Although Western medicine can trace its roots to classical antiquity, the medical profession was still very much pluralistic and poorly organized at the beginning of the nineteenth century. In England, the monopolies of the Royal College of Physicians, the College of Surgeons, and the Society of Apothecaries – each with its own privileges and responsibilities – were beginning to break down in the face of new societal pressures. The influence of Continental patterns of medical education, pioneered in early nineteenth-century France and Germany, were challenging traditional pedagogies; younger British practitioners chafed at the elite and exclusionary practices of the College of Physicians, who had the right to police and fine other members of the medical profession in both London and the provinces. New medical journals – like *The Lancet*, established in 1823 – challenged existing medical authority and mocked the lack of scientific knowledge of Oxford- and Cambridge-educated practitioners. Meanwhile, younger medical trainees were seeking and gaining double qualifications – in surgery and in apothecary – becoming "surgeon-apothecaries" and acting in the capacity of general practitioners to the non-elite population, particularly outside of the major cities. Some of these surgeon-apothecaries became the first generation of medical officers of health in the English industrial cities, providing much-needed statistical surveys on deaths and disease. Meanwhile, alternative practitioners in popular healing traditions, such as homeopathy, vied for a growing demand in popular remedies in what was becoming a crowded medical marketplace.[29]

Part of the claim of superiority made by mainstream medical practitioners was based on recognized degree qualifications, something that fostered the growing alliance between independent, proprietorial medical schools and an emerging network of universities offering degree programs. Although the Scottish medical schools had long been recognized as having the leading formal curriculum in medical education in Britain, English institutions were now hurrying to catch up. The university medical degree – the MD or equivalent – became the standard by which self-styled "orthodox" medical practitioners attempted to distinguish themselves from a myriad of healers who were competing for paying clients. After several failed attempts, the medical profession in Britain agreed to a uniform set of professional regulations – including educational qualifications, licensing, and self-regulation – in the landmark 1858 Medical Registration Act. Within this generations-long process of medical professionalization and unification, hospitals became increasingly important as places of medical training, conferring practical experience and professional connections to young trainees and senior consultants alike. As medical curricula evolved in the nineteenth century, the new specialist hospitals – eye hospitals, lying-in hospitals, lunatic asylums, and fever hospitals – became useful locations for young medical staff to develop their own areas of clinical and research specialization. They, in turn, fostered a belief in the need for specialist (as opposed to generalist) skills and a growing predisposition to see the primacy of ever-specialized medical knowledge and clinical practice.[30]

The establishment of specialist hospitals, therefore, cannot be seen narrowly as merely a response to some pre-existing demand that operated in society at large. Rather, the emergence of Great Ormond Street and other children's hospitals needs to be understood as a complicated interaction between the epidemiological reality of nineteenth-century society, a new view of childhood, and the aspirations of groups of medical practitioners eager to carve out a professional niche. The process was thus reciprocal and interactive. Children's hospitals would shape the attitudes of families and communities towards the need for institutionalization and specialist care; in turn, the medical and surgical challenges of children with ill health or disabilities would inform how these hospitals would develop, whom they would admit, and whom they would exclude. Medical staff working in these new children's hospitals would publish medical texts and clinical papers on the diseases of children, all engendering and validating the specialist care in the first place and reinforcing the trend towards specialization.

This process can be seen in the publication of medical treatises on children's diseases. For example, George Armstrong, who had established the children's dispensary in London, authored *An Essay on the Diseases Most Fatal to Infants* in 1767. In 1793, Michael Underwood published the longer-lasting and influential *A Treatise on the Diseases of Children*, in which he appears to have described the first clinical account of poliomyelitis. His book would become the standard reference work for medical practitioners in Britain for the next half century. The American William Dewees contributed his own compendium, *A Treatise on the Physical and Medical Treatment of Children*, in 1825.[31] In an era before bacteriology, late eighteenth- and early nineteenth-century medical texts on childhood illnesses and disorders were largely descriptive and exhortative, discussing the physiology of diseases and establishing benchmarks of "normal" physical and intellectual development. To be sure, medical practitioners had some practical knowledge to dispense, such that bottle-fed and wet-nursed children faired particularly poorly in terms of infant survival. Medical men emphasized breastfeeding, good nutrition, daily bathing, and exercise. In general, however, these early medical texts were largely concerned with taxonomy and rather circumspect in terms of the medical profession's ability to deliver cures for the most important maladies of the era.

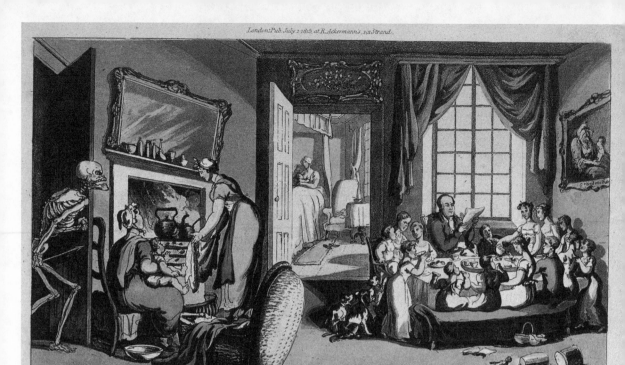

London Pub. July 1 1815, at R. Ackermann's, 101 Strand.

'Twere well to spare me two or three
Out of your num'rous Family.

1.4 In this Victorian caricature, Death (far left) lurks behind a door, ready to snatch away an unsuspecting child from a family overflowing with youngsters. During the second half of the nineteenth century, two out of every five children would die before their fifth birthday.

Despite the limited ability of formally trained medical practitioners to combat many of the worst scourges of the time, advances outside of academic medicine (as much as it can be called that) helped imbue the medical approach to childhood diseases with some social and cultural validity. Inoculation, and later vaccination, for smallpox, pioneered in England by Edward Jenner in 1796 and adopted throughout Britain and British colonies (such as Canada) in the first decades of the nineteenth century, may well have saved tens of thousands of young lives. Controversial, and indeed mocked, as it was in its early years, vaccination won over many educated members of the middle class, even if its compulsory imposition by the state in the middle of the nineteenth century was resisted by many communities. A lot of other interventions, by contrast, were ineffective, and some were outright harmful. An Edinburgh doctor, for example, taken with the apparent success of vaccination, attempted to inoculate poor children against measles but found – after many accidental deaths – that "it did not work."[32] Even the growing anatomical knowledge that was central to medical education during the "Age of Reform"[33] was achieved concurrently with a growing mistrust in the way that medical schools procured corpses – something particularly pronounced in Upper and Lower Canada. Rumours of medical "graverobbing" – whereby young medical trainees would illegally procure corpses from welfare institutions and public cemeteries – only hardened parental anxiety about handing their children over to medical institutions. Put simply, some poor families simply did not trust members of the medical profession, questioning the aims of their interventions, their effectiveness, and their eagerness to achieve monopoly status. Nevertheless, the spirit of innovation and experimentation was ascendant at the dawn of the Victorian era. The discovery of anaesthesia transformed surgery in the 1840s, paving the way, several decades later, for the emergence of orthopaedics. The creation of the ophthalmoscope, the invention and dissemination of the portable microscope, these were all tangible and, for some, magical, manifestations of the potential of what some were calling, from the 1870s onwards, "scientific medicine."[34] Scientific inquiry was taking hold within the professional middle class, leading to a slow, and at times begrudging, acceptance of the utility of medical authority and medical institutions.

The Charitable Legacy

By the time of the establishment of The Hospital for Sick Children in Toronto in 1875, Great Ormond Street had transformed into a purpose-built facility with 100 inpatient beds, solidifying its reputation as the flagship children's hospital of the British world. Its size and recently constructed surgical amphitheatre, however, were anomalous. Almost all of the rest of children's hospitals in the Anglo-American world and British Empire were of modest size, concentrating on outpatient (non-surgical) care. For example, the children's hospitals in Washington, Albany, and Detroit, all established in the 1870s, had fewer than a dozen beds in their early years, as had the other five lesser-known metropolitan children's hospitals founded in London by the end of the 1860s.[35] In the wider British Empire, small children's hospitals were also opened in the 1870s in Melbourne, Brisbane, and Adelaide. Some sprang from the philanthropic efforts of groups; others emerged as offshoots of children's wards in general hospitals.[36] In addition to their modest size, children's hospitals were few in number relative to general hospitals and children's asylums. By the First World War, there were only twenty-five children's hospitals in the United States, compared to over 4,000 general hospitals. By one estimate, even by 1930, children's hospitals treated only "10 per cent of all hospitalized children."[37]

As this chapter has suggested, the early children's hospitals in the English-speaking world were as much about moral uplift as medical therapeutics. These nascent institutions were an uneasy alliance of social reform and clinical practice. Identified as blameless and malleable, children were thought to be most susceptible to the influence of Christian charity. Educational and reformist texts introduced crippled children "as emotionally resonant figures, using the melodramatic mode as an effective way to promote individual institutions or particular causes."[38] In such an emerging cult of benevolence, the pathos of crippled children functioned to elicit the sympathy of the middle and upper classes. A vertiginous multitude of overlapping charities would emerge in Britain and throughout the Empire. After the publication of Dickins's *A Christmas Carol* in 1843, a Tiny Tim Guild was begun "to relieve the plight of crippled children in England."[39] "Drooping Buds," published in 1852, is said to have inspired the opening of a children's hospital in Norwich. In response to Dickens's works, the Lord Mayor of London began the Lord Mayor's Little Cripples' Fund, an appeal to support a countryside home for urban children. Several years after Dickens's death in 1870, the introduction of mandatory public education made "crippled children" more visible, and in the 1880s and 1890s more organizations, such as the Guild of the Brave Poor Things, emerged specifically for their needs.[40]

Toronto inherited this British legacy of medical charity. A good proportion of the population in Victorian Ontario had been born in the British Isles. Many prominent medical men had been trained in the leading British medical schools. The religious traditions of charity were transported to the colonies, as was the cultural preference for charitable assistance over state entitlement. Educated members of the middle class in both Toronto and elsewhere in English Canada were deeply cognizant of the developments in medicine, and in medical institutions, happening in the mother country. They too saw around them the disorder and vice of urban living, the privation and despair that had animated writers and social reformers like Dickens. Toronto had its own slums, its own epidemics, its own "crippled children." Torontonians, no less than Londoners, embraced the new and emerging view of childhood and the desire to combat unnecessary childhood mortality. Of course, these traditions and preoccupations would be adapted in particular ways in what was still, largely, a white settler society in the process of political union and still in the early stages of industrialization. The founders of the hospital in Toronto received support from the apparent success of Great Ormond Street, as exemplified in a letter from the hospital's secretary encouraging a group of Baptist women who had been lately organizing to establish Toronto's own hospital for sick children:

> I have much pleasure in sending our reports and some papers describing our work here which will be useful to you in your project at Toronto, which I sincerely trust will be eminently successful, and the Canadian Hospital for Sick Children prove a real blessing to numberless poor little ones in the same way as this Hospital during its twenty-three years has been to the poor of our great city.[41]

As the next chapter will demonstrate, the original project for Toronto's Hospital for Sick Children was one pioneered by educated, middle-class women. This appeared to be part of a broader pattern. While voluntary hospitals for children in Victorian Britain were largely male initiatives, many of their North American counterparts were founded and operated by female philanthropists. The children's hospital in St. Louis, Missouri, for example was founded in 1878 by a mixed team of four doctors and seven women civic leaders. In Sydney, the children's hospital board of management boasted two female vice presidents, one of whom, Lady Allen, served for over two decades.[42] So when a small group of Toronto lady visitors began to discuss openly the possibility of a hospital for sick children in Toronto, they were drawing upon a long heritage of medical charity and reflecting a culturally validated role for educated women who were largely restricted from medical education and professional schools. However, tensions would quickly emerge, ones that drew lines between the original founders and their vision of Christian charity and a growing cohort of medical men eager to transform the institution into a hospital that was secular and scientific.

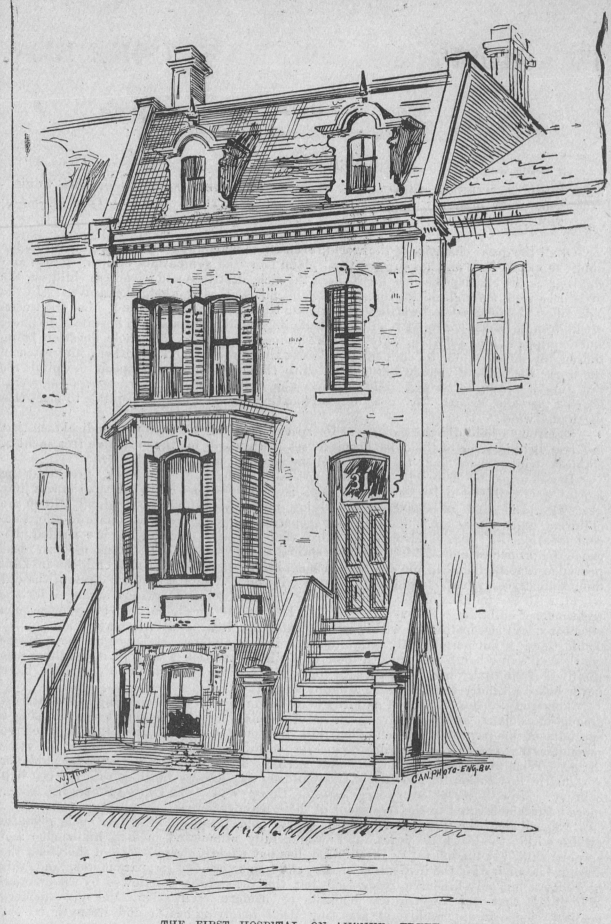

THE FIRST HOSPITAL ON AVENUE STREET.

TWO

The Sweetest of All Charities

More than fourteen years ago, two Christian women, belonging to Toronto, became deeply impressed with the very great necessity which existed, for the establishment of a Hospital for Sick Children. In visiting the poor and sick, they found many little ones, languishing and dying for the want of pure air, good nursing, and proper nourishment. After many months of waiting on God in prayer, at length, led as they believed by the Holy Spirit, they resolved to publish in the city newspapers a plain statement of the needs of these sick children and await results.[1]

Annual Report of The Hospital for Sick Children, 1887

This account, in what may be considered one of the first historical reflections on the origins of The Hospital for Sick Children, articulated clearly the central compelling principle of the new charity. The author framed the hospital as a religious initiative, ordained by God and guided by prayer. It was established and run by women as part of a larger movement of charitable initiatives directed towards assisting, and uplifting, the urban poor. Indeed, the initial organizing meeting was held in December 1874, under the auspices of the Young Women's Christian Association, as part of ongoing

2.1 The first rented home of Toronto's own Hospital for Sick Children, as published in an early history of the institution. Situated on Avenue Street, it had room for eight cots and did not, at first, have running water or a working boiler.

discussions on how to better relieve poverty in the slums of Victorian Toronto.[2] Although there had been rumours of such an initiative for two or three years, the establishment of a Ladies Committee in 1874 gave organizational expression to these hopes. By March 1875, sufficient donations had been received to rent a row house and celebrate the formal opening of the hospital, despite the fact it did not yet have any patients. The *Daily Globe* described the small dedicatory service, at which several reverends read scripture and offered their own prayers.[3] At the service, "a little band of praying women" joined the celebration and, thereafter, met every Friday morning at the institution for religious congregation.[4] The reporter encouraged readers to support the organizing committee "in furthering the interests of this institution — which certainly should command the sympathy and help of all — so that the institution may meet the demands which will undoubtedly be made upon it."[5]

Local newspapers and medical journals reported that the new charity met with a "hearty and sympathetic" reaction.[6] An individual from Fergus, Ontario, anonymously donated $20, enabling the organizing committee to publish a pamphlet declaring, without apparent irony, "that such an Institution was to be opened in full dependence upon God alone for its support."[7] Printed circulars generated further offerings, ranging from 21 cents to $20, all of which were couched in the language of Christian charity. Donations would soon arrive from Sunday schools, the society of Oddfellows, and even other "sick children."[8] "Several prominent physicians" agreed to attend the small number of potential patients on a rotating basis.[9] Yet, despite the appellation of a *hospital*, the early annual reports emphasized that the institution was as much a religious as a medical enterprise:

> We are especially anxious that this work should be recognized as the Lord's Hospital, and we earnestly desire that all who look upon it as one of the agencies by which the Lord would comfort and heal many little sufferers who cannot plead for themselves, will speak of it among their christian friends [sic], and give it a place in their prayers. It is particularly requested that ministers would make its existence and principles known, that children may come, as does the support we have received, from all parts of the Dominion.[10]

The Ladies Committee rented a two-story red-brick house on 31 Avenue Street, a road adjacent to what is now College Street, whose block of residences were later razed to make way for a new building of the Royal College of Dental Surgeons. The rental, as depicted in image 2.1, boasted eleven unfurnished rooms, no running water, and a small backyard. By March, the Ladies felt confident enough in the future to hire a matron, a nurse, and a servant. The home was equipped with six iron cots and a second-hand oil stove. Two young women brought quilts, and the house was outfitted with, among other gifts, "six beautiful illuminations framed; ½ dozen towels; 27 pairs of woolen socks; 27 night-gowns, and innumerable other articles of clothing." Two additional cots were given in May, bringing the inpatient capacity to eight.[11] The first patient, a scalding victim named Maggie, was admitted on 3 April 1875, being the first of forty-four inpatients treated by 1 July 1876.[12] Her arrival, now an iconic moment in the collective memory of the hospital, was the symbolic beginning of the medical attention that one contemporary trumpeted as the "sweetest of all charities."[13]

Moral Reform and Its Medical Manifestations

The establishment of The Hospital for Sick Children in 1875 reflected a fascinating intersection of charity, religion, and medicine that informed late Victorian Canadian society. Upper Canada, upon its foundation in 1792, did not implement a comprehensive structure of poor laws for the relief of destitute individuals. As a consequence, people experiencing severe privation had no "legislative right" to welfare, as they did in England. Not that there was universal lament over the absence of the poor laws in what had also been known as Canada West in the twenty-six years leading up to Confederation in 1867. Voluntary charity was thought by many to create a stronger bond between donor and recipient and to be more effective at remedying poverty than "the giving of relief as a legal entitlement mediated by a state functionary."[14] Private organizations – some religious, others non-denominational – knitted an imperfect patchwork of services in response to the social problems unleashed by industrial capitalism. They operated in a semi-independent manner amidst a ceaseless discourse of "voluntary" charity, even though many organizations would ultimately become dependent upon government subsidies and subject to statutory regulation.

Provincial governments in Canada retained constitutional responsibility over medical and charitable institutions after Confederation. However, the initiatives in Ontario were constrained by resources and by custom. Legislation tended to be reactive, limited to empowering acts passed in response to local social and epidemiological crises, such as the cholera outbreaks that had menaced Toronto as recently as 1866. It fell largely to local munic-ipalities to provide welfare services, in conjunction with, or through, private charitable organizations. Some smaller municipal governments in the prov-ince did take modest direct measures to alleviate poverty in their communities. By contrast, in larger urban centres like Toronto, charitable relief was primar-ily a religious prerogative carried out by a large number of denominations. Although the city would establish a permanent department of public health in the early 1880s, organized charity was the "visible face of relief" for Ontario's poorest subjects, an awkward and uneasy alliance between church – or in this case, churches – and state.[15]

Sectarian tensions would animate welfare services throughout the latter decades of the nineteenth century.[16] While Protestants organized most charitable initiatives in Toronto, half of those accepting poor relief were Catholic, although they made up only 21 per cent of the urban population. As a consequence, there was ongoing anxiety among Catholics that Protes-tant-led charities and institutions, particularly those working with children, were being used to convert poor and vulnerable youth. For example, in nearby Hamilton, a controversy erupted in 1852 when Catholics accused the Ladies Benevolent Society of proselytizing children in the city's orphan-age.[17] Partly in response to these anxieties, the Catholic Bishop Charbonnel initiated a comprehensive set of parallel Catholics charities and services in the province, which in part led to a system of Catholic hospitals in the major cities of Ontario, such as Toronto's St. Michael's Hospital, founded in 1886.[18] These sectarian sensitivities would lurk in the background of any municipal projects that involved the care or treatment of children.

Organized charity was informed not only by tensions between Protes-tants and Catholics; it also reflected changing power relations *among* Protestant denominations in Victorian Toronto, most notably between the elite Anglicans and Presbyterians on the one hand, and the non-conformist congregations, such as the Baptists and Methodists, on the other. A tide of social activism was energizing Protestantism during this era, particularly among the upwardly mobile members of the middle class.[19] Most activists were "evangelicals" – an ambiguous term that was used to capture a height-ened religiosity, a dedication to welcome (and convert) new members into one's faith, and an emphasis on the involvement in community works. Evan-gelicalism underpinned what historians refer to as the period of "moral reform" in late nineteenth-century urban Canada. Moral reformers hoped to address what they considered to be major social, political, and economic problems of the time – including poverty, disability, crime, and sickness.[20] Whilst traditional charity sought to "relieve the immediate need of the recipient while earning virtue points for the giver,"[21] moral reformers criticized this older model "for fostering continued dependency."[22] The new context of moral reform necessitated that groups striving to "save the social" did not wish to simply meet the material needs of the poor, but also to improve the moral character of those who received aid.[23]

A central theme in Protestant charitable activity in this period was thus a tension – almost a psychological angst – between the perceived Christian duty to aid the poor and a persistent fear of "promiscuous giving."[24] How could one truly distinguish between the deserving and the disingenuous? To add to the uncertainty, it was believed that the most worthy recipients were those who were most reluctant to seek aid, which occasionally made middle-class philanthropists suspicious of those who availed themselves too easily of assistance. Prominent organizations, such as the Toronto Women's Christian Association, strove to prevent individuals from obtaining aid from multiple sources, and carefully scrutinized applicants. Over the middle decades of the nineteenth century, a common method of evaluating potential recipients was through home visiting, a practice whereby middle-class women went among poor homes to dispense material relief and offer unsolicited advice on how the poor could improve their familial situation. Unsurprisingly, the households of the poor themselves became targets of reform and the perceived causes of many social and medical problems. Moral reformers increasingly turned to extra-domiciliary solutions – middle-class substitutes for impoverished domestic environments – where individuals could attain "the disciplined autonomy required by liberal society."[25]

Participation in charitable initiatives thus became deeply embedded in the social and cultural lives of upwardly mobile middle-class households and, particularly, the lives of intelligent and ambitious women. In an era before universal suffrage, when women were denied access to careers in medicine, law, politics, and the ministry, philanthropic activity became a means through which women gained access to, and dominance in, public spaces. By freely offering their labour, women acquired organizing experience in a socially validated manner, given the constraints of gender expectations in the Victorian era. Indeed, some historians have argued that the invocation of "divine endorsement" – replete in the early annual reports of the children's hospital and other charities – was used strategically by women as a "means by which to convince the public of the significance and rectitude" of their work and provide ideological justification for their public presence and administrative responsibilities in a male-dominated society.[26]

Elizabeth McMaster and the Ladies Committee

It is within this social context that we can best understand Elizabeth Jennet Wyllie, the daughter of two Scottish immigrants to Canada, George Black Wyllie and Mary Ann Reid. Born in 1847, Elizabeth was baptized at St. Paul's Anglican Church, where her father – a man who had "achieved modest prosperity" as a woollen draper and dry goods merchant – had been a church warden.[27] At the age of seventeen, Elizabeth solidified the middle-class aspirations of her family by marrying Samuel Fenton McMaster, who worked at A.R. McMaster and Brother, also in the dry goods business. Samuel was the nephew of William McMaster, whose wealth would make him an influential civic leader and who would become one of the first Canadian senators appointed at the time of Confederation. The senator's own philanthropy would lead to the establishment of a Baptist college in Toronto, perhaps as a counterbalance to the dominant Anglican Trinity College, the Presbyterian Knox College, and the Methodist Victoria College. Samuel Fenton McMaster's prominence in the Baptist community in Toronto is demonstrated in his acting as the official witness to the 1870 marriage of Humphrey Ewing Buchan to Jemima Fisher Cameron; Buchan, perhaps not coincidentally, would be one of the first six consulting physicians to the children's hospital. Elizabeth had grown up "just on the fringe of Toronto's high society."[28] Her own marriage in 1865 brought her into a kinship network that included, among others, Edmund Osler (the brother of William Osler) and, more distantly but no less notably, John Ross Robertson, with whom she would engage in an epic battle over the future of the hospital itself. A year after marrying, and shortly after the death of her devout Anglican father, Elizabeth joined the McMasters at the Bond Street Baptist Church and, over time, embraced the evangelical drive of the Toronto Baptists of the 1870s.[29]

The precise events leading up to the establishment of the first hospital remain unclear, with early histories of the institution portraying Elizabeth McMaster very much as the materfamilias to the institution, with her portrait (see image 2.2) conjuring up contemporary images of Florence Nightingale. We have no private diaries or correspondence that would illuminate her character beyond the more official documents of the hospital's archives. We do know that she was still in her twenties and the mother of three children when she organized, and later became secretary of, a "Ladies Committee," probably sometime in 1874. Elizabeth's position in the respectable – if second – tier of Toronto society provided her with an expansive social network that was engaging in home visiting of the poor.[30] And it is notable that several newspapers alluded that she was part of a small group of active lady visitors in the city who had already been distributing relief and advice to the poor for several years. She made the first symbolic donation, and was secretary of the Ladies Committee from 1875 to 1883 and president from 1883 to 1891, becoming the active force behind the early years of the hospital.[31]

Despite her formidable presence in the formation of the hospital,

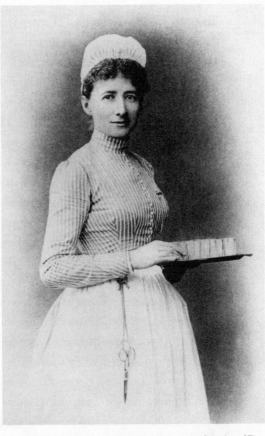

2.2 Elizabeth McMaster, widely regarded as the founder of The Hospital for Sick Children. She organized a Ladies Committee to visit sick children in their homes and, later, to manage a "hospital" that would treat those unable to pay for medical care.

Elizabeth could not have managed the founding of a new medical institution on her own. The annual report of 1877 stipulates that sixteen ladies were to be committee members; by December of 1878 this figure had grown to twenty-two.[32] Minutes of the early Ladies Committee still exist, giving us an insight into its composition, which included some prominent Toronto Anglicans and Presbyterians, despite the characterization, in some early publications, of the original committee as being made up entirely of "Baptist ladies." Such grandees included Lady Agnes MacDonald, whose husband, "reputedly one of the wealthiest men in Toronto," was also a founding member of The Haven.[33] Joining her was Mrs. Clara Boddy, wife of the Archdeacon of Toronto, and Mrs. Howland, whose husband briefly held the position of mayor ten years later (1886–7) after being president of the

Toronto Board of Trade.[34] Other women, such as a Mrs. Walter Lee and Mrs. Henry O'Brien,[35] were inscribed in the 1881 census enumerator's schedules as wives of merchant bankers and lawyers. Although Lady Agnes MacDonald was clearly one of the grand dames of Toronto society, periodically lending her spacious gardens on St. George Street to the children for a "day of recreation,"[36] many of the Ladies Committee who could be traced in contemporary census records appear to be of more modest standing, mostly upper-middle-class mothers with young children. Mrs. C.S. (Maria) Gzowski, for example, whose husband was a city broker, was the mother of six children, having lost two children in infancy.

The Ladies Committee performed multiple functions, facilitating political influence within the municipal, provincial, and federal circles of political power; contributing monies of their own; and dedicating innumerable hours of unpaid volunteer work. The first order of business was financing the new charity, for the newly proclaimed hospital had no significant tangible resources or endowments: "no capital, no collectors, and no subscription list."[37] Although the lady visitors had hoped to charge 20 cents per day for their "little patients," they found that even that modest sum was too much for many of Toronto's poorest households.[38] They therefore pursued a policy of not charging for care. From June 1875 onwards, funds were acquired through collection boxes placed in the house itself, as well as in Rossin House Hotel, a gas office, a mechanics' institute, and Fulton and Michie's grocery store.[39] Considerable support arrived as gifts in kind; indeed, the donation of hundreds of minor household necessities comprises page upon page of the early annual reports, all gratefully acknowledged by the managers of the fledgling institution. One anonymous donor left a box of soap; another, upon seeing an appeal at church, promised a company gift of a large cooking stove. The ladies were particularly grateful for a "parlour organ," which aided the children in their rendition of "Safe in the Arms of Jesus."[40]

Committee members themselves supplied many of the early sizeable monetary donations to the hospital. As mentioned in chapter 1, Great Ormond Street in London, England, had pioneered the clever practice of sponsoring cots (inpatient beds). This tradition continued in Toronto. Nine volunteers agreed to collectively sponsor a cot for $100 per year – the estimated cost of care for one patient per year – thereafter known as the "The Consolidated Cot."[41] In 1877, Mrs. Edward (Margaret) Blake then individually sponsored the "Ethel Cot," Mrs. Aikins the "The Morley Cot," and Mrs. Howard "The Children's Cot." By 1881, eleven cots had ongoing sponsorship, paid for

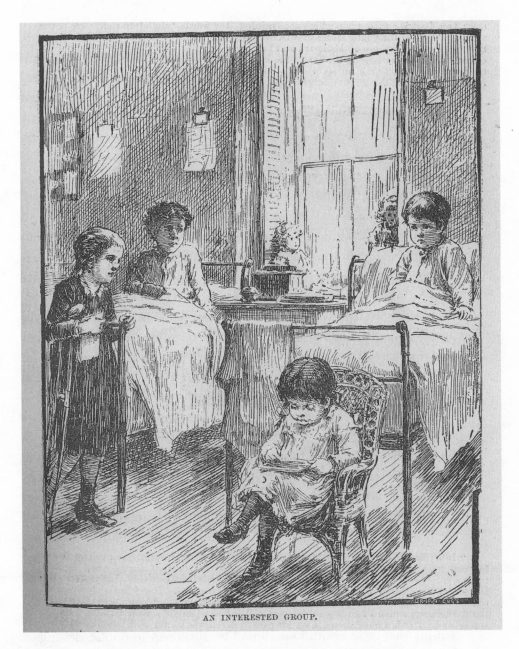

AN INTERESTED GROUP.

through quarterly contributions of $25. Such regular subscriptions provided some degree of ongoing financial security and tied the bene-

2.3 One of the few drawings extant depicting children in the rented homes, prior to the construction of the first permanent hospital. Note the patient charts hanging on the wall and make-shift crutches supporting the boy.

factor to the well-being of individual patients and the success of the institution. Supplementing this guaranteed revenue stream were fundraising events, such as Mrs. Edgar Jarvis's garden party, which raised $187.50, and a bazaar at the home of her uncle, which yielded a substantial $378.[42] In 1875, the charity raised just shy of $1,000 from individuals or families, $458 from special events, $186 from schools or church congregations, $37 from charitable collection boxes, and only $30 from patient fees from families judged to be able to contribute a nominal amount. These revenues all trebled by 1886, with an income exceeding $9,000 per annum, facilitating a transfer in 1876 to a second hospital on Seaton Street, and a move again to a third home on Elizabeth Street in 1878.[43]

The Ladies Committee in Toronto retained an unusual amount of authority during the early years of the hospital. The committee oversaw all aspects of the institution's operation. Committee membership required attendance at monthly business meetings, and the secretary and treasurer attended additional weekly meetings "to look over the accounts."[44] Elizabeth McMaster opened most meetings with prayer; in October 1878, weekly devotional meetings were added.[45] The committee supervised hospital operations through "visiting ladies," who toured the hospital, in pairs, on a rotating basis. The women volunteers reported to the committee on all aspects of the institution, ensuring that children were admitted according to the regulations, their linen was changed, the diet was appropriate, and they were all "tenderly nursed, fed, washed and cared for" and surrounded by Christian practices and influence.[46] Ladies volunteered for additional duties as needed, such as forming a committee "to read and sing with the children," or meeting weekly "to assist the Matron in the sewing department."[47] They held themselves responsible for the spiritual welfare of their patients and even formed a separate committee to attend to the religious instruction of the children. Minutes indicate, however, that the committee had difficulty finding sufficient volunteers to attend in pairs, particularly during the summer months, and later appointed only one visitor at a time.[48] This managerial method mirrored other cultural practices of late Victorian society, including the importance of external "inspectors" of public institutions and the convention that civic institutions should be also open to public viewing at specified hours of the week. The women were, in some respects, inspectors of their own institution, each with a vested interest in the probity of its internal affairs.

The Ladies Committee held itself responsible for both the physical and *moral* condition of their charges. Special emphasis was placed on cleanliness, comportment, and religious instruction. At the dedicating services, one speaker observed that "not only was the body treated," but so was the mind "at a time when [it] was peculiarly susceptible to good impressions."[49] The ladies undertook to provide for the religious instruction of patients, and to ensure the daily observance of "family prayer" and weekly attendance at "divine service."[50] The annual reports expressed disquiet when patients displayed a "disinclination for religious instruction," and attempted to guard children from "evil companionship" and "evil influence" in the form of disagreeable fellow patients and "unauthorized" books.[51] Many women who were not formal committee members also "spen[t] many a useful and happy hour in reading or singing to the little patients, in some cases teaching those who are well enough to like a little easy schooling, or playing with small sufferers confined to their little iron cots, the sliding trays of which are often covered with toys."[52] Such volunteering was crucial to the internal culture of the hospital, where middle-class ladies were providing moral instruction to the sick and disabled children of poor, urban Toronto. On an individual level, the ladies were performing multiple administrative and informal nursing duties, as their presence was considered indispensable to "enliven a little life not overflowing with pleasure."[53]

Sick Children in Victorian Toronto

Medical services for sick children were certainly known in Toronto before the establishment of a hospital dedicated to their care, but they existed in a fragmented and uncoordinated manner among a dizzying array of institutions. From its origins in 1829, Toronto General Hospital constituted the principal hospital in the city. Reflecting the British tradition of medical philanthropy, it was intended to benefit the "sick poor." The insane, pregnant women, and incurable cases were excluded.[54] In the late 1840s, the epidemics accompanying large-scale immigration prompted the city government to build sheds and provide basic care near the institution for immigrants suffering from typhus and cholera, in an effort to control the spread of disease. Temporary sheds continued to be erected and used for cholera victims and arriving immigrants, but by the 1870s the sheds' main purpose was immigrant reception, with the sick being sent on to the General Hospital for treatment.[55] After 1856, the institution, now in a new building on the eastern edge of the city, began to differentiate itself from other charitable organizations, as "the more specialized function of the hospital – involving cure and treatment, in addition to custodial care – was starting to become more apparent."[56] However, Confederation precipitated a financial crisis for the hospital, which had depended on "unpredictable annual grants" from the provincial government. Patients were discharged and the hospital actually closed from August 1867 to August 1868. By the time of the opening of the children's hospital in 1875, the general hospital had recaptured its pre-eminent role among medical institutions in the city, attending to almost 8,000 outpatients on an annual basis.[57]

The desire to have medical institutions concentrate on cure, rather than safe custody and nursing care, animated debates over the other principal medical institution looming over pre- and post-Confederation Toronto – the lunatic asylum. The Toronto Lunatic Asylum was a *provincial* institution, supported and managed by the government from its inception. The cornerstone for the impressive new building was laid in 1846, and the facility on Queen Street West, then one of the largest non-military buildings in North America, admitted its first patients in 1850.[58] Built to accommodate 250 patients, by the end of its first year the asylum contained over 300, the majority of whom were funded by the province.[59] Conditions, at first, were dismal. The overcrowded asylum had bad ventilation, bad drinking water and overflowing drainage pipes, and stood upon a massive cesspool. Dr. Joseph Workman, superintendent from 1853 to 1875, worked assiduously to improve the conditions at the institution, introducing a classification system for his patients in order to emphasize curative rather than merely custodial services.[60] Over time, regional lunatic asylums would be constructed in Kingston (1853), London (1867), and Hamilton (1875), bringing the inpatient psychiatric capacity to over 2,000 residents. All of the principal cities in the province would host lunatic asylums, except for Ottawa, which was to become the permanent home of the House of Commons and the Senate.

Children were largely excluded from both of these large medical institutions in Toronto. The general hospital discouraged the admission of children but provided emergency care and some outpatient services throughout the mid-Victorian period. The provincial asylum formally refused those with what we would now call developmental disorders, advocating instead for a separate asylum for children. Such an institution would ultimately be established in Orillia, 130 kilometers north of the city, notably within months of the founding of The Hospital for Sick Children itself. This latter provincial facility for "idiot and imbecile children," to use the medical and legal term of the time, would act as a relief valve to divert children with epilepsy and developmental disabilities to a residential setting.[61] This important rupture between "mental" and "medical" services for children would continue for at least another fifty years; psychological services would not re-emerge in general and children's hospitals until the 1930s.

The admission of children for inpatient medical treatment was uncommon in the 1870s. Rather, children who were already institutionalized might receive medical or nursing care *incidental* to their residential situation. For example, Toronto witnessed a proliferation of homes and hospices for orphans at mid-century, including the Orphans' Home and Female Aid Society, the Girls' Home and Public Nursery, Protestant Orphans' Home, and the Boys' Home. The Roman Catholic House of Providence, run by the Sisters of St. Joseph from 1857, fulfilled a similar function. Other large welfare institutions, like the House of Industry, wrestled with the question of what to do with sick residents, including children. Both "Houses" were as large as the Toronto General Hospital, serving the indigent of all ages and performing multiple functions, from housing the elderly to treating the victims of infectious disease.[62] The House of Refuge itself, adjacent to the Don Jail, was actually transformed into a smallpox hospital after the 1869 epidemic in order to contain citywide scourges that would reoccur until the end of the century.[63] Each of these institutions received some form of weekly medical and nursing attendance, including treatment and attendance of poor children. And most of these welfare institutions dwarfed the new children's hospital in size: by 1879, the Roman Catholic Orphan Asylum, for example, housed 256 children; the Toronto Orphans' Home and Female Aid Society (also known as the Protestant Orphans' Home) had 100 residents, and the Toronto Girls' Home reported 115 residents.[64] Compared to these institutions, the new children's hospital, with its inpatient capacity of eight beds, was very modest indeed.

Many impoverished mothers avoided the stigma associated with residing in a welfare institution by taking their children to hospitals for dispensary services. The Toronto General Dispensary, for example, which shared many medical officers, trustees, and patients with the Toronto General Hospital was one such institution.[65] The Toronto Free Dispensary was founded by Dr. Abner Mulholland Rosebrugh in 1863 and offered free medical care to the poor. Shortly after, Rosebrugh also established the Toronto Eye and Ear Infirmary, which "soon developed into one of the city's most specialized medical care institutions."[66] Other medical institutions came and went, stimulated in part by the University of Toronto's inaugural Faculty of Medicine (1843–53), together with competing academic and private medical schools. The 1851 census of Canada West (Ontario) enumerated three lying-in (maternity) hospitals in Toronto, all of which merged to form the Burnside Lying-in Hospital, which itself became affiliated to the Toronto General Hospital in 1877.[67] Within such a varied and complicated picture of medical and welfare institutions, then, the singularity of the new children's hospital was not so much in the medical attendance of children – which was clearly happening inside and outside of all sorts of environments – but rather the dedication of an institution that was built *solely* for the reception of children for the ostensible purpose of medical treatment.

Medical Attendance

The early annual reports of The Hospital for Sick Children list eleven to fourteen honorary medical staff, including five to six consulting medical officers (the more senior staff), five to six younger attending medical officers, and one to two consulting eye surgeons. Anchoring the consultants were two of the most powerful medical men in the province. The first was Edward Mulberry Hodder, who studied medicine in London, Paris, and Edinburgh, joined the Royal College of Surgeons in 1834, and practised in London and France before immigrating to Toronto. Hodder was already on staff as an obstetrician and gynaecologist at the Toronto General Hospital, and was credited as a founder of the Upper Canada School of Medicine, the *Upper Canada Journal of Medical, Surgical, and Physical Science*, and, among other accomplishments, the Toronto Boat Club. One biographical entry suggests that he was the leading ovariotomist[68] of the time, and the acknowledged "father" of Canadian obstetrics and gynaecology. In the very year of the establishment of The Hospital for Sick Children, he was the president of the Canadian Medical Association. He continued as a part-time instructor at the Toronto School of Medicine, and later was dean of Trinity College Medical School from 1871 until his death in 1878.[69]

Hodder was accompanied by William Thomas Aikins, who began his medical training at John Rolph's Toronto School of Medicine before gaining his MD at Philadelphia's Jefferson Medical College in 1850. Aikins is described as an "exceptionally wealthy physician" who was involved in medical politics, gave generously to the Wesleyan Methodist Missionary Society, and attended at several city charities in addition to the new children's hospital.[70] Aikins flourished in Toronto as an eminent surgeon and medical educator for nearly fifty years, affiliated with Rolph's school and the Victoria College school of medicine. Among his many accomplishments, he participated in the proprietary Toronto School of Medicine until 1887, at which point he became dean of medicine at the University of Toronto (1887–93). Hodder and Aikins were instrumental in fostering alliances with both the Toronto General Hospital and the emerging power centre of the University of Toronto.[71]

Prominent Baptist medical practitioners could also be seen in the early medical attendants. Humphrey Ewing Buchan, mentioned earlier in the chapter, was born and raised in Ontario and received both a BA and MB in medicine from the University of Toronto before spending two years at the "leading hospitals of London and Glasgow."[72] He too was a physician to the Toronto General Hospital and represented the University of Toronto on the College of Physicians and Surgeons of Ontario. A deacon of the Jarvis Street Baptist Church in the 1870s, he also served as president of the Ontario Baptist Missionary Convention and was involved with the Toronto Baptist College, the Baptist Union of Canada, and various religious publications. Buchan began as an attending medical officer in 1875 and continued as a consulting physician from 1877 to 1882. He left to take up the position of resident physician at the provincial asylum on Queen Street in the mid-1880s, yet he continued his affiliation with the children's hospital, being reappointed to the consulting medical staff in 1891.[73]

Starting off as a junior (attending) medical staff member, Buchan would have been responsible for visiting the hospital once a week for a few hours. The other attending medical men appear to have been even more junior, in their late twenties and thirties, including the twenty-six-year-old Irving Cameron, as well as F.H. Wright, the son of one of the other senior consultants. We know comparatively little about these junior attending physicians; they were members of a rapidly expanding group of medical practitioners in Ontario, whose numbers had quadrupled from 400 in 1840 to about 1,600 in 1870. Notwithstanding the increase in the general population, this augmentation represented an increase in the density of practitioners, resulting in a competitive medical marketplace. Indeed, some researchers have associated the perceived oversupply of medical practitioners with multiple attempts to close the ranks of the profession in the 1850s and 1860s, making it harder for non-Canadian trained physicians to become licensed. A combination of factors may well have motivated these young medical practitioners to volunteer their time: a professional interest in a particular medical specialty, a religious compulsion to provide free services, as well as a financial incentive to widen their own private practice (through interaction with the charity-giving elite of a particular city). It should come as little surprise that there were no female medical practitioners. Historians have identified only three formally trained female practitioners in all of Ontario in the 1870s, all of whom were trained outside of the province and whose credentials were contested by the medical elite of the time.[74]

Although the clinical records have not survived from the early years of the hospital, it is clear that this tension over medical traditions had already emerged at the children's hospital. Formally trained "orthodox" or – to use the contemporary term – *allopathic* practitioners in Victorian Ontario repeatedly tried to restrict the clinical practices of those who practised alternative therapies. The lay public tended to perceive such moves as an attempt to impose a monopoly over medical services, and thus dramatically hike medical costs and restrict freedom of choice. In the context of the 1850s and 1860s, the orthodox medical practitioners could not make a compelling case for the inherent superiority of their own techniques over competing therapies. Ultimately, a Medical Act passed the legislature in 1869, which established a formal register of practitioners and a regulatory agency (the College of Physicians and Surgeons of Ontario) but notably continued to recognize certain groups of alternative practitioners, such as the homeopaths. These tensions over medical modalities lingered on in the 1870s and could be seen in the confusion over the therapeutic orientation of the new children's hospital. One delicately worded response to a reporter's query in December 1874 suggested, "In order also to meet the wishes of parents as much as possible, there will be one section for treating children homeopathically and another allopathically."[75] It may well have been the presence of Hodder, Aitkens, and other luminaries within the orthodox medical elite that pressured McMaster to backtrack in a letter just one day later: "The allopathic system has been adopted as in the meantime the only one to be followed in this hospital," explained Elizabeth McMaster, adding, "We hope that in time a homeopathic branch may be established under the same management, but with different nurses."[76]

With an inpatient capacity of only eight beds, there were necessarily great constraints on the admission of new patients and, for that matter, the duties of the medical staff. The attending medical officers each visited the hospital on one (different) afternoon per week, usually at 2 p.m., to see inpatients, outpatients, and potential new admissions. During the first fifteen months, they admitted only forty-four patients in total, thirty-seven of whom were from Toronto.[77] Consistent with other children's hospitals at the time, only those over age the age of two were admitted as inpatients, though some infants were occasionally treated as outpatients.[78] The inpatients presented with a diverse array of conditions, including urgent cases such as Alice, who was "frightfully burned by the explosion of a coal oil lamp" and a boy brought in by cart and horse with a broken leg. One little girl – four years old – had accidentally swallowed lye and after eight months of treatment at the hospital was still only able to take lime water and milk. The patient profile from 1875 until 1882 reveals over one hundred discrete presentations, from anal fistula to a gunshot wound to the foot. Some clusters of diseases, however, can be identified. A significant minority of patients were suffering from Pott's disease, a form of extrapulmonary tuberculosis affecting the thoracic part of the spine. Sometimes known as "consumption of the spine," this debilitating condition often affected children through a degeneration of the spine leading to vertebral collapse and spinal damage. The circumstances leading to admission of these patients is unclear, though we do have hints of the emerging relationship to other medical institutions and welfare institutions discussed above. Among the first patients were transfers from the Toronto General Hospital, including a six-year-old girl with hip disease, who underwent the hospital's first operation, and two brothers brought from a Hamilton hospital both suffering from "inflammation of the lungs."[79] Another "bonnie little lad of 12" came from the Boy's Home in Toronto with the same condition.[80]

Throughout its first half century, The Hospital for Sick Children treated far more outpatients than inpatients, and consistently treated more boys than girls. Ladies Committee minutes indicate that Dr. Cameron first requested the opening of a designated "extern department" (outpatient care) for poor women and children in October 1876.[81] The number of patients treated through the dispensary increased more rapidly than the number accommodated within the hospital; in 1880, nearly ten times as many cases (617 compared to 66 inpatients) were treated externally, causing some tensions within the Ladies Committee and medical team.[82] Small donations trickled in for the dispensary, but expenses mounted and the work was limited by financial constraints. The explosion of outpatient care may reflect many factors, not the least of which was the restricted physical space of the early rental homes. However, it may also have indicated the continued ambivalence about the efficacy and desirability of inpatient care. Indeed, a retrospective of the hospital, written in 1881, recalled, "We had gone to many places in Toronto, telling the poor all about the contemplated work; and from them we had received the promise of nine little sufferers. But when the House was opened, *not one of them came.* Again and again we went, begging the parents to send them, but all to no purpose; till at last we betook ourselves to prayer concerning the suffering little ones, and very soon came answers."[83]

The annual reports felt compelled to repeatedly make the argument for the admission of children, employing justifications that one could see in other national jurisdictions, including the persistence of high child mortality rates, the inappropriateness of mixing children and adults in general hospitals, and the need for specialized nursing care. A circular in 1876 entitled "Facts Illustrative of the Need of a Children's Hospital," made the case to the general public. The appeal made clear that children's hospitals already existed in European and American cities, the implication being that Toronto needed to show that it too was a world-class city.[84] In addition, the plight of the poor working mother was repeatedly cited to demonstrate an economic, as well as medical, need for admission:

> It is intended for the children of those whose homes, means and occupations may not allow proper attention, care, nourishment and medical attendance to the suffering little ones ... Take such a case as that of a poor woman who goes out washing, necessarily leaving her children all but untended during the day. If any of these fall sick it is not possible for the mother to stay at home and nurse her child without cutting off entirely her slender means of living. If the disease, however, is not of an infectious character, she can, for a payment not beyond her own means or those of her friends, get the little one transferred to this hospital for sick children, where it will be better cared for than at home, and be far more likely to recover health speedily and permanently, while the mother can pursue her ordinary avocation with the full confidence that her little invalid is well cared for.[85]

Indeed, the historical memory of Maggie, retold numerous times in hospital publications, was not *just* a memorialization of the first-ever patient; it can be read as a morality tale of the plight of poor families and their inability to care for their own children:

> Our first patient was little Maggie, aged three years, who had fallen backward into a tub of hot water, and was badly scalded. She had been left in the care of an elder sister while the mother was earning bread for the family. This case seemed an answer to the oft put question, "Are

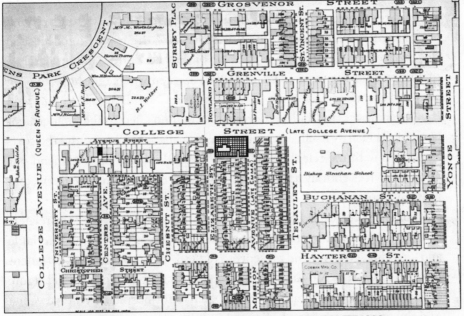

Location of The Hospital for Sick Children Year ■ 1875 ☐ 1878 ▦ 1892

Map Source: Goad's Fire Insurance Plans for Toronto, Plate 15, 1894   0 25 50   100 Meters

not the mothers the best ones to care for their children when sick?" Our hearts would say "yes," but our experience too often says "no," they have neither the skill nor time to nurse the little ones, and hence the latter often suffer from severe accidents or grow up cripples, and a large percentage of them perish before they are able to take care of themselves.[86]

2.4 The location of some of the early rented homes superimposed on a contemporary fire map. The image shows the remarkable density of the downtown core, before whole blocks were razed to make way for some of the most famous medical institutions in Canada.

Despite the multiple moves from Avenue Street to Seaton Street to Elizabeth Street and to Jarvis Street, the ability to secure and finance greater capacity for inpatients while remaining in the heart of the city remained a challenge (see image 2.4). Indeed, the growing financial problems may have been, in part, a result of the unusual stance taken by McMaster and the original Ladies Committee. The founders of the proposed hospital set themselves apart from other institutions by adopting a principle of relying on voluntary donations rather than making direct public and individual appeals for money. Contributions were supposed to be "voluntary and spontaneous," occurring only when the giver was moved by God.[87] The first circular printed declared, somewhat implausibly, "We do not intend to solicit help from any one, further than to give information relative to plans, purposes and wants ... There will therefore be no canvassing the city for funds, contributions will be voluntary in the fullest sense of the word."[88] Indeed, the *Ottawa Free Press* reported, in 1875, "One of the peculiarities of the charity is that no subscriptions are to be asked, but all their wants they hope to have supplied by making them the subject of prayer."[89] This approach may well have been novel, and indeed devout, but it almost led to the financial collapse of the charity itself. The escalation of outpatient services and the costs associated with the relentless demand forced the hospital to suspend outpatient services entirely as of January 1881, cease to give free medicine, and publicly announce their desperate need for new funds.[90]

Somewhat obscured in this financial crisis and debate over the relative merits of outpatient treatment and dispensary services, was an appreciable and growing government presence. By 1886, the provincial government, through its Charity Aid Act of 1874, was contributing to the hospital a figure of $1,900 per annum, or just over 20 per cent of the hospital's yearly revenue. And the proportion of funds directed from the government would increase steadily to almost 50 per cent by the turn of the century.[91] It may well be that the hospital flourished, in Elizabeth McMaster's words by "prayer alone," but it was prayer generously underwritten by the taxpayers of the province.

Conclusions

The establishment of the first hospital for sick children in Toronto was an auspicious confluence of an environment increasingly sympathetic to children's charities, the specific efforts of a small group of dedicated lady visitors and the support of the medical elite of Toronto. It is true that other children's hospitals were being founded elsewhere in the British world, such as the first home in Melbourne, which had opened a few years earlier. However, the mere identification of the need for a separate medical institution did not always result in tangible outcomes. In 1869, for example, the *Montreal Gazette* reported on the first meeting of an organizing committee for a hospital for children in Canada's other principal city, but it took over thirty years before the Montreal Memorial Children's Hospital was actually founded. Of course, sectarian tensions loomed even larger in Montreal, but there also appears to have been resistance from within McGill University and the English-speaking medical community to a separate institution for children.[92] In Toronto, by contrast, the most senior men of the medical community were convinced, at an early stage, that the hospital was not a threat to their own project of medical professionalization. Medical luminaries like Hodder and Aikins acted as conduits to the Toronto General Hospital, to the University of Toronto, to the newly established College of Physicians and Surgeons, and to the provincial and federal legislatures. Their support, even if it was largely nominal, would prove invaluable.

The hospital started life as a series of small rental homes strategically located in the heart of Toronto. As this chapter has demonstrated, the charity emerged from a tradition of visiting poor children in their own homes. Yet, instead of *visiting* and reforming the poor in their own home environments, the ill and disabled of the poor were invited to be cared for, and reformed, in a respectable, middle-class environment. Ladies acted as surrogate mothers, supervising the moral upbringing of children in a home that was a model of middle-class domesticity. In the era just before bacteriology would radically change the understanding and treatment of diseases, founders regarded the *environment* of the hospital itself as therapeutic and uplifting, and many "were convinced that physical removal [of children] from the impure domestic environment, in which everything from the water and air to the bedding and language was polluted, would not only cure them, but would enable them to become better citizens."[93] Providing "moral training" by immersing the objects of charity in the routine of a model home environment, female philanthropists sought to teach their patients rules of health and hygiene. It was hoped that patients would then share these values and habits with their families.[94] In this way, medicine and moral reform were inseparable.

Elizabeth McMaster would later claim that her decision to spearhead a hospital for sick children was divinely inspired. Her religious zeal should not be taken as disingenuous or contrived. McMaster led prayers at the opening and close of Ladies Committee meetings, and initiated weekly devotional meetings in addition to monthly business meetings, upbraiding the matron, and even the medical men, for their poor attendance at Sunday services held at the hospital.[95] This insight into Elizabeth McMaster's world – the belief that the hospital was, in effect, fundamentally a *religious* mission run by women – is central to understanding the struggle that would ensue over the future of the hospital itself and the schism that would occur between her and the powerful newspaper magnate John Ross Robertson. For all of his shortcomings – and he had many – the ascendancy of the "Paper Tyrant" would propel the somewhat unremarkable children's hospital to the attention of the medical world.

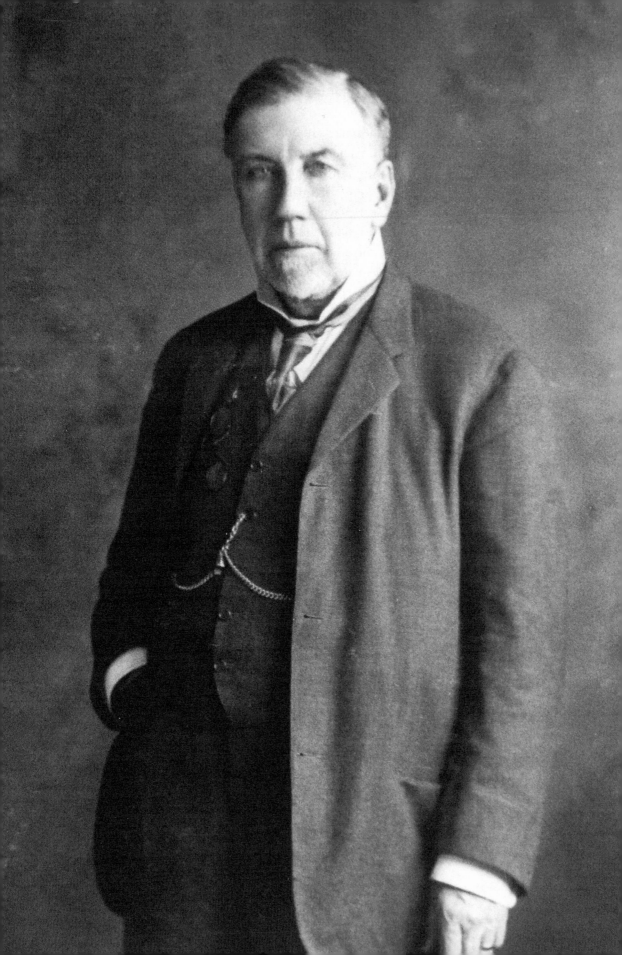

THREE

The Paper Tyrant

You are a singular character and possess marked traits peculiarly your own ... [You] are remarkable for excesses and deficiencies ... You lack self-restraint ... [and] are so likely to go to extreems [sic] that you haz-zard [sic] your health. You care very little about what others say or think of you ... Your religion what little you have consists simply in kindness, generosity, a willingness to share whatever you possess with others and who have no claims upon you ... It is hard for you to refuse and roughly to say "no" when appeals are made to your sym-pathy and your pocket ... [you] cannot endure to be opposed.[1]

Excerpts from a phrenological analysis of John Ross Robertson, 1871

During a trip to New York, John Ross Robertson, then the co-proprietor of the *Daily Telegraph*, an upstart broadsheet in Toronto, ventured to have his phrenological profile conducted by the most famous firm in the United States – Fowler and Wells. The thirty-nine-page handwritten analysis reflects an admixture of personality traits and predictions that, despite their often critical nature, must have satisfied Robertson to the extent that he would later have his son submit to a similar examination. Phrenology, by the 1870s, was losing its lustre as a science of the mind and morphing in the final decades of the nineteenth century into one of a host of theatrical side-show amusements – along with for-tune tellers, astrologers, and palm readers – for urban tourists and audiences at travelling fairs. Whether or not Robertson put much stock in the sometimes unkind conclusions and prognostications, it is hard

3.1 A photograph of John Ross Robertson, the "Paper Tyrant" and proprietor of the *Evening Telegram*, who almost single-handedly bankrolled the new hospital on 67 College Street.

not to read with some degree of wonderment the insights embedded in this rather benign New York diversion. Robertson was indeed a remarkably generous, if authoritarian and ill-tempered, newspaper magnate who would leave his mark indelibly on a host of Canadian institutions, not least of which was Canada's first children's hospital.

John Ross Robertson was born in Toronto in 1841, the son of dry goods merchants who had emigrated from Scotland in the previous decade. He attended the elite prep school Upper Canada College, where he first demonstrated his lifelong passion for journalism, being credited with starting the first student paper in Canada. The precocious John Ross later registered in the Model Grammar School in downtown Toronto, where he founded the serial *Young Canada*. Robertson's rise to prominence in formal journalism began as city editor of the Toronto newspaper, the *Globe* in 1865 and then continued as co-proprietor of the aforementioned *Daily Telegraph*, a paper that prided itself on uncovering political corruption. When the *Daily Telegraph* folded in 1872, Robertson returned to the *Globe* as "resident correspondent and business representative" in England for three years, after which he became the business manager of the weekly journal *Nation*.[2] In 1876, the historian and political commentator Goldwin Smith provided Robertson with start-up funding of $10,000 to begin publication of the *Evening Telegram*.[3]

Robertson publicly declared that the *Evening Telegram* was a newspaper with "no patron but the public,"[4] a clear indication that he sought to position the broadsheet as independent, in contrast to the *Globe* which had long been seen as a Reformist and Liberal newspaper under the leadership of George Brown. The *Telegram* published local news and had a sensationalist style, emphasizing investigative journalism. Its commercial success was partially attributable to Robertson's strategic decision to halve the rate for want ads and to slash the price of an issue to one cent. Such cost-cutting measures were facilitated by Robertson's suppression of labour costs, including his denial of the right to organize to his printers. As a consequence, he was able to pay below-union-scale wages. "He was notoriously domineering and tight-fisted," concluded one biographer, "believing that low pay and long hours kept his employees virtuous."[5] By the 1880s, the *Evening Telegram* had a wide-ranging readership and the largest circulation of all Toronto papers. With this success came wealth and political influence. The *Telegram*, and for that matter Robertson himself, gained "the reputation of being able to make and unmake civic politicians."[6]

Robertson's political views, however, are harder to characterize. His *Evening Telegram* editorials certainly reflected opinions associated with Tory Protestant Toronto, including the defence of Canadian nationalism, imbued with a thinly concealed anti-American and anti-Catholic bias. He was initiated in 1861 as an Orangeman in Temperance Lodge No. 301, with which he marched in fifty-three annual parades. Indeed, rumours had it that one "had to be a Protestant and an Orange Tory" to be hired at his paper.[7] At the age of fifty-five he made an unexpected foray into politics, elected to the House of Commons in 1896, representing Toronto East as an "independent Conservative."[8] Amidst the debate over the Manitoba Schools Question, which bitterly divided the federal Conservative Party, he opposed, as most Orange Order leaders did, the publicly funded instruction of children in French in that province.[9] He clearly regretted his decision to join formal politics, and despised parliamentary life, declining to run for re-election in 1900, "believing that he could have more influence on public affairs through the pages of his newspaper."[10]

Yet, an independent streak in Robertson often made him strike out against his natural supporters; he was constantly displeased by Tory politicians, and his paper critiqued the actions of all parties. Despite being a member of the Temperance Lodge, he continued to advertise alcohol in his newspapers. Occasionally he adopted positions that appeared to be inconsistent with his conservative constituency, including the public ownership of utilities, such as Toronto Hydro. Robertson thus cut a complicated figure in late Victorian Toronto, positioning himself as the consummate outsider,[11] even to the Protestant Tory community that most represented his own views and with whom he most often socialized. His temperament, above all, kept people at a distance. Even apologetic biographers paint an impetuous man, who cared little about personal appearance, was quick to temper, and whose views were regarded by some as bigoted, even for the times. At work, he was understood as impatient and aggressive, a man once known as the Paper Tyrant. And yet, despite all this, he gave most of his life's fortune to the children's hospital, visiting on a weekly, and at times daily, basis throughout his life and every year dressing up as Santa Claus and driving a sleigh full of toys, pulled by a pony, into the wards.[12] One contemporary named him an "irascible philanthropist" and "the grand crank of benevolence," proclaiming that "[a]bsolutely and petulantly impressive, totally democratic and simple, bigotedly a friend of the people, and always favourable to a rumpus — this self-engendered interpreter of a restless democracy never could have been conventionally cribbed in a common sanctum."[13] Little wonder that the phrenologist discovered the strange mixture of generosity and authoritarianism captured in one of few portraits of Robertson, taken by a photographer whom he himself had hired to record for posterity the early years of the new hospital that he would be so instrumental in founding (image 3.1).

Personal tragedy complicates further our understanding of John Ross Robertson. In March of 1881, his one-year-old daughter, Helen, died of scarlatina (scarlet fever) at the family home in Toronto. To compound the family's despair, his two-year-old niece, Grace, died the very same day. The two young cousins were buried together in the family crypt in the Necropolis. Three years later, Robertson's wife, Maria, would also perish prematurely, from causes that are not entirely clear but may well have been complications from a ruptured appendix. Although the widower Robertson would later remarry, it is clear that the loss of his daughter, wife, and niece had a devastating emotional impact on him and guided many of his later philanthropic endeavours, which would become more and more consumed by the children's hospital. Not known to do things by half measure or accustomed, as the phrenologist sensed, to share power or "be opposed," Robertson didn't just *support* the fledgling hospital for sick children; he effectively took it over, building a secondary hospital on the Toronto Islands, marginalizing Elizabeth McMaster and the Ladies Committee, and constructing the magnificent new facility on College Street in 1892.

The Enchanted Island Abode

Robertson's first major contribution was to bankroll a seasonal convalescent home on the Toronto Islands in 1883. As cherished as it became, the Lakeside Home was far from unique, and in fact reflected a practice widely employed in the English-speaking world at the time. As chapter 1 illustrated, children's hospitals emerged in the middle decades of the nineteenth century, funded by charities for the urban poor. Although the main hospitals would be constructed in major industrial cities, there persisted a long-standing anti-urban bias within medical and lay opinion. In essence, observers believed that the ill health of the urban poor was a reflection of the deleterious health effects of the crowded slums, of the environment of urban living. Many social commentators and health practitioners waxed lyrical about returns to the countryside. Indeed, it was a common occurrence for the propertied classes themselves to travel to the seaside to convalesce during the summer. Such prejudices about getting out of the city and enjoying the therapy of open air (and bracingly cold water) can be seen in the spas and sanatoria that emerged in the 1880s and 1890s in Europe and North America.[14] There was also a turn-of-the-century notion of "getting back to nature" that would figure large in the summer migration of those who could afford it to country homes and, in the case of Ontario, the cottage district of Muskoka.

Children's convalescent homes, which sometimes also referred to themselves as "sanatoria," became frequently seen adjuncts to children's hospitals by the close of the nineteenth century. As Eduard Seidler observes, "There was hardly any children's hospital which did not ... have its own salt-water spa, seaside hospital, or high altitude health resort."[15] Indeed, by 1890 there were over fifty convalescent homes for children in England and Wales alone. Great Ormond Street itself opened a convalescent home at Cromwell House in Highgate in 1868, and from 1874 on the Ladies' Aid Association of the Boston Children's Hospital funded and managed a convalescent home in Wellesley.[16]

Before Robertson's arrival, the Ladies Committee in Toronto had already sent a few children to a private home in Barrie, more than 100 kilometres outside of the city, for short periods of convalescence, but the long trip north was a hindrance and the use of the home had to be negotiated around the personal travels of the owner.[17] At some point, interest was raised in using the near-pristine Toronto Islands as a proximate haven from the ill effects of industrializing Toronto. In the hospital's annual report of 1882, the Ladies Committee publicly announced their intention:

> God willing, to establish a temporary Convalescent Hospital on the island opposite our City; not only for these poor little mortals who have passed through their period of sickness with us, and are on the road to recovery, but for the children of any who have not the opportunity of taking their ailing ones away for [a] change of air.[18]

After they had announced this ambition at the hospital's annual meeting, Robertson contacted the Ladies Committee and suggested that, if the city would grant the land, he would offer a substantial $1,000 donation towards constructing a summer home. The city obliged, leasing several acres of land in the name of Elizabeth McMaster. The home, which over time was increased to nine acres, was located on Gibraltar Point, the southwestern corner of Toronto Island, just north of the government fog signal, 100 yards from the Lighthouse and a twenty- to thirty-minute walk from Hanlan's Point. An architect and construction supervisor offered their services freely, and the modest wooden Lakeside Home was ready for habitation in the summer of 1883.[19]

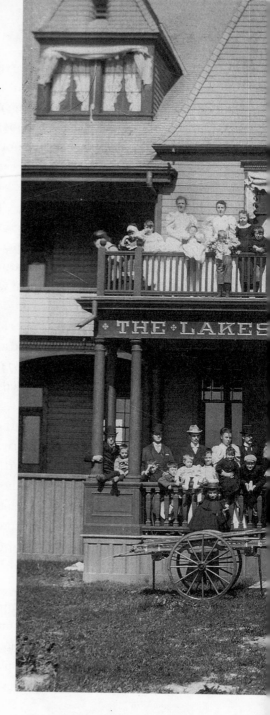

Almost single-handedly, Robertson funded the construction and much of the maintenance of the Lakeside Home facilities over the next quarter of a century. The total expenditure, for its time, was massive. The 1883 structure ultimately cost $3,000; two years later Robertson spent another $2,500 to build a second wing at the home, doubling its bed capacity.[20] Renovations in 1891 proved the most extensive ($16,000), transforming the appearance of the home, which was subsequently compared to a "chateau" or, tellingly, a "summer resort" of the affluent.[21] These additions increased the main building's square footage sixfold, completely enveloping the old home, and increasing the bed capacity to 200 patients, instantly making it one of the largest medical institutions in the city (see image 3.2).[22] Robertson's generous philanthropy, however, came with conditions. He insisted that the "sick children of Freemasons" be admitted to both the Lakeside Home on the island and the main Hospital for Sick Children itself free of charge.[23] Later, he would secure other prominent Masons to form a separate board for the Lakeside Home, which began to

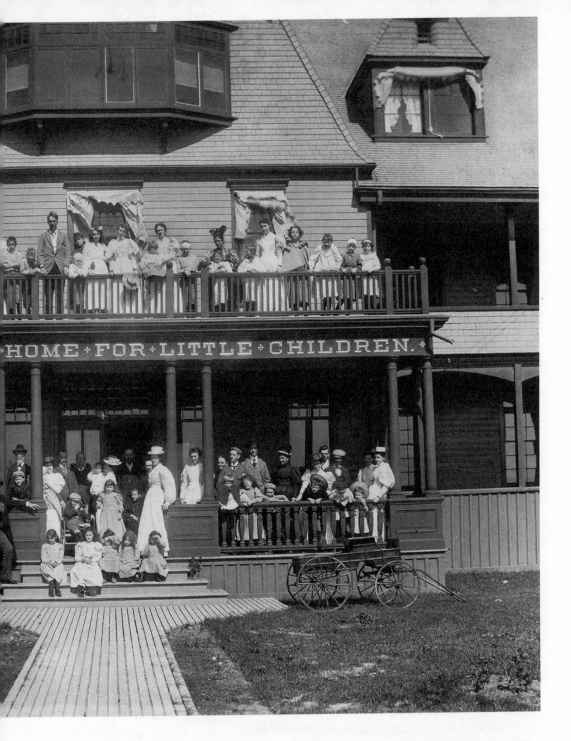

HOME • FOR • LITTLE • CHILDREN •

meet independently and without notification to the pre-existing hospital board. More controversially, he attempted to prohibit any "[v]isits of the Roman Catholic priests or nuns for the purposes of religious conversation with the children."[24]

3.2 The Lakeside Home was one of Robertson's most beloved projects. Running for over three decades near Gibraltar Point on the Toronto Islands, it received most of the College Street patients for the summer months.

The Toronto Island itself was rapidly becoming a seasonal site of open-air leisure. In the late nineteenth century, Ward's Island was populated by tents pitched by families of modest means, while Centre Island hosted the grand summer homes of the wealthy, and the hotel and carnival amusements of Hanlan's Point attracted crowds of day-trippers.[25] Contemporary fund-raising appeals of The Hospital for Sick Children portrayed the Lakeside Home as a "paradise,"[26] an earthly idyll, where "poor little mortals" could enjoy all of the fun of a true childhood despite their real poverty and illness. In addition to playing on the beach, paddling in the water, gathering shells, riding in boats, playing games on the lawn, and picking flowers, children learned to work with clay, draw, sew, and knit. Such innocent pleasures and carefree existence were contrasted with the bleak circumstances from whence many children came:

> One little child, brought into the Lakeside from one of our city's worst slums, after being bathed and placed in a comfortable cot in the ward, was observed looking around her with a strange, excited, almost unearthly expression on her face. On being questioned and soothed by the nurse, she asked if this was "Heaven."[27]

Hospital publications described the Lakeside Home not as a hospital but as "one great play-house,"[28] declaring "Lakeside" to be "a word of magic" to patients, and extolling "the marvellous joys of this enchanted island abode."[29] Promotional materials emphasized the love children had for the summertime retreat: "Weeks before the time for leaving, the little ones are asking the question, 'When are we going to The Lakeside?'"[30]

Hospital management and medical staff praised the home for its trans-formative climatological benefits, with the fresh air and gentle breeze of Lake Ontario credited with therapeutic effects complementing, and at times exceeding, medical or surgical interventions. Reports boasted that children who had been carried to the wharf in June could be seen walking or running back to the docks in September. Accounts endlessly praised the "health-giving properties" of the home's location on Lake Ontario. Every ward opened onto a veranda,[31] and many of the children slept outside on open balconies, with curtains drawn during poor weather. Nurses were instructed to keep the children outside as much as possible. Nourishing food and fresh air were paired with physical therapy, and after the addition of a gymnasium in 1891, many patients spent a half hour per

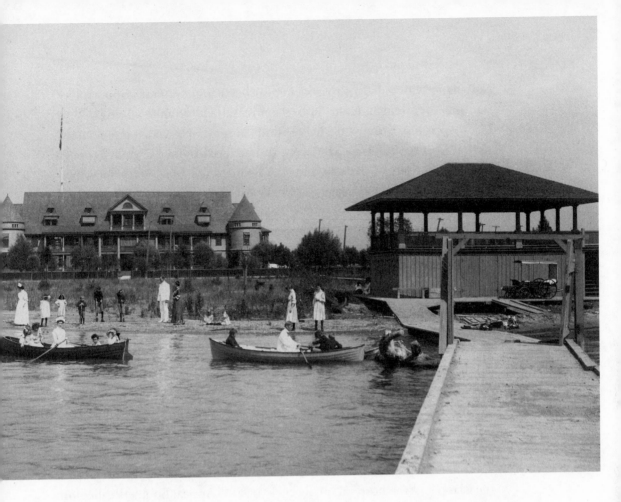

day exercising. In the early twentieth century, helio-therapy, or the "sunshine cure," was thought to be a highly effective treatment for convalescents and tubercular patients. Children were exposed to the direct rays of the sun until "the whole of their bodies were tanned to almost a mahogany hue."[32] The out-come of a patient's stay on the island was most often measured according to weight gain, transformed pallor, and the strengthening of their overall "constitution." Appeal booklets bragged of miraculous recoveries: "One youngster for a time at death's door picked up 7 lbs. – will soon be [a] baby athlete."[33]

3.3 The Lakeside Home became a retreat not only for patients, but also for the medical staff, many of whom relocated there for part of the summer. Here, a doctor and nurse row patients off the main dock.

Robertson is often credited as having the flair of a showman, and he soon took full advantage of the seasonal pilgrimage, turning the semi-an-nual transfer of patients to and from the island home into a civic parade engaging Torontonians of all different backgrounds and eliciting the sup-port of local businesses and hopeful politicians. The initial cohort of forty-nine patients was moved to the wharf with the assistance of the Queen's

Ambulance Corps.[34] In subsequent years, sensing the photo opportunity that this event engendered, Robertson recruited "prominent citizens" to lend "open horse-drawn carriages" and "larger horse-drawn ambulances" to transport the children, as journalists memorialized the dramatic procession.[35] At the wharf, patients and staff boarded the *Luella* ferry, for which they were given free passage, and later season passes, by the Ferry Company.[36] In 1905, the donation of a "beautifully fitted-up" motorboat eased the journey from the Point to the home, which had previously been a twenty- to thirty-minute walk. In that same year, at the request of the trustees, the City expanded the bay and installed a dock so that the *Luella* could make regular summer afternoon (and occasionally morning) trips to the island.[37] The caravans often had police escorts and public onlookers. As an early hospital staff and chronicler recounted, they "elicited many words of pity and sympathy, with words of congratulation that the sick and suffering children were on their way to a place of rest and relief from the heat and confusion of the city."[38]

In time, the Lakeside Home became a popular site for summertime visits of supporters, for urban tourism in general, and for hospital events. Robertson himself visited every Sunday during the summer "with very few exceptions,"[39] and in the 1880s Ladies Committee members visited both the island and the hospital on a weekly basis.[40] Appeal booklets called on readers to tour the facility, asking "Did you ever visit The Lakeside Home for Little Children?"[41] and advising "When in Toronto pay it a visit."[42] In the summer of 1904, the home welcomed around 1,000 visitors per month, as well as 3,200 "friends who visited on Wednesdays and Sundays."[43] By 1906, reported visitors had increased to around 4,000 per season.[44] Robertson cleverly built on the popularity of the island retreat, by concentrating institutional events there, such as the nursing school graduation ceremony, various concerts, meetings of medical associations, and fundraisers. In an era before medical opinion turned against the widespread public visitation of medical institutions, children's hospitals from Boston to Toronto used the seaside institutions to raise much-needed funds and win over public sympathy and support. The Children's Seashore House in Atlantic City, and Coney Island's Sea Breeze Hospital, were also well-visited convalescent institutions for poor children that became "tourist destinations" in their own right.[45]

In practice, the Lakeside Home was as much a seasonal transfer hospital as a convalescent facility. From June to September it accommodated all children who could be moved, regardless of whether they were truly "convalescent" or not. In June 1894, for example, forty-eight children were at the Lakeside Home, and only eight remained in the new hospital on College Street.[46] Through the first decade of the twentieth century, over three-quarters of the nursing staff and patients remained at the Lakeside during the summer. On two occasions, in 1886 and 1912, patients and staff remained at the island later into October while the "mother hospital" underwent a move or renovations. It appears that one argument for locating the new hospital, which opened in 1891, at 67 College Street rather than in leafy Rosedale was that the patients were nearly all out at the island during the hot summer months anyway. For a quarter of a century, even after the main building of the island hospital burnt down in 1915, the Lakeside Home would occupy an ambiguous status as a parallel hospital and summer retreat, while embedding itself deeply in the cultural and social history of turn-of-the-century Toronto.[47]

Training School for Nurses

The Lakeside Home reflected the growing influence of John Ross Robertson, who insisted on establishing an independent trust, controlled by him, to administer the seaside institution. Yet, the rise of Robertson's group brought with it a clash of cultures and management that put him into direct conflict with Elizabeth McMaster and the Ladies Committee. Children's hospitals had, after all, based their appeal as distinct institutions on a commitment to middle-class caring, which, it was believed, only women could properly provide. Part of this appeal relied on a sense of children's care and supervision being a feminine domain, both in terms of management by women and in the central role occupied by female nurses. Nurses, overseen by ladies committees and, later, by matrons or lady superintendents, were expected to offer kindness and patience of "saintly" proportions.[48] By the 1880s, nurse training in paediatric hospitals began to become formalized in the English-speaking world, as, for instance, in Sydney, Australia, where a formal program began in 1883.[49]

In Toronto, the employment and status of paediatric nurses in the early 1880s had been capricious, due, in part, to the unsatisfactory nature of the small rental buildings in which the charity found itself. In addition, with a nurse training program recently started at the Toronto General Hospital, there was a sense that a parallel nurse training program might prove redundant. Nevertheless, in the autumn of 1886, the Ladies Committee hired Hannah Cody as lady superintendent when the children's hospital in Toronto moved to what was its fourth location, at the corner of Jarvis and Lombard Street.[50] Cody, a Quaker, was a member of the second graduating class of nurses from the Toronto General Hospital, and her employment was a signal that McMaster wanted to professionalize the nursing care at the institution. Her arrival prompted the Ladies Committee to formalize the salaries of nurses at $12 per month for trained nurses, and $8 month for night nurses and probationers. Cody herself was paid $25 per month as matron/superintendent.[51] Although the children's hospital did not announce a nurse training program, Cody was soon joined by someone who may be regarded as the first nurse trainee: Josephine Hamilton. Hamilton was instructed to follow doctors on their rounds, pose questions, and record notes. Effectively, she served a two-year apprenticeship, "following the example of the few graduate nurses and community ladies who worked in the wards."[52] Hamilton "graduated" after two years in December 1888, receiving a parchment certificate signed by Elizabeth McMaster herself. The document certified that Hamilton was "qualified to nurse cases of medical and surgical diseases in children."[53]

In 1887, four more nursing candidates entered, followed by subsequent classes of three or four students in the years 1889–92.[54] Reports suggest that in these early years, training was largely by apprenticeship, supplemented by occasional lectures. Miss Cody interviewed applicants as they arrived and sent promising prospects to join staff. The 1888 annual report explains that trainee nurses served one month's probation, after which, "if they prove suitable, they are provided with our uniform, and allowed eight dollars a month the first year, and ten [dollars] the second." They were to have regular lectures, "given three times a week" by the medical staff, on "subjects bearing upon their work."[55] Despite this intention, the 1889 report confessed to the inconsistency of instruction: "These lectures, owing to the large demands upon the time of Miss Cody, our Superintendent (herself a trained nurse), have been somewhat irregular during the past year." As a consequence, Miss Kesiah Underhill, a matron with two years' experience at Lakeside Home, was hired as assistant matron to enable Cody "to pay more attention to the training-class, as well as to other matters which require her efficient supervision."[56] The 1890 report stated that pupils received weekly lectures from medical staff on "surgery, fevers, obstetrics and bandaging," and studied "various textbooks on nursing and physiology."[57] The authors of an annual

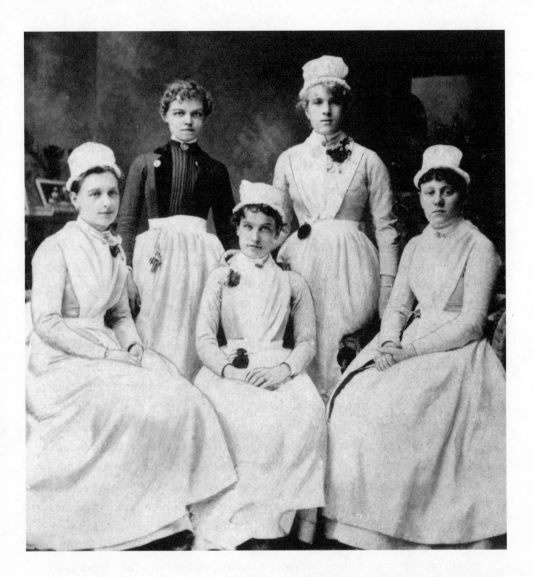

report indicated that life as a nurse trainee was far from cosy: "It is almost impossible for one to conceive the amount of self-sacrifice required to carry out what seems to us a noble resolution. It involves separation from children and friends, hard – almost menial – work, long hours, restraint, conformity to discipline, besides many other things connected with the profession of nurse, which are both unpleasant and difficult."[58]

3.4 An early photograph of Nursing School trainees. Once the school took roots, it flourished, receiving applications from young single women eager to join a respectable middle-class female vocation.

With the success and expansion of the Lakeside Home, and growing tensions between Robertson and McMaster, something quite extraordinary occurred, the specifics of which may be forever lost to posterity. In 1889,

Elizabeth McMaster herself chose to leave the hospital to undergo formal nurse training in Chicago. Upon her return from the two-year program, McMaster replaced Cody as lady superintendent and pushed hard to expand nurse training at the institution. However, her return in 1891 only renewed tensions about the future of the hospital and the relative power of the Ladies Committee and the board of trustees. Clearly, the presence of trained nurses in the hospital and the power that they gave to the lady superintendents became the flashpoint for divergent and clashing priorities. McMaster appears, by many accounts, to have been a personality no less formidable than Robertson himself. Now with her own degree in nursing, she began to advance the issue of an independent nurse training school at the hospital, against opposition from the male board of trustees.

The board did not initially target nursing training itself, but rather began by criticizing the conduct of McMaster and the resident medical officer for accepting infectious cases, contrary to hospital policy.[59] McMaster had sent nurses to aid the staff of the Isolation Hospital on the Don River during an epidemic, without consulting the trustees. The board of trustees chastised McMaster for "overstepping" her authority and for her efforts to formalize a nurse training school. In their minutes, they stated flatly that it was *not* the intention of the trustees to establish a "Training School." In particular, they opposed the Ladies Committee's efforts to train nurses to do outside work in private homes or other institutions.[60] The trustees' minutes thundered against the "injudicious" establishment of a training school managed by nurses and a lady superintendent. They added, unkindly, "that nurses who have rec'd so called training in the Hospital for Sick Children have not proved an unqualified success in adults so much so that their employers have sometimes been compelled to dispense with their services."[61] They would subsequently issue an ultimatum, advising that those who transgressed the institution's rules ought to resign.[62]

The year of 1891 thus proved to be a watershed in the history of the hospital. In May of that year, the Ladies Committee surrendered complete financial and governing responsibility for the hospital to the board of trustees. The ladies were left to attend to internal "household" matters and only to make recommendations to Robertson and his allies. Robertson was in the process of consolidating his power, and he now moved to circumscribe further the prerogative of Elizabeth McMaster and the Ladies Committee. In December, Robertson and the trustees suspended operations of McMaster's nurse training program altogether. Minutes of a Ladies Committee meeting six days later stated simply, "Minutes of last meeting read, also letters from Trustees as to diet, Training School, & other matters. There is to be no Training School. No nurses are to go out to nurse, & no infectious cases taken in."[63] McMaster resigned from the hospital in May 1892, having surrendered legal title to the Lakeside Home to the board of trustees a few months earlier.[64] During the meeting in which they accepted McMaster's resignation, the board of trustees further amended the by-laws and regulations to express complete authority over hospital nurses: "[that] the By-Laws and Regulations be amended by striking out the words 'They shall hold office' and substituting 'They shall all, except the nurses hold office' and that to the Sec[tion] VII Clause 2 the following be added 'The nurses shall be engaged for a period of two years at wages to be fixed by the Trustees, said nurses being subject to dismissal for incompetency or improper conduct without notice.'"[65]

The schism between Robertson and McMaster appears to have been less about nurse training than a struggle for power over the hospital itself. For after McMaster's resignation, the board promoted the thirty-four-year-old Kesiah Underhill to lady superintendent and granted her responsibility for the continuation of a training school, which accepted over two dozen new applicants in 1892 and 1893. As of June 1893, the Hospital had twenty nurses in various stages of training who received lectures from surgeons and physicians and completed their training with examinations by those physicians and Underhill.[66] That month, the board of trustees announced the first graduation ceremony held at the Lakeside Home, where Edmund Osler, one of the trustees, "presented the medals of the Training School to the following nurses who had passed the medical examinations."[67] We do not know a great deal about the young women who graduated from the program. The *Nursing School Register* indicates that most applicants and graduates in the 1880s and 1890s hailed from Ontario, and all recorded applicants were clearly identified as Protestant.[68] Subsequent annual reports of the hospital show that by 1896, twenty-nine of the forty-seven graduates were working as private nurses, three as head nurses, four "at home," and three as lady superintendents. One had died, one had married, one was working in the operating room at the Royal Victoria Hospital in Montreal, and three had undertaken post-graduate courses.[69] Even with this relative success, the board of trustees remained ambivalent about nurse training and in 1896 dismissed Underhill, whose management of the school they concluded to be poor and liable to endanger the reputation of the hospital. At a board meeting, John Ross Robertson identified the training school as "the weak spot" of the hospital, one that had to be addressed "if the Hospital expected to attain that success at which they had aimed since its foundation."[70]

Financing the Hospital

Considering the dominance and investment of Robertson during this period, it would be easy to conclude that he single-handedly financed the hospital during the last two decades of the nineteenth century. To be sure, his monetary contribution was enormous. But, as mentioned in chapter 2, medical charities in the late Victorian era were both private *and* public, with independent charities increasingly regulated, and subsidized, by the state. The principal piece of legislation in Ontario was the 1874 Charity Aid Act, which intended to create a more consistent and transparent system for the distribution of provincial grants to social welfare institutions. The act designated institutions as Schedule A (hospitals), Schedule B (refuges for the destitute), or Schedule C (homes for dependent children and single mothers).[71] The annual aid that an institution received was calculated on a per diem rate. The province subsidized Schedule A institutions by twenty cents for each day's actual treatment of every patient; Schedule B homes received five cents "for each day's actual lodgment and maintenance therein of any indigent person"; and, finally, Schedule C homes were afforded one and a half cents "for each day's actual lodgment and maintenance therein of any orphan or neglected and abandoned child."[72] This sliding scale thus reflected the perceived relative "medical" and "welfare" function of each institution. As a result, institutions like The Hospital for Sick Children had direct financial incentive to emphasize the curative and acute dimensions of patient care and to protect against perceptions that it was little more than a welfare institution for the destitute. Moreover, the legislature cleverly designed the Charity Aid Act to cap expenditure and leverage private funding. For example, it promised an additional rate of provincial support "contingent upon the institution receiving aid from sources other than the province."[73] In effect, Schedule A, B, and C institutions could all receive an additional subsidy of up to one-quarter of the amount that they raised from sources separate from the provincial government. This requirement provided an incentive for institutions to solicit outside funds. The act thereby provided institutions with consistent funding, and was also meant to "stimulate and encourage" municipal, corporate, and individual support of local institutions.[74]

In return for provincial funding, the Charity Aid Act required that facilities be externally inspected and report their annual returns in a public and transparent manner. To achieve this, the province expanded the duties of the provincial inspector, a position originally created through the 1868 Prison and Asylum Inspection Act. The inspector was responsible for identifying, inspecting, and reporting on all welfare institutions, recommending which ones should be added to the act's list of funded institutions. The Charity Aid Act required the inspector to examine supported institutions "from time to time" with an eye to "the maintenance, management, and affairs thereof; and by examination of the registers and such other means he may deem necessary, particularly satisfy himself as to the correctness of any returns."[75] He was to report his findings to the lieutenant governor in council, who could order that aid to a particular institution be discontinued or recategorized. Standards were particularly important for hospitals: "[I]f at any time, upon report of said Inspector, it shall be found that any institution of the character named in Schedule A, is insufficient, or without the necessary and proper accommodation or requirements for one of its nature and objects, the Lieutenant-Governor in Council shall thereupon make such order [to discontinue aid]."[76] In addition to inspection, the Charity Aid Act empowered the lieutenant governor to request financial returns from institutions and instituted "a penalty of one thousand dollars" in the case of false returns.[77] More intrusively, the act extended provincial influence over administration, requiring that managers of Schedule A and B institutions "enact by-laws or regulations for the government and management of such institution, prescribing the method and terms of admission thereto, and defining and regulating the duties and powers of all officers and servants of such institution, and the salaries (if any) of such officers and servants." Before taking effect, institutional regulations had to be approved by the lieutenant governor in council.[78]

The provincial inspector during the first two decades of the hospital was John Woodburn Langmuir, who firmly believed that the purpose of provincial support of institutions was not to promote indigence and dependency through long-term institutional care, but rather to return individuals as quickly as possible to the workforce. Pursuing the spirit of the Charity Aid Act, Langmuir emphasized the duty of hospitals to limit patient stays to the period of *active* treatment. In his reports, he observed that hospitals often inappropriately admitted non-treatable patients, and he called for the government to restrict the "maximum period for which patients will be paid for at full hospital rates." The original act in 1874 did not define "actual treatment" or place limits on the length of institutional stays that the province would subsidize, but mindful of the increasing cost of hospitals, an 1879 Order in Council specified that patients hospitalized for over nine months (270 days) would be regarded as Schedule B for purposes of subsidies, thereby meriting the lower, "refuge"-level rates.[79] In one historian's opinion, Langmuir "identif[ied] aged, chronic patients as a particular problem," and hospital managers, such as those at the Toronto General Hospital, "transferred out older, chronic patients to houses of industry."[80] In 1896, the limit on patient stays for Schedule A hospitals was dramatically reduced from 270 to 120 days; The Hospital for Sick Children was, notably, exempted from this new limitation.[81] Over time, more conditions were attached to public financial support. As the inspector stated in his 1898 annual report, hospitals "receiving Government aid are required to admit all who apply and who are proper subjects for hospital treatment, without regard to nationality, religion or their ability to pay."[82]

Within this emerging framework of regulation and government funding, The Hospital for Sick Children posed particular challenges. Langmuir first formally visited the hospital in July 1881,[83] but was unable to make up his mind as to whether it was a Schedule A or Schedule B institution. In a report in 1882, he disclosed his ambivalence:

> It is, to all intents and purposes, an Hospital. It receives aid and cares for children suffering chiefly from chronic diseases, who cannot well be received either into the General Hospital or a regular Orphanage. It combines the character of the General Hospital and the Home for Incurables, but for children alone, hence the large comparative cost of maintenance. [84]

He recommended that the hospital receive only two cents a day per patient during its first year of provincial support because he was unable to obtain full financial returns, a problem complicated by the fact that the hospital continued to pursue a policy of not formally soliciting for private funds. Earlier in the year, Langmuir had informed the provincial secretary about the children's hospital, requesting provincial aid on its behalf. Despite its title as a "hospital" and Langmuir's musings that it was "to all intents and purposes" a hospital, he added it to Schedule C of the Charity Aid Act, granting it a sum of $100, as well as future aid "at the rate of two cents per day for each child treated and cared for in the Hospital."[85] This rate was substantially lower than the twenty cents per day allotted to Schedule A institutions, yet slightly higher than the one and a half cents given to other orphanages in Schedule C.[86]

The Charity Aid Act shaped the composition and experience of the patient population over the course of the 1880s and 1890s. The early mission statements and annual reports of the 1870s explicitly claimed that "the incurable" could not be admitted: "No child suffering from SMALL POX, or other infectious, or any incurable disease, call be admitted into the Hospital."[87] There are signs that in the 1880s, in response to the growing importance of provincial grants, the non-treatable were indeed quietly excluded. The 1881 report, for example, tells of the ladies struggling to transfer a patient into the Hospital for Incurables. Initially excluded from that institution because of her "idiocy" (developmental disability), she would have otherwise had to return to England.[88] The 1884 and 1885 annual reports proposed a "special ward" "where we can take all the sorely afflicted ones, the odds and ends of tiny humanity, in short, the cases that are refused by all other Institutions, keeping it a separate work, maintained by a separate fund and having special Nurses."[89] The 1893 report identified incurable children as both an underserved population and a problem population occupying the space of deserving, treatable sick children.[90]

The evolving provincial regulations and the growing dependence of the hospital on provincial grants (see chart 3.1), also shaped attitudes to curability and payment. In 1880–1, as the hospital began to receive government funding, the regulations for attendance and admission were elaborated beyond specifications of age and illness. The regulations explicitly listed the "classes of children" admitted to the hospital:

1. Sick children, destitute and friendless.
2. Sick children whose parents, owing to poverty, are unable to care for them.
3. Sick children, who, from various circumstances, cannot receive the necessary care and attention at home, but whose friends are willing to contribute somewhat towards the expense actually incurred in their maintenance.

An additional sentence added that the Committee, "unwilling to foster pauperism," was becoming more strict in extracting payments from those who were able.[91] By 1893, the trustees reminded the public that the hospital,

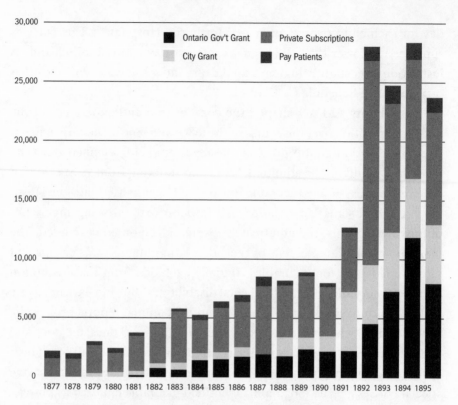

Chart 3.1 Sources of revenue, The Hospital for Sick Children, 1877–95
Source: Annual Reports of The Hospital for Sick Children

in response to the new Charity Aid Act, *had* to accommodate all sick children whose parents could not afford to pay. Partly in response to this, they were adopting a more vigilant stance against incurables: "The cases offered must be acute, such as can be cured or relieved. No chronic or incurable case is under any circumstances admitted." Further, they were encouraging parents of moderate means to contribute something to their child's treatment: "For parents who can afford to pay a rate of $2.50 is made for the public wards, $5 for the semi-private wards and $10 for a private ward. The Trustees desire that all should contribute something towards the hospital."[92]

By the 1890s, the trustees' minutes display ongoing concern about the number of days for which the province would subsidize patients. Minutes from November 1892 reveal that the hospital contacted the inspector when a chronic case sought readmission after a two-year stay. The inspector stated that the government would not subsidize such a case at 30 cents per day, and instructed that "the surgeons and physicians attached to the Hospital should be specially requested to exercise the greatest care in the admission

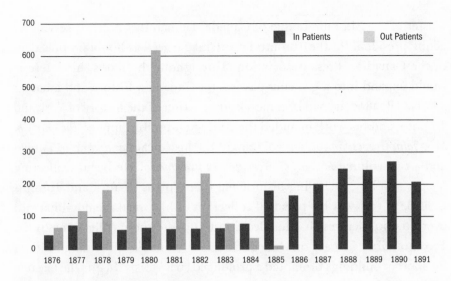

700
600
500
400
300
200
100
0

In Patients   Out Patients

1876 1877 1878 1879 1880 1881 1882 1883 1884 1885 1886 1887 1888 1889 1890 1891

Chart 3.2 Total annual number of inpatients and outpatients treated prior to the opening of the new hospital on College Street (1892)
Source: Annual Reports of The Hospital for Sick Children

of patients, as the Hospital was intended for acute and not for chronic cases."[93] Annual reports were emphatic that the hospital did not retain long-stay patients: "Chronic cases are admitted only when there is a hope that treatment will effect improvement or a cure, and are discharged when this result is attained."[94] In 1896, the annual report tried to further convince its audience that this policy meant shorter patient stays: "The shifting character of the patients is another tribute in the same direction. Children do not remain long, because no incurable cases are received."[95] The hospital's statistics do show that the average stay declined from 88 days in 1888 to 66.7 days in 1893 and 53 days in 1900, bringing it closer to non-paediatric hospitals of the time. [96] Over time, these length-of-stay calculations were presented not just in tables of the medical reports but in the text of the annual reports themselves.[97] By 1894, it was proclaimed, "Every year our Hospital for Sick Children is steadily changing from a permanent 'Home' for ailing children, to a 'Hospital' for the treatment of sick children."[98]

Conclusions

By the time of the construction of the new hospital on College Street in 1891, John Ross Robertson had reached an unparalleled level of wealth and influence in a diverse array of fields. A year earlier, he had become Grand

Master of the Masonic Lodge of Canada. He had just finished serving as acting president for the Toronto Press Club, as well as honorary president of the Canadian Press Association. Throughout the 1890s, his interests would expand into a growing passion for Canadian history and amateur sports.[99] By 1899, he had become a leading writer of the history of York and Toronto, and his work included the editing and publishing of *The Diary of Mrs. John Graves Simcoe*, six volumes of the historical *Landmarks of Toronto*, and a two-volume *History of Freemasonry in Canada*. He began collecting images as a boy, including historic maps and plans of York and Toronto. Indeed, so vast was his personal collection of historical memorabilia and over 20,000 pictures that his decision to donate these collections to the Toronto Public Library on College Street (without also providing funding for another building) prompted a prolonged space crisis. In 1914, he became a fellow of the Royal Society of Canada, and two years later he became the first and possibly only person in Canadian history to reject both a senatorship and a knighthood on the same day.[100]

Robertson is chiefly remembered for his work as a philanthropist and primary benefactor of The Hospital for Sick Children. In his lifetime, he gave the hospital over half a million dollars. In addition to the Lakeside Home, Robertson funded the addition of a five-storey nurses' residence in 1905 and, as will be discussed in the next chapter, the establishment of a milk pasteurization plant in 1909. At his death, his will stipulated a special endowment fund for the hospital based on profits from the *Telegram*. After the death of his second wife in 1947, the hospital received approximately $10 million from his estate and the sale of the newspaper. In 1949, the John Ross Robertson Endowment Fund was established, and in the next two decades the hospital received an additional $6,522,000.[101] Although comparisons across generations are fraught with difficulty, the 1947 sale and the additional funds would approximate the equivalent of over $200 million today.

By the time workers were arranging the pink sandstone blocks for the new hospital on 67 College Street, Robertson had assumed complete control of the charity. In April 1891, he had gained sufficient influence to push through a new incorporation of the hospital, placing the board of trustees firmly in charge. These trustees included powerful men from all walks of life in Toronto and the province. The earliest trustee was Justice Christopher Salmon Patterson, who had also been chairman of the Toronto General Hospital. He resigned in 1888 upon being confirmed as a chief justice of the province. He was joined by William Gooderham, an eccentric Methodist financier and railway magnate who almost single-handedly funded the move of Victoria College to Toronto. Another trustee was Henry O'Brien, a leading lawyer and editor of the *Canadian Law Journal*, whose wife was one of the founding members of the Ladies Committee. Justice John Alexander Boyd, the second-ranking justice in Ontario, who was related to hospital physician Buchan by marriage, was also a member for several years. Unlike Robertson, Body accepted his knighthood (in 1899). Finally, there was Edmund Osler, the supremely wealthy financier and land speculator (who would later be a member of the board of governors of the University of Toronto and had managed the transaction of 245 Elizabeth Street, part or all of which he had owned). After Robertson, Osler appears to have been the most involved in the decision-making of the institution.

Within this powerful group, however, Robertson was primus inter pares, perceiving of the hospital as, in effect, *his* hospital. He would reign as chairman of the trustees for over a quarter of a century, until his death in 1918. As one contemporary suggested, "Here also he is boss. No nurse and no doctor, no parent or guardian must interfere. The self-centred benevolence of the man who created the hospital and the greatest nurses' home in America must be permitted to play the genial despot."[102] The nature of the intense conflict that arose between himself and Elizabeth McMaster may never be known. No doubt, it was in part Robertson's conservative, but hardly unusual, attitude towards women in positions of power in the late Victorian era. Robertson and Goldwin Smith (the editor of *The Nation*) were both in agreement that "a drink and a vote were male prerogatives" and that, reflecting on the growing demand for women to have the vote in the early years of the twentieth century, "[they] haven't the faintest idea what they would do with the franchise even if they had it."[103] Such attitudes were reinforced by the disposition, so skilfully dissected by the phrenologist, that he could "not endure to be opposed." Nevertheless, after a quarter century of his chairmanship and sponsorship, The Hospital for Sick Children would be utterly transformed from an underfunded charity in a small rental home in Toronto to one of the most recognized paediatric institutions in the Western world. Although the romanticism of the island home would continue to charm reporters and well-wishers, it was the construction of a new purpose-built hospital on College Street that would become the focal point of the new medical science of the 1890s.

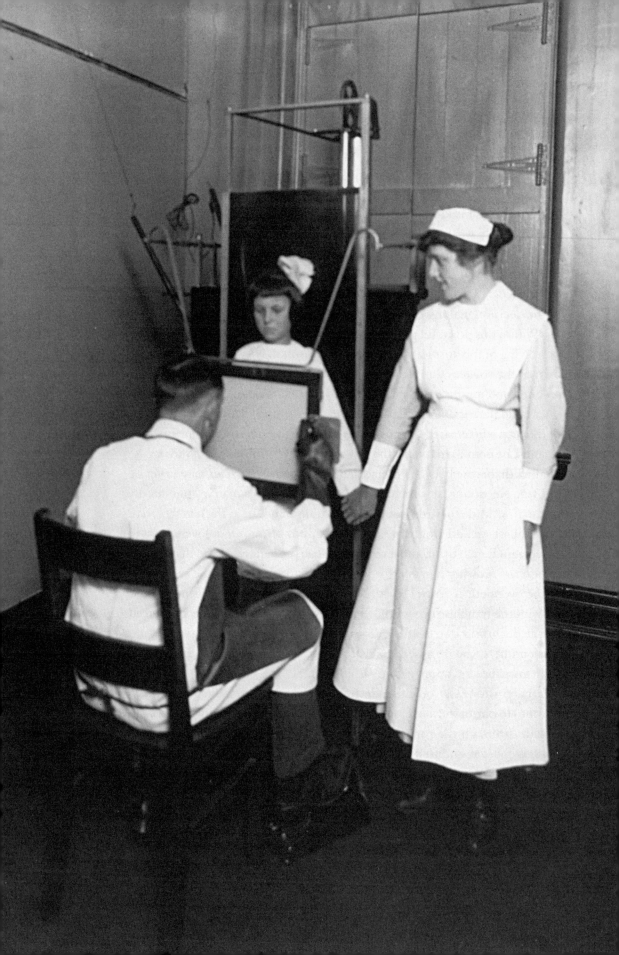

FOUR

Club Feet and Crooked Limbs

Frail little limbs, distorted until one would imagine they could never be put into their proper shape again, are now inactive no more. Heads and arms that were maimed figure in the playground and street, where before they were bandaged and encased in surgical appliances, and it is the same with the little feet.[1]

> "For Deformed Feet. An Appeal for Little Ones with Club Feet and Crooked Limbs" (Appeal Booklet), 1902

Eleven-year-old Thomas J.[2] was admitted to The Hospital for Sick Children in September, 1890. His family circumstances are hard to determine. He was described as being one of a family of fifteen, where at least three other siblings had died in childhood. At the time of admission, he was living with another family, headed by a painter, and alongside five lodgers, one of whom was his brother. Thomas was born with the bottom of his feet turned upwards, a condition that rendered walking virtually impossible without assistance. Remarkably, he was not the only child of his family who was suffering from *talipes equinovarus* or "club foot." His fifteen-year-old brother, Samuel, was also admitted concurrently for the same condition, while an older brother had chosen not to submit himself to surgery. Thomas had little mobility

4.1 John Ross Robertson made much of the new technologies that he acquired for the new College Street hospital. The Hospital for Sick Children claimed to be the first medical institution in Canada to operate an X-ray machine.

in his ankle joint and his Achilles tendon was extremely tense due to his trying to compensate for his feet while trying to walk.[3]

On September 13, a surgeon, Dr. McKenzie, divided Thomas's Achilles tendon in order to correct the angle of his foot, a procedure known as tenotomy. Next the doctors cut the *plantar fascia* – the thick connective tissue that supports the arch of the foot – and the *abductor hallucis*, which is the muscle below it. This created a one-inch wound, which was dressed with gauze and held in place by a flannel roller. The foot was then encased with a plaster of Paris cast. In the days following the surgery, extension[4] was applied. When the toes appeared to darken, the plaster cast was removed and a new, less constrictive one was put in place. By the end of October the right foot had improved; by December, Thomas no longer needed a cast. His Achilles tendon had healed and he was able to flex his right foot to the point that he could continue with only a splint. In early December the doctors began the same surgery on his left foot. On 1 April 1891, after eight months in the hospital, he was discharged as cured from the hospital wearing splints made by the orthopaedic shop. While Thomas still required some aid in walking, his feet were much straighter.[5]

Thomas's surgery reflected an important new era for children's hospitals. What had been small rental homes across the Western world, with volunteer "lady visitors" and limited medical interventions, became laboratories – both physically and figuratively – for some of the most exciting advances in medical science. No longer were these institutions well-meaning, if somewhat ineffective, hospices for children of the sick poor. In late-nineteenth-century Britain and North America, the paediatric hospital was being remade as a site of science and research, which slowly raised its appeal over three decades among a middle-class clientele. The visual imagery of the hospital reflected this transformation, with sterile wards, white nursing uniforms, and long laboratory benches representing order, professionalism, and the emergence of bacteriology. In no other domain of children's treatment was the rise of what is known now as the new "scientific medicine" felt more acutely than in the field of orthopaedic surgery, transforming not only what *could* be done, but, as importantly, what *ought* to be done to reconfigure "crippled" bodies into healthy ones.

John Ross Robertson travelled annually to Europe, during which time he regularly visited institutions and consulted with hospital staff and architects in various British and European cities, gathering ideas about the physical layout of a new children's hospital in Toronto. He would later construct his own two-volume scrapbook entitled "Round the World Hospitals" with pictures, postcards and written notes on his observations.[6] It is likely that he would have seen first-hand the novel medical laboratories that were being constructed on the Continent, particularly during his visits to Berlin, Vienna, Paris, and Munich. Robertson continued to have strong family and cultural ties to Scotland, which remained an important centre of medical education, with Glasgow and Edinburgh producing generations of medical graduates who would spread across the British Empire.[7] It was while in Scotland that Robertson was attracted to the structure of Glasgow's Hospital for Sick Children as a model for his vision for Toronto. He hired John Sellars, a Scottish architect who had worked on that hospital, "to prepare plans for a new Hospital for Sick Children in Toronto."[8] Robertson then passed these preliminary designs onto the well-known architectural firm of Darling and Curry with a request to make the potential building more "rugged and monumental."[9]

By 1886, a building committee had been established with Robertson as the Chair, though there was some debate over the location of the permanent, purpose-built institution. From 1878, the trustees had owned property near the corner of Elizabeth Street and College Street, deep in the heart of the city and still surrounded by tenement housing. As the hospital moved between locations in the 1880s, there was discussion over whether to expand the Elizabeth Street site or refurbish a mansion in Rosedale, in the leafy north of the city that was being populated by grand houses of the city's well-to-do. The trustees originally decided on the bucolic surroundings of Rosedale, but a municipal building grant of $20,000 to commemorate the Queen's Golden Jubilee in 1887, was contingent on the hospital being situated more centrally and its name being changed to the *Victoria* Hospital for Sick Children. Despite these legal conditions, the Building Committee seemed confident that they could locate the new hospital in Rosedale; they rather rashly proceeded to purchase property there for the eventual construction of the hospital. It was only when legal opinion confirmed that the municipal money could not be used for a Rosedale site that the trustees relented to both the College Street location and the revised name, which, though it was only used for a few years in hospital publications, is still visible above the archway to the first permanent hospital.[10]

Building on the College Street site had always been favoured by the medical staff, who feared the difficulty of commuting between their hospital duties and their own private practices if the institution moved northward.

Samuel Blake, the University of Toronto Senator and social gospel reformer, made the most of College Street as a juncture between two Torontos in his speech of maudlin metaphors at the ceremonial turning of the sod in September 1889:

> Toronto did herself great honour in 1887, on the 50th anniversary of Queen Victoria's accession, by voting a grant to this Hospital. I am sure that many blots on the record of the City Council, and many entries of misdeeds, will be wiped out by a tear from the recording angel as his hand writes down their grant towards this building. I am glad that the building is situated just where it is – in St. John's ward, where so much of the city's wretchedness and squallor [sic] are gathered – but also on one side of this fine avenue fronting the costly residences of rich people. Let it be a symbol of how the hearts of the rich should go out to the poor, and the hearts of the poor beat back to the rich ...[11]

Construction of the building was scheduled to be completed by the summer of 1891, but delays forced the trustees to move the children into the constructed, but largely unfurnished, building when the Lakeside Home was closed for the season in late October. After a winter of final touches and donations, the ceremonial opening of the renamed Victoria Hospital for Sick Children was held in May 1892.[12]

The style and scale of the new building reflected architectural trends in Canada and the northeastern United States in the final two decades of the nineteenth century. The distinctive Credit Valley stone, a ruddy-hued sandstone, and the emblematic arched entrance ways could be identified in dozens of contemporary residential and governmental buildings in the core of city, most notably in the magnificent new Parliament buildings, which had been completed only months before the ceremonial sod turning of the children's hospital. Keen observers could detect other prominent Toronto landmarks constructed in this Romanesque Revival style, such as the new (and third) City Hall, as well as the principal building of the relocated Victoria College of the University of Toronto. Although relatively few medical buildings bear this imprint, the Ontario Medical College for Women (1890) was also said to have been constructed in this style.[13] Peculiar to the Toronto hospital and its sister buildings was its distinctive colour. Above the pinkish stone base and rounded portage entry stood "very dark, hard-burned,

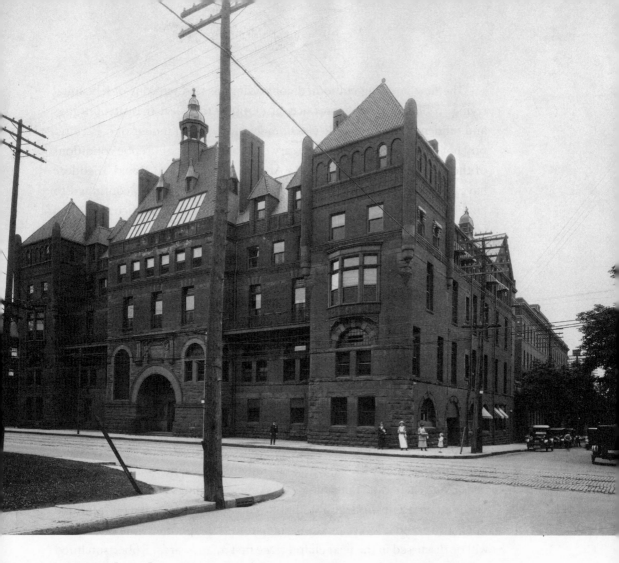

red brick [walls] laid in mortar tinted with Cabot's mortar stain." Hospital advocates suggested, somewhat unconvincingly, that the overall dull red shade "convey[ed] an impression of rest and comfort so the dead material structure seems to harmonize with the benevolent purpose for which it has been erected."[14]

4.2 A photograph of the College Street hospital, looking south from Elizabeth Street. The arched front entry is on College Street (left), emblazoned with the title Victoria Hospital for Sick Children.

Perhaps there was some degree of irony in constructing a children's hospital with a hue that appeared so close to blood red, a double irony now that the building is the headquarters of Canadian Blood Services. Nevertheless, on a streetscape that was still dominated by shanties and lodging houses, this four-story dedication to medical science must have cut an immensely impressive profile, its architectural similarity to the nearby Parliament buildings and Victoria College signifying its position as an important civic institution and symbol of learning and modernity.

The new building embodied contradictions and tensions of a hospital trying to be many things at once, attempting to reflect the surroundings and refinements of a middle-class home, imply the grandeur of contemporary hotels, and provide the necessary environment for antiseptic conditions of the new era of bacteriology. As Annmarie Adams and David Theodore have observed, the College Street hospital, despite its size, continued to emphasize a late-Victorian preoccupation with domesticity, "accomplished largely through the hospital's massing, roof type, materials, scale, historicist imagery, plan, and furniture[.]"[15] The domesticity abutted new spaces of scientific medicine. Sterile operating environments were configured around the corner from mosaic floors and feminine vestibules, "decorated in the spirit of middle-class consumer tastes."[16] In addition to this tension between science and sensibility, the sheer scale of four floors and "steeply pitched roofs ... lent the institution an aristocratic air, conjuring up the obvious associations of European castles."[17] Indeed, the 1891 internal history of the hospital somewhat imaginatively affirmed that it had the "suggestion of [a] French chateau."[18]

Fronting College Street and encompassing an entire block between Elizabeth Street and Emma Street, the internal structure was shaped as a four-story letter E, with the wings embodying long, open wards with metal beds along each wall. Tall windows and curved ceilings emphasized the late-Victorian preoccupation with sunlight, ventilation, and "air flow."[19] Multiple "open air verandas" were incorporated around the perimeter, including, as will be discussed in the next chapter, the first infant wards. Robertson hired a photographer to take scores of images of the new building and patient care, providing an iconography of the College Street building that continues to adorn the hospital to this day.[20] These photographs of the wards suggest a physical environment very similar to that of other turn-of-the-century hospitals in transition to a new aesthetic of sterility, save for the small clusters of toys and the unusual placement of an open-air playground on the second floor. The architecture reflected that another salient feature of the building's design was the avoidance of "sharp angles and edges" on the wards: "the wood work is all rounded, the ceiling is coved, and there are no sharp points and lines to weary the eye of the little sufferers."[21]

New technologies permeated the day-to-day operations of the Victoria Hospital for Sick Children and became a source of immense pride. As the inpatient capacity skyrocketed to over 140 patients,[22] the hospital depended upon a state-of-the-art industrial washing room. The mechanized facilities

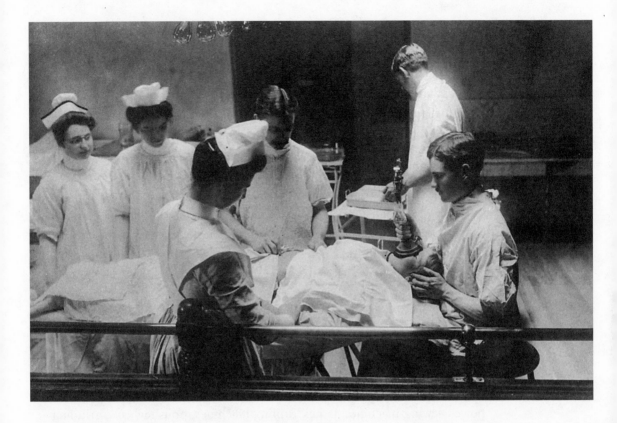

were supervised by a "laundry man" and staffed by five women "helpers" who operated an array of machinery: a steam mangle, a starcher, a centrifugal wringer, a damping press, an ironing table, a range of steam dryers, body and collar ironers and a collar shaper. The facility's importance lay in its role in "preventing the spread of infectious disease,"[23] though apparently it made so much noise running at full throttle that the surgeons, on the floor above, had difficulty communicating with each other.[24]

4.3 Despite the emergence of bacteriology, aseptic and antiseptic techniques were employed somewhat idiosyncratically. Note here the white smocks and the bowls of iodine in the background, but the absence of gloves or facemasks.

In contrast to the hospital's earlier dwellings, which lacked even piped water in the late 1870s, 67 College Street contained numerous technological efficiencies, including expensive elevators and mechanized heating and ventilation. The electric lighting, fans, and laundry were powered by "motors supplied from an electric plant on the premises."[25] An engineer and electrician joined the paid staff to address the "heating, plumbing, gas and electrical challenges" of such a large institution.[26] Within the first decade of operation, the hospital also acquired its own X-ray equipment and in-house photographer (1896–7), bacteriological room (1897), and orthopaedic machine shop

(1899). In that same year, a gymnasium was begun "with the very latest apparatus for the treatment of lateral curvature of the spine and other deformities."[27] In 1896, the trustees boasted about the institution's modern medical and scientific trappings, in particular the purchase of the X-ray machine, apparently the first of any children's hospital in North America:

> To show that the trustees are keenly alive to the progress of science, as applied to the healing art, it may be stated that the most improved surgical apparatus is introduced and used by the best surgical and medical skill available. An X Ray equipment has just been imported from Europe, and this wonderful evolution of the scientific genius of the 19th century is added to the fine mechanical appliances at hand. It will be sure to add to the marvelous cures already effected in this Hospital.[28]

In 1899, an orthopaedic shop and surgical appliance shop were established in a cottage on hospital property in order to provide more efficiently and economically the necessary apparatus (supports, trusses, crutches, braces) for in- and outpatients. Reports emphasized the industrial, mechanized nature of shop work: "All the machinery is run in this Department by electric power, sewing machines, lathes, drilling machines, polish wheels, grinding stones, etc. And thus this constant work by our expert orthopaedic machinist goes on every hour of the day."[29] Annual reports indicate that surgeons sent their "designs and measurements" to workmen, who were directed by "a highly qualified mechanical specialist," supervised by the surgeons themselves.[30] In praising the new building, a correspondent to the *Lancet* in Britain concluded that it was probably the "most complete" children's hospital in all of North America. However, he regretted that the enormous cost of the new facility left the trustees with an unaddressed debt of about 20,000 pounds, which, he feared, might well "cripple its usefulness."[31]

Paediatric Surgery

Over the next two decades, the hospital's new self-image would emerge from the operating theatre, originally a modest twelve-by-twelve-foot room leading from one of the principal waiting rooms on the ground floor in the east wing.[32] Surgery had long been the backwater of medical practice, a tortuous and much-feared ordeal of amputation, dental extractions, bone-setting, and minor invasive procedures. However, the discovery and application of anaesthesia from the 1840s – first in the form of ether and later chloroform – helped to transform the gruesome spectacle into one of comparatively painless wonderment. Freed from the nightmare of inflicting surgery on poorly anaesthetized patients, clinicians became more adventurous in their procedures, even if, as in the case of Caesarian sections, the outcome was often a higher rate of maternal mortality than that which existed before. While there was some debate over the risk of anaesthetizing the young, Martin Pernick, the leading historian of anaesthesia in the nineteenth century, has argued that "[f]or children too little to be restrained by reason, yet too big to be restrained easily by force, anesthesia was especially valuable."[33] Indeed, the first "guidelines" to paediatric anaesthesia were published as the soil was being turned on College Street, in 1889. However, some historians claim that a persistent issue with childhood surgery was the fear induced by the administration of anaesthesia itself. Sedation would eventually be employed just prior to the First World War, because up to that time many children had to be restrained before anaesthesia was administered.[34]

Surgery, of course, continued to be constrained by the fear of septic infection, which contributed to persistently high rates of post-operative mortality during the Victorian era. The advent of antiseptic techniques (the killing of "germs" during the surgical procedure) and asepsis (the establishment of sterile environments before and after surgery) helped to diminish these threats. Although pioneered in the 1840s, antisepsis has long been associated with the Scottish surgeon Joseph Lister, who experimented with a range of antiseptic sprays and "disinfection" techniques in late-1860s Glasgow. Lister built upon Louis Pasteur's experiments in fermentation and hypothesized that septic infection was due to microorganisms that were too small to be seen by the naked eye. He experimented, as did Pasteur, with various agents that would control putrefaction and sepsis, ultimately embracing the deployment of carbolic acid (phenol), an agent that had been used in contemporary agriculture. His technique, known popularly as Listerism, was controversial among contemporary physicians, many of whom were skeptical of the efficacy of washing their hands with various chemical agents prior to surgery or having carbolic acid sprayed on the operating table during procedures.[35]

British and North American medicine subsequently witnessed two decades of debate over what is now known by medical historians as the "germ theory of disease" – that is, the contention that specific diseases (such as tuberculosis or cholera) were the result of infection from specific micro-organisms. It was a radical idea – and not one readily accepted by all practitioners. Although Ontario's Abraham Groves reputedly performed the first antiseptic operation in Ontario as early as 1874, the widespread adoption of the technique in Canada probably did not occur until the 1880s, and even then there were differences of opinion as to what Listerism actually meant in practice.[36] J.T.H. Connor suggests that the 1878 appointment of Fred LeMaitre Grasett (who trained under Lister and has been credited with introducing antiseptic methods to Canada) explains that hospital's "smooth transition to this new surgical era."[37] Grasett, who had also a brief association with the children's hospital in 1877–8,[38] returned to the Active Medical Staff of College Street between 1897 and 1901, the year that the bacteriological room was opened. Even then, as one can see from photographs of surgery in the new children's hospital in the early twentieth century (see image 4.3), antiseptic techniques might well be employed in a variety of ways, such as surgery without the use of gloves or masks, which many surgeons complained compromised their technical accuracy. As the historian of surgery Thomas Schlich has demonstrated, "local cultures" of aseptic practice operated concurrently in the final decades of the nineteenth and first two decades of the twentieth century.[39] Clearly, at The Hospital for Sick Children in Toronto certain new standards – surgical smocks, white nursing uniforms, techniques of sterilization – had been adopted whilst other aspects were largely not observed until the 1920s. Nevertheless, with the identification of the tuberculosis and anthrax bacteria in the 1870s, the era of bacteriology was slowly taking hold and transforming medical practice and the hospital.[40]

Medical literature of the Victorian era reveals a multitude of childhood conditions that could, theoretically at least, be treated by surgery. In 1860 the Englishman Athol A. Johnson gave a series of lectures, later published in the *British Medical Journal*, that included operations for newborns with fusion of lips, imperforate anus, colostomy (the Littre operation), vaginal atresia, cleft lip, and congenital joint dislocations. The same year, John Cooper Forster authored the first English textbook of paediatric surgery, *The Surgical Diseases of Children,* one of the first works to discuss the use of anaesthesia with children. Translations of European texts soon followed, such a key work by Paul Louis Benoit Guersant (Paris), who authored a text on childhood surgery (in 1864), which was translated into English in 1873. Guersant included chapters on conditions and interventions such as gum lancing, eye cancer and cataracts, hernia repair, ear foreign bodies, burns, chronic arthritis, anal prolapse and rectal polyps, cysts, vascular tumour, cervical adenitis, phimosis, fractures, tracheostomy, hypertrophy of tonsils, and ozaena (nasal ulcerations).[41]

Despite the wide variety of *potential* interventions, surgery was relatively rare and used sparingly with children at mid-century. At Great Ormond Street in the 1850s, bladder stone removal and emergency tracheostomy were the most common surgical procedures. The only serious surgery consisted of "a few amputations of diseased and tuberculous joints, where otherwise the child would have inevitably died."[42] Yet as antiseptic techniques began to be generalized in the 1880s, orthopaedics quickly rose to the forefront of the new paediatric surgery and operations became more invasive. Medical men slowly turned their main attention from life-saving surgery to the alteration of bodily deformities. Indeed, when introduced in the eighteenth century, the term *orthopaedia* itself referred to the straightening of *children*'s bones (ortho – paedia) by mechanical apparatus and surgery. Robley Dunglison's *Medical Lexicon* (1842), defined orthopaedics as "the part of medicine whose object is to prevent and correct deformity in the bodies of children" though he added in 1853 that the term was "[o]ften used, however, with a more extensive signification, to embrace the correction or prevention of deformities at all ages."[43]

New surgical procedures transformed the treatment of compound fractures, osteomyelitis, and joint infections, which formerly could only be treated by amputation. For example, the 1860s witnessed the development of a major form of surgical intervention, subcutaneous osteotomy (the technique of cutting and dividing bones by making insertions under the skin). Osteotomy was performed primarily on children, at times to treat "knock-knees" and legs bowed by rickets. By the 1880s this was replaced by what was called "open" antiseptic osteotomy. Procedures involving tendon and muscle transfer were introduced in the 1890s for patients with infantile paralysis, who were also treated with myotomy and fasciotomy. The repeated opening and excision of diseased glands also became common by the 1890s. By the end of the century spinal surgery was becoming a realistic procedure, and in 1909, the invention of the motor bone-saw initiated a "new era in bone grafts."[44] Most of these procedures were incorporated into De Forest Willard's *The Surgery of Childhood*, the first American surgical textbook specifically concerning children, which was published in 1910 and focused on fractures and orthopaedic deformities.[45]

Surgery at The Hospital for Sick Children

The Hospital for Sick Children in Toronto was well positioned to be at the forefront of this revolution in paediatric surgery. Its proximity to the University of Toronto figured as an important factor. The Department of Surgery at the University of Toronto had been founded just a few years earlier in 1887 by William T. Aikins, who was a consultant to the children's hospital from its early years and was then dean of the Faculty of Medicine. With such personal connections to the university elite, it was little surprise that medical students began to receive some instruction at the children's hospital from 1894, with the first formal university teaching of paediatrics beginning in 1899. With the recruitment in 1894 of Clarence Starr, who had trained at the Hospital for Ruptured and Crippled Children in New York, orthopaedic surgery had a new champion. By 1906, orthopaedic surgery became the first surgical specialty offered by the university, and orthopaedics was then overwhelmingly concerned with children.[46]

The earliest extant medical casebooks from the children's hospital, dating from the years 1889–92, or just at the period of transition to the new hospital, provide a rare opportunity to examine early cases of paediatric surgery and place them within the context of the broader patient profile. Cross-referencing names and addresses (when given) to the 1891 census of the province of Ontario also contributes some basic socio-demographic information on the patients and their families. In total, 220 patients appear in the medical casebooks that date from 1890 to 1892, of whom 45 per cent were girls and 55 per cent boys, all aged between two and fourteen.[47] Of these, approximately 80 per cent of patients came from Toronto itself. The patient population was part of the working poor of the city – with fathers whose occupations (in the 1891 census) included labourers, blacksmiths, carpenters, shoemakers, and rag peddlers.

The hospital admitted children for a variety of environmental and congenital conditions. Formal diagnoses were attributed to only two-thirds of the patients, but one can still make some general statements. Of the acquired, or what one might more accurately call "environmental" conditions, tuberculosis reigned supreme, implicated in as many as one-third of all admissions. The White Plague, as tuberculosis was then often called, may well have been the primary infection for osteomyelitis and the principal cause of Pott's disease. The largest clusters of "complaints" – as the *pro forma* header on the medical case records referred to them – were hip-joint disease, attributed to at least 10 per cent of admissions at this time, with another 10 per cent suffering from *talipes* (club foot), knee-joint disease and other deformities of the leg, hip and spine. There were also smaller groups of patients who were suffering from nutritional deficiencies, such as "rickets" (a condition due to malnutrition resulting in, among other things, skeletal deformities) and "marasmus" (a more general term referring to severe malnutrition and loss of body fat). Rickets may well have been the cause of the "knock knees" and "bowed knees"

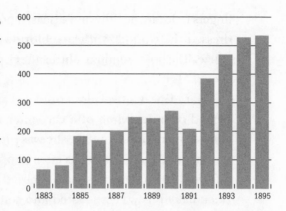

Chart 4.1 Total number of inpatients treated annually, The Hospital for Sick Children, 1883-95
Sources: AR 1883-95

described in some of the surgical cases. The hospital, like other children's hospitals, tended to prohibit the admission of children with infectious diseases, which accounts for the very small number of children (compared to the city as a whole) who were suffering from enteric and typhoid fevers (no more than a dozen in the sample). A small number of children suffering from various "ophthalmia" were also seen, some for cataract surgery.

A few case studies illustrate some of the dimensions of clinical care at the time of the construction of the new hospital. Patient William P. was a six-year-old boy, the son of a marble cutter, suffering from acute osteomyelitis (inflammation of the bone or bone marrow). The boy first became ill with a swollen and painful right ankle, fever, and delirium. Once admitted to the hospital, the patient was repeatedly chloroformed, and both deep and superficial incisions were made to release pus and "purulent matter" from swellings on his thighs, knees, calves and ankles. The cavities were washed out, drainage tubes inserted for discharge, and the wounds dressed antiseptically. This type of procedure was carried out at least five times by mid-September. On November 6 and 10 Dr. Peters operated twice again, excising portions of necrosed bone as well as "unhealthy gelatinous material" from the tibia. These operations entailed a long recovery: At the end of March 1892, it was noted that the patient was discharging less pus and was "lately ... able to get about a little in chair" and go to school. Another operation was performed in early May 1892 and early June 1892. In June, Dr. Féré administered chloroform. The physician explored the sinus and excised "small scale of bone" from the left tibia, using a probe and his own fingers to locate healthy and diseased bone. He inserted drainage tubes and dressed the wounds with perchloride gauze and sinuses with Iodoform gauze. The boy "vomited a little after operation, but there were no signs of shock."[48]

Mary F. was a twelve-year-old girl suffering from hip-joint disease, the second of six children of a carpenter in St. Matthews Ward.[49] After her admission in March of 1891, she was placed in bed "with the limb between sandbags." About five weeks later an operation was performed under chloroform: "an incision was made behind the great trochanter," from which "thick flaky pus was evacuated and some gelatinous tissue scraped away." The cavity was thoroughly irrigated, a drainage tube introduced, and a dressing applied. The tube was removed three weeks later. She began wearing a Thomas Modified Hip Splint at the end of October, and began to learn to walk with the splint, boot, and crutches. A small amount of discharge continued to emerge from the sinus left by the drainage tube in November. Nevertheless, she was discharged by the end of the month, cured.[50]

By contrast, patient Beatrice C., a six-year-old girl, died in the hospital from the same condition. She had been "lame" for three months, complaining of pain in her knee. Her condition worsened despite Dr. Watson administering her cod liver oil. Although she had suffered from measles three years prior, apart from the pain in her legs, her overall health appeared good. Her pain came from the fact that her long bone (femur) was too large for her hipbones. The doctors tried to treat this by using a technique of extending her legs with a four-pound stocking and then putting sand bags around them. She was kept on bed rest for nine months. During the summer months she was moved to the Lakeside Home, where her health appeared to improve. When she returned to the hospital, despite feeling better, there was renewed swelling over her hipbone. On 27 November 1890 Dr. Cameron and Dr. Primrose made an incision from the girl's spine to the neck of her femur. They removed the pus from the area and then proceeded to take a keyhole saw and cut through the large part of her trochanter, which is the part of the femur that connects to the hipbone. During surgery the doctors had difficulty moving the muscles in order to perform the bone removal. Her acetabulum, the concave surface of the pelvis where the head of the femur meets with the pelvis, showed signs of extensive disease. The doctors irrigated the area and set about disinfecting the wound. After a two-and-a-half hour operation on this area, the patient went into shock. Her pulse decreased rapidly. The staff administered Brandy beef tea through her rectum and surrounded her with hot water bottles. Although she regained consciousness and recognized her doctor for a few minutes, her temperature rose to 104 degrees. Nineteen hours after the operation she died.[51]

Despite tragic outcomes in some patients, the total number of operations rose dramatically during the first quarter century of the hospital, from half a dozen in 1875 to close to 200 in 1891, surpassing the 500-operation milestone by 1906. In that last year, there had been 518 surgical operations: 82 for adenoids/tonsils, 49 for club feet, 36 for diseases of the bone, 31 for concussions, 20 for abscess incisions, 17 for hernias or ruptures, 11 for cleft palates, 10 for wounds and injuries, 9 for catarrhs, 8 for mastoids, 6 for cyst incisions, and 1 for hammer toe.[52] Of these, club foot took on a totemic presence in the institution during the period from the opening of the new hospital in 1892 until the First World War. Hospital publications were flooded with the photographs of dozens upon dozens of club foot cases (sometimes entire groups of club feet). Routinized surgical cures for club foot, in particular, would become of visual and symbolic importance to the hospital of scientific surgery. As one 1905 appeal pamphlet proclaimed the transformative effects of the new era of orthopaedic surgery and invited more and more applicants:

> It means a lot to a crippled youngster to have his feet straightened, for then he has a fair chance in the race for life.
>
> Scores of cases can be found in the Hospital books where boys, who were absolute cripples, to all external appearance incurable, are now doing well at manual employment
>
> ... There must be many cases of club feet in Ontario that could be corrected if sent to the Hospital.
>
> Can you send us the name of the any parent who cannot afford to pay for his child's correction?[53]

Surgery for club foot thus operated on emotional and instrumental levels. Certainly, it restored functioning to children, but that restoration was not based solely on returning a happy true childhood to children from poor backgrounds, but also on rendering them healthy and productive and thus (although not always stated) compliant working-class citizens. It also suggested something far more subtle and complicated about changing attitudes to physical disability. Rather than something "natural" and inevitable, and indeed ubiquitous within industrial societies, physical deformity was slowly being reconceptualized as stigmatizing and pitiable. There emerged a palpable sense that correcting physical deformity was not just a scientific possibility, it was a moral and economic obligation.

The growing emphasis on surgery also led to a major medical spat in 1894 involving Dr. B.E. McKenzie, the orthopaedic specialist who was the surgeon in the opening case of this chapter. Two staff members objected to McKenzie using the outpatient clinic as a vehicle for his private practice and complained to the trustees about their concerns. McKenzie was alleged to have claimed "full charge of the Orthopaedic Surgery both in-door and out"; he denied this but asserted that he and John Ross Robertson had agreed that the surgeon would begin a Friday afternoon outpatient orthopaedic clinic. His correspondence reveals the unclear distinction between gratuitous hospital care and its relationship to private income in the decades before state health insurance. McKenzie identified to the board of trustees thirty-three patients whom he had privately treated.

> Of this number thirty either consulted me at my own office previous to admission to the Hospital or came to the hospital for the definite purpose of consulting me. More than ten of the number came to consult me as private patients and were paying me as such, when owing to various circumstances they sought admission to the hospital, in several cases not by my advice. Under these circumstances it was impossible that the condition should exist that the surgeon should not accept a fee from a ward patient under his care. I have lived up to the letter and spirit of the hospital regulations in this regard, which in my opinion is a proper regulation, while at the same time due care is exercised by the hospital not to interfere with private practice. [54]

The two complaining resident surgeons – Frank Martin and J.T. Robinson – protested McKenzie's attendance at the outdoor clinic and alleged that he "conduct[ed] that part of it which is of most interest [to him], viz: deformities, bone diseases and the like, leaving the medical cases to our care or to their own devices." Further, they claimed he had been seen accepting fees from outdoor patients, that multiple families were unable to pay fees due to contracts with McKenzie, and that he treated his nurses in a "discourteous and ungentlemanly" manner. McKenzie retorted that he had not accepted fees from clinic patients, but that he had accepted payment merely for "boots and other appliances." The trustees resolved to settle the dispute by completely separating the work of the outdoor and indoor medical staff, and by articulating a payment policy for private patients admitted by staff members. A separate outdoor staff of five was appointed.[55] Later, in 1906, the outpatient and inpatient staff were merged, and "physicians attending a case in the dispensary follow it to the ward."[56]

This rather minor dispute reflected the growing importance of the hospital as a locus of surgical care. Although minor operations had, in the Victorian era, been performed in a host of environments, including people's homes, this practice was fading quickly. By the 1890s, the hospital was the centre for modern, aseptic procedures. Who had access to the hospital's facilities, and most importantly, the supporting infrastructure and nursing staff was becoming of cardinal importance to medical livelihoods. The Hospital for Sick Children, with its rising success of surgery and its attachment to the University of Toronto became increasingly coveted. However, it was not just the techniques and the physical site of surgery. The new era of surgery and patient care also required a new supporting staff of trained and experienced nurses. As Ulrich Tröhler argues, "Antisepsis, and particularly asepsis, required a strict set of rules, and became instrumental in transforming surgery to a form of teamwork."[57] What is more, experienced nurses were needed for the long and arduous period of rehabilitation after surgery. In order to achieve this, the hospital would bow to the inevitable, and overcame its ambivalence by establishing a robust and ultimately successful training school for nurses.

A New Profession for Women

The new era of "scientific medicine" required not only the regulation of the medical profession itself; it also encouraged the professionalization of nursing. There had been women who had self-identified as nurses for hundreds of years, an occupation that was often barely distinguishable from the duties of domestic servants. There were no regulations as to who could call themselves nurses or indeed what practice they might entail. All was done by reputation, local custom, and word of mouth. With the rise of the Georgian and Victorian hospital systems, however, the demand for *institutional* nursing increased dramatically, as did the sense that nurse training should be somehow formalized. Within the British world, the professionalization of nursing has, rightly or wrongly, been associated with Florence Nightingale and the establishment of nurse training schools in the 1860s and 1870s. "Nightingale nurses" – educated, predominantly middle-class women – were contrasted with a caricatured traditional nurse, who was uncouth, lacking dedication and, too often, drunk. The new role models were young women receiving institutional training – usually based in hospitals – in the new science of medicine and receiving salaries, however modest. Formal periods of apprenticeship emerged, as well as curricula, uniforms, and nurse residences.[58] "A New Profession for Women" had been established, trumpeted the *Canadian Independent* in 1883.[59]

By the 1880s, nursing schools were becoming increasingly common in Canada, as evidenced by the establishment of one at both the Toronto General Hospital and Montreal General Hospital.[60] Despite the falling out of Elizabeth McMaster and John Ross Robertson, ostensibly due to the nature of nurse training, the 1893 annual report of The Hospital for Sick Children offered an upbeat and optimistic vision of their own nurse training at the College Street site: "Our Nurses' Training School, under the care of the superintendent and members of the medical staff, has been specially successful in the new building. The training given is of a high order, and with the many illustrative appliances at hand, our nurses are sent out at the end of two years well equipped for nursing, not only diseases of children, but for general work."[61] Reversing his objections to nurse training in the children's hospital a few years earlier, Robertson proclaimed that, "We have endeavoured to place our trained nurses on a par with those who graduate from the best training schools on this continent." In a direct contradiction of his earlier contention that nurses trained in a paediatric institution would not have sufficient skills to be generalized to community work, he emphasized the graduates' professional competency "to undertake any kind of work in a sick room, from the charge of sick people, be they babies or adults."[62]

The appointment of Superintendent Louise C. Brent energized nurse training at the hospital. Brent had graduated from nursing at Brooklyn City Hospital in 1890 and was superintendent of Toronto Grace (Homeopathic) Hospital until she joined The Hospital for Sick Children in 1896. Over the next four years, Brent helped systematize training, in part by expanding the training school curriculum from two to three years.[63] Brent taught a class weekly, and, from October 1899 to May 1900, "the active and special staff of the Hospital" gave a series of 28 lectures to the nursing students (see table 4.1). In keeping with many nursing schools of the 1890s, nurses resided on site, crammed into the top floor of the hospital, unless they were seconded to the Lakeside Home during the summer months.[64] Indeed, the living quarters of the nurses seemed to fluctuate from season to season, with certain wards taken over by excess nursing students and then converted back to patient wards during periods of high demand.

Table 4.1 Course of lectures delivered to the nurses during the year 1 October 1899 to 30 September 1900[65]

Anatomy (4)	Dr. D. J. G. Wishart
Gynaecology (4)	Dr. R. J. Wilson
Surgical Appliances (2)	Dr. F. N. G. Starr
Anatomy of Eye and Ear (1)	Dr. J. M. MacCallum
Diseases of the Ear and Eye (1)	Dr. J. M. MacCallum
Dietetics (4)	Dr. Harold Parsons
Pneumonia, Rheumatism, Erysipelas, Malaria (4)	Dr. W. B. Thistle
Obstetrics (4)	Dr. H. Crawford Scadding
Surgery (4)	Dr. A. Primrose

By the turn of the century, the new curriculum and new hospital began to attract significant numbers of applicants. In 1900, there were 450 applications, of which "less than five per cent were accepted."[66] By 1907, the school boasted a cohort of 53 nursing students: 9 head nurses, 9 senior nurses (in their third year), 9 intermediate (in their second), and 12 junior (in their first year), and 14 probationers.[67] Like other hospitals with training schools, the hospital relied heavily on the labour of probationary and pupil nurses. In addition to caring for patients on the wards, nurses were assigned an array of housekeeping, dietetic and administrative tasks, from preparing patient meals to recording and maintaining records of patients in the admitting and outpatient departments. In March of the same year, the training school appointed its first full-time instructor and created the first "preliminary" training course in Canada, where probationary students were taught full-time before working on the wards. Miss Annie Kinder instructed these students until she became assistant superintendent in 1913.[68]

Nurses were central to both the new surgical reality of the College Street hospital and the complementary rehabilitative treatments that addressed physical deformity. Surgery occurred in conjunction with a range of pre- and post-operative interventions that were gaining traction, so to speak, from the 1880s onwards.[69] As mentioned in the previous chapter, much stock was put in open-air treatment – either on the verandas of College Street or at the Island home. Nutrition was to take on an increasingly important role, as evidenced by the training in the new science of dietetics at the hospital by 1900. The training school added a course in dietetics, taught by dietician Mrs. George MacBeth, for "[m]uch emphasis was placed on the cooking and serving of food and on the diet needs of patients, including infants."[70]

New splints and frames were being constructed in Toronto, Boston, and London to allow for total immobilization of diseased parts of the body. These methods required prolonged bed rest and were "characterized by an array of metal appliances, plaster-of-Paris casts, splints, and bandages[.]"[71] One new device, an iron pipe and canvas frame – aka the "Bradford Frame" – became a standard piece of orthopaedic equipment in children's hospitals at the turn of the century, named after Edward Hickling Bradford of the Boston Children's.[72] Other non-surgical approaches to treatment involved techniques such as "medical gymnastics, massage, and mechanotherapy, electrotherapy, galvanotherapy and hydrotherapy ..."[73]

By 1907, the consolidation of the nursing program was more or less complete. In February, a nurses' residence formally opened with 70 bedrooms for nurses and 21 for domestics, as well as a suite for the Superintendent.[74] Funded by Robertson and named after his late wife, Maria Louisa, the five-floor red-brick Colonial building residence was constructed at a cost of about $140,000 on ten lots owned by the trustees, located roughly 300 feet south of the hospital. It was outfitted with modern amenities including a sewing room with two electric sewing machines, a "vacuum cleaner electric plant" in lieu of brooms, and a refrigeration room equipped with a sanitary "arctic" dry air refrigerator. The residence also contained a lecture room, demonstration room, reference and fiction libraries, a roof garden, gymnastics room, parlour, writing room, and even a heated swimming pool.[75]

The introduction of nurse training schools was a core part of the larger transformation of the late nineteenth-century hospital. Residential, apprenticeship systems of nurse training supplied hospitals with an increasingly skilled, constant, and flexible labour force enabled hospitals to accommodate greater numbers of patients at minimal cost. Average monthly stipends for nurses ranged from $8 to $12, and hospitals could hire out student nurses

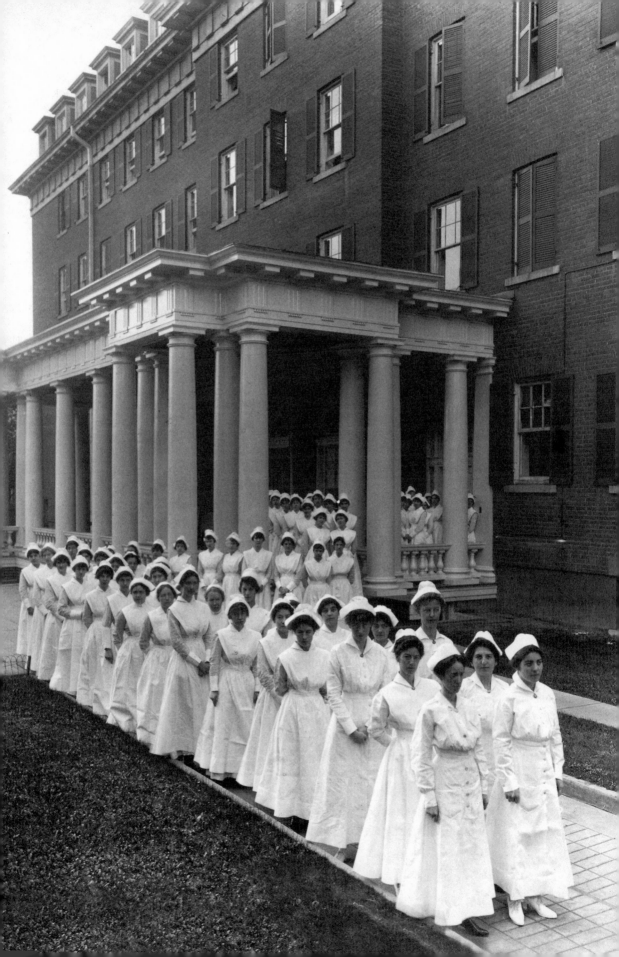

for private duty nursing, for which the institution received payment. Strict schedules and codes of conduct governed nurses' behaviour. As Kathryn McPherson suggests, training school managers "implemented codes of dress and behaviour designed to desexualize apprentices and enhance the social status of nursing and hospital care."[76] Moreover, trained, uniformed nurses were the guardians and guarantors of the moral environment and quality of care. Children's hospitals led the reform of nursing's image "because of their pressing need to convince parents and subscribers that the young patients were getting the very best in care."[77] Exalted as heroically devoted, self-sacrificing caregivers, they occupied a central, often angelic, role in The Hospital for Sick Children's photographic collection.[78]

In the wake of the regulation and monopoly of the medical profession, nurses occupied an interstitial space in hospitals at the time; male doctors – and they were all male doctors at The Hospital for Sick Children in its first three decades – were eager to have highly trained women who acted in a professional but also a subordinate manner. Women's presence reinforced the modern nature of the hospital and its appeal to middle class clientele, but at the same time the nurses' subordinate position did not challenge male medical authority. This tension might account for the rambling ambiguities of the 1894 commencement speech to nurses from the then provincial inspector, Mr. Chamberlain, who attempted to emphasize both their professionalism and their subservience:

> You could not have chosen a calling which requires greater patience, greater diligence, perhaps self-sacrifice. While you have learned, and faithfully, I believe, to follow the directions of the medical man under whose charge you act without having recourse to any suggestions of your own, – because you know that is strictly forbidden, but while I say strictly forbidden there are cases – no doubt you have met with them here – in which that rule cannot be strictly followed and to do so would exhibit your ignorance more than to obey it would prove your devotion ...[79]

Despite the patronizing tone of the provincial inspector, the quotidian pressures of the children's hospital must have been emotionally draining, the reality of medicine in the 1890s suggesting a parallel narrative to the much-publicized success stories of the orthopaedics department. Take, for example, the case of ten-year-old Harry J. He lived all of his life at a Girls'

Home until he was eventually transferred to the Victoria Industrial Home and later the hospital. He was described as "stupid" and "slightly deaf." When he was first admitted to the hospital in 1890, his generally physical condition was fairly stable, despite having a past history of seizures. His temperature, heart rate, and bowel movements were regular, however, he suffered a constant frontal headache. Over the next three months, his physical state deteriorated. Beginning only a week after being admitted, he began to suffer convulsions with increasing regularity. Food began to make him feel nauseous and he began to vomit more often. His face would become flush, his body would shake, and his eyes would roll from side to side. By the end of February he had completely lost the ability to see. He began to lose control of his bowels and the nurses would find him covered in his own excrement. Soon he was unable to walk unescorted and eventually felt too weak to leave the bed. In the final days his breathing became more and more irregular. He would froth at the mouth and his convulsions, which had previously only lasted a few minutes continued for hours. On his final day, after an epically long seizure, he ceased breathing and died at 9:00 a.m., less than two months after coming to the hospital. The autopsy showed that his sarcoma (tumour) was the size of a hen's egg and had filled the anterior notch of the cerebellum. The archives record details of the medical state of the child; it only hints at the emotional world of the nurses in whose care he was placed and who would oversee his tragic demise.[80]

Conclusions

Over the fifteen years between the opening of the new hospital in 1891 and the establishment of the paediatric specialty of orthopaedics at the University of Toronto (in 1906), surgery had become the defining image of the new hospital on College Street. Surgical success stories dominated the hospital's public appeals for support, with the ubiquitous "before and after" photographs transforming public sensibilities of what could be achieved through the miracles of scientific medicine. This dominance of orthopaedic surgery was transatlantic. Great Ormond Street, Boston Children's, and Children's Hospital of Philadelphia were likewise becoming known for their orthopaedic work.[81] Orthopaedic surgery altered not only the self-image of the children's hospital at the turn of the century, it also affected popular attitudes to disability — to the "crippled child." Crippled children became the objects of charities that sought to render them "useful and independent."[82]

Over time, Clarence Starr and the other staff surgeons at The Hospital for Sick Children became a new generation of medical heroes. Orthopaedic surgery was about reconfiguring the body, performing miracles that had, a generation before, been entirely unanticipated. This represented a remarkable transformation for a field of medicine that was a gothic drama of amputation and excruciatingly painful interventions. From the dawn of the twentieth century, surgeons would be characterized as pioneers, venturing daringly into uncharted territory. Surgery also contributed to a tendency in twentieth-century medicine towards "localism" – the physical identification of diseased body parts that could be either excised or reconfigured largely apart from the patient as a whole. Notably, some medical images thus began to disassociate the operation or the "disease" from the person, as evidenced in the many contemporary images of club feet, photographed apparently without any complementary body attached. There was also a subtle financing incentive: surgery was perceived as a fundamentally acute *medical* intervention, and thus requiring full provincial funding. As one author suggests, "the decision to operate for chronic diseases [often] depended on social rather than medical motives, since in the absence of public-health insurance long-lasting conservative treatment was accessible for the well-to-do only."[83]

After years of working in a noisy and cramped room on the main floor, and complaints from 400 medical students,[84] surgery soon so dominated inpatient care that the entire upper floor of the College Street hospital was reconfigured in 1912 into an operating *department*, consisting of "two large well lighted and equipped operating rooms, general and emergency; surgical dressing room ; sterilizing room ; instrument room ; nurses' workroom, for making supplies ; surgeons' locker and dressing room, with shower bath; surgical supply room, and dental room." The old operating space on was refitted as the X-ray department.[85] To finance this, the trustees approached the city again, this time for a loan for a staggering $250,000. It is an indication of the growing popularity of the hospital that, although the modest 1887 city loan (of $20,000) only passed narrowly by a margin of eight votes, the vote on the expansion in 1912 was overwhelmingly supported by a 4:1 margin, a greater plurality than the votes on a slew of other massive municipal expenditures ($6.6 million for water works, $1.3 million for water filtration, and $2.5 million to extend Bloor eastward and construct a viaduct).

Surgery, in some key psychological respects, became all about control. The routine and ritual of antisepsis, the precise attention of the new era of surgery in closed, sterile environments, contrasted with the mayhem of the streets outside. The Dispensary – the window onto the wider community – was coming under incessant pressure, as mothers with infant children begged for help with infectious diseases and nutritional conditions. By the first decade of the twentieth century, the hospital acknowledged that there had been over thirty annual deaths due to "diarrhoea with inflammation [alone]."[86] Hundreds more were occurring every year in the neighbouring streets, children dying, sometimes literally, at the doorsteps to the hospital. To make matters worse, infant mortality was actually *worsening* in Toronto during the first decade of the twentieth century. As a public hospital receiving almost 40 per cent of its annual funding from the taxpayers, there was little choice but to confront infant illnesses. The hospital could no longer confine its attention to the sterile wards of the operating theatre; it needed to go out into community.

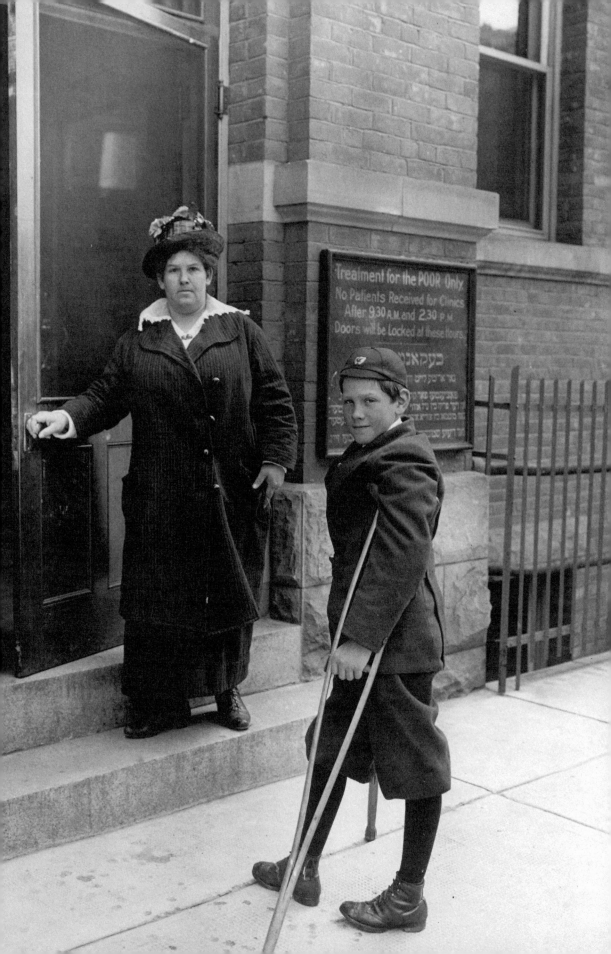

FIVE

Milk Sewage

If the truth were known the epitaph on the vast majority of the tomb-
stones on this continent marking the graves of children under two
years of age would be "poisoned by milk."[1]

      Dr. Charles Hastings, Toronto's Medical Officer of Health, 1912

The Ward

The College Street hospital was a beacon of medical technology in the heart
of Toronto. Its new surgical wards reflected the stripped-down sterility that
typified turn-of-the-century medical institutions. In 1914, one of Robertson's *Evening Telegram* reporters described the sanitary environment in
futuristic terms:

> ... a large room flooded with white light, where, instead of a wall on
> one side, was ground glass that threw no dazzling glare of sunshine nor
> deep contrasting shadow on the operating table in the centre. Three
> wall basins opposite this window were equipped with elbow pushers for
> the taps, and foot pedals for the liquid soap, so that the immaculately
> clean hands of the surgeons may stay chemically free from any germs
> lodged on the metal. Nearby was fixed the bichloride
> immersion bowl filled for the further cleansing pro-
> cess of the hands before skilled fingers felt for disease
> with knife probe and lancet ... The Operating room's
> atmosphere differed from that of a merely clean room.
> It felt like the concentrated essence of cleanliness.[2]

5.1 By the early twentieth century,
the hospital was serving thousands
of outpatients from across the city.
Behind the boy, the dispensary
plaque describes hospital regulations
in English and Yiddish.

However, if one passed down the sanitized corridor of the fifth floor of the new hospital, away from the pristine surgical theatres to the south end of the building, and looked out the Romanesque windows towards Lake Ontario, the contrast could not be greater. The Hospital for Sick Children stood on the edge of St. John's Ward, a dirty, ramshackle neighbourhood, now erased from Toronto's urban landscape, "where so much of the city's wretchedness and squallor [sic] are gathered," to borrow the words of Samuel Blake, a prominent social gospel reformer.[3] This six-block by four-block downtown district was Toronto's public health disaster, an urban shantytown which stretched southward from the hospital to the "new" City Hall on Queen Street. This quarter, known in short as simply "The Ward," has been characterized as a slum, a veritable "red light district" surrounding the vagrants who milled around, or lived in, the House of Industry. Regardless of the appellation, within this densely packed community of decrepit single-family dwellings were gathered the newest, the poorest, and most vulnerable of Toronto's citizens.[4]

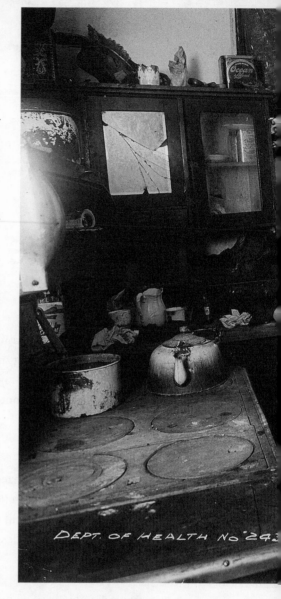

At the turn of the century, The Ward swelled in size and changed dramatically, as Eastern European Jewish immigrants poured into city. Until this point, Toronto's Jewish population had been small and dispersed, mainly British or German, and middle class. The new arrivals, by contrast, were impoverished Yiddish-speaking families fleeing the pogroms of Eastern Europe. They flocked to The Ward for its cheap rents and proximity to the city's commercial centre. Toronto's Jewish population trebled from 534 in 1881 to 1,425 in 1891, doubling again to 3,044 in 1901.[5] By 1921, it had

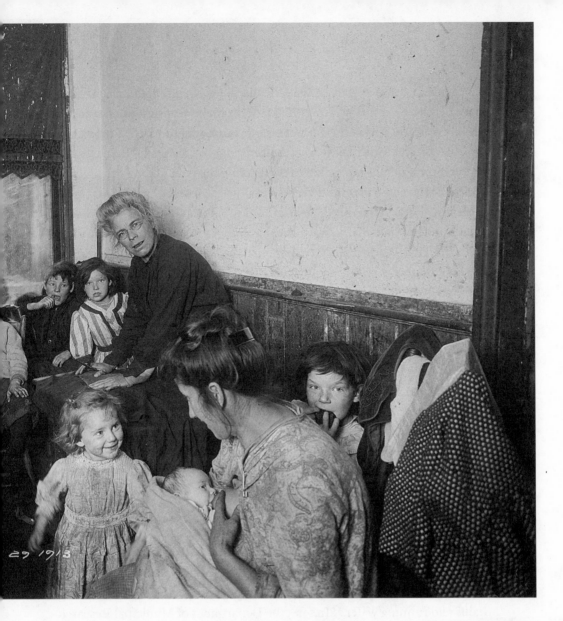

27 1913

increased tenfold to almost 35,000.[6] Jews quickly became the principal community in what was sometimes also dubbed "St. John's Shtetl." Indeed, the 1911 census returns suggested that The Ward's population was officially recorded as 68 per cent Jewish.[7] Charles Hastings, the medical officer of health, who often decried the state of The Ward, counted 1,207 "Hebrew" households, dwarfing the next largest "national" group – the 180 Italian families.[8] By that time, in the words of Stephen Speisman, The Ward "had become virtually a self-contained community as regards Jewish services and cultural, religious and educational facilities."[9]

5.2 This image, by renowned urban photographer Arthur Goss, captures the sheer density of some of the downtown slums, as well as the (multigenerational) women attempting to feed and clothe many children despite extreme poverty.

Lacking capital to start businesses, many Jewish immigrants worked as street peddlers or, at best, struggling storekeepers. Jewish women workers became concentrated in the garment trade, labouring for the T. Eaton Company, whose factories lay at the eastern edge of district. The changing socio-cultural demographic led to predictable disquiet among the predominantly Christian Scottish and English middle classes who saw, in their heart of the city, a shantytown and "foreign" culture. Public and private criticism of Jews and the state of The Ward became more frequent in the years leading up to the First World War. Newspapers, particularly Robertson's *Evening Telegram*, regularly publicized negative news related to the Jewish community and associated it with the public health challenges of the slum conditions. Indeed, the *Evening Telegram* had become so vitriolic in its attack on the Jewish quarter of Toronto in the years leading up to the First World War, that Edmund Scheuer, a prominent philanthropist and leader of the city's Jewish community, reputedly approached John Ross Robertson himself to ask that his journalists tone down their anti-Semitic coverage.[10]

Toronto's medical officer of health directed city photographer Arthur S. Goss to document the unsanitary living conditions of The Ward and other impoverished areas of the city, thus leaving an impressive visual remembrance of a part of the city that has largely vanished (see image 5.2).[11] In 1911, as one of his many duties as medical officer of health, Charles Hastings completed a report on slum conditions in the city. In the "Central" or City Hall District – which more or less corresponded to The Ward – he visited 2,051 families and found 108 homes in a condition that he declared "unfit for habitation." He reported higher rates of infectious disease and poorer physical conditions of inhabitants, many of whom lived in homes lacking drains and running water.[12] In 1918, the Department of Municipal Research conducted a second study of "undesirable living conditions" in The Ward. This report presented case studies to illustrate the various afflictions "piling up on this community."[13]

The proximity of the district of tenement housing meant that The Hospital for Sick Children began to treat more and more Jewish children suffering the multiple effects of urban poverty and inadequate sanitation. And while it would be too much to suggest that the outpatient department became an unofficial Jewish children's dispensary, the statistics during the first two decades of the twentieth century are striking. Annual reports listing the religious backgrounds of patients demonstrate that, in 1905, only 3 per cent were neither Protestant nor Catholic; by 1915, this figure rose to 15.5 per cent.[14]

By 1921, an appeal for funds that appeared in the *Canadian Jewish Review* claimed that Jewish patients comprised a remarkable 45 per cent of out-patient attendances, and 25 per cent of all inpatients.[15] This religious composition of patients represented a startling transformation for a hospital that had been founded by devout Baptist women and whose powerful Chair-man, Robertson, had tried to restrict the attendance of Catholic clergy at the Toronto Island home. Unsurprisingly, then, the growing presence of poor Jewish children from The Ward figured prominently in the subculture of medical practice. As a 1920s "Songbook" of the Nursing School remi-nisced: "OH – How we all loved the dear old Outdoor / And all the Jews from Elizabeth Street."[16] Yet, despite the disquiet over the Jewish presence, the hospital persisted in its long-standing policy to be non-denominational in terms of its clientele. Even the signage on the outpatient department came to be written in English and Yiddish (see image 5.1).

Infant and childhood mortality arising from poverty was not, of course, something singular to the Jewish community. Rates of death and disability remained remarkably high across all religious and ethno-cultural groups during the last decade of the nineteenth century, despite the scientific advances that were being conducted in the rarefied confines of European and North American scientific laboratories. Although great strides had been made in areas such as surgery, the chance of dying in the first years of life had barely budged in the sixty years following the first Canadian Public Health Act of 1848.[17] Indeed, as Michael Piva demonstrated in his history of the working class in Toronto, during the first decade of the twentieth century the city's infant mortality rate rose "from a low of 141.4 (per 1,000 live births) in 1902 to an appalling 179.7 in 1909."[18] This paradoxical juxta-position of worsening infant mortality rates amidst the advances in the bacteriological understanding of infectious disease presented itself as the major challenge to public health reformers. The medical community was all too aware that gastrointestinal ailments were the largest single cause of infant and early childhood mortality. In Hamilton, just around Lake Ontario, for example, "[d]iarrheal diseases were far more prevalent than either typhoid fever or scarlet fever" and were responsible for the largest single proportion (nearly one-third) of deaths.[19] In the poorer sections of Ottawa, diarrheal conditions accounted for nearly two-thirds of all infant deaths in 1901. Many terms were used by practitioners at the time, including "cholera infantum," "gastro-enteritis," "enteritis," "gastritis," "dysentery," and "indiges-tion."[20] Despite the varied nomenclature, infants typically succumbed to "acute electrolytic disturbance and circulatory failure brought on by severe dehydration."[21] Contemporaries were also aware of the seasonality of infant illness and death, with peaks of mortality emerging in the summer months, giving rise to names such as the "summer complaint" and "summer diarrhea." In Montreal, one of the filthiest cities in the Western world in the first decade of the twentieth century, 71 per cent of annual intestinal deaths took place in the summer months.[22] In an odd allusion to French tourist landmarks, Helen MacMurchy, one of the few women doctors in Toronto at the time and a rising star in eugenics and child welfare reform, declared that "August forms the Eiffel Tower of the infant mortality year."[23]

As public health officials looked frantically for the cause of worsening infant mortality, their attention was drawn, perhaps inevitably, to breast-feeding practices and the quality of milk given to infants. A growing body of data was suggesting that babies being weaned off the breast in the summer months were the most likely to succumb to the "summer complaint."[24] Moreover, public health nurses in the community recognized that breast-feeding practices varied between different cultural groups, with French Catholic mothers breastfeeding for the shortest period. Since deaths were more common among weaned infants and during the summer, seasonal infant mortality due to gastrointestinal diseases has been attributed to the "unsanitary feeding of babies."[25] Historical geographers, conducting sophisticated retrospective studies of infant mortality, have reinforced what contemporaries observed: namely, that in cultural groups where breast-feeding was not attempted or was discontinued early – such as Catholic Francophone communities – there existed the highest rates of infant mortality. By contrast, Toronto observed comparatively lower levels of infant mortality among the Jewish families who, despite the poverty of The Ward, were observed to have breastfed the longest.[26]

Despite these cultural differences, weaning young children was a dangerous undertaking for any family. Many physicians blamed, rather unsympathetically, "improper bottle-feeding resulting from maternal ignorance" as the source of deaths from digestive ailments.[27] Armed with turn-of-the-century knowledge of bacteriology, British and American research connected scarlet fever, typhoid, and cholera infantum to tainted cow's milk. In Toronto and Montreal, dairy inspections revealed filthy conditions, and bacteriological analysis of milk samples in the late 1890s revealed contamination with "dirt and tuberculosis bacilli" and intentional adulteration "with water, boracic or salicylic acid, and annatto (a yellow dye)."[28] As infant mortality rates worsened in the years leading up to the First World War, public health officials began to focus on the contentious debates over breastfeeding and the quality of cow's milk. Clean milk became a rallying cry for reform groups in urban centres in Canada and elsewhere, a cause that provided The Hospital for Sick Children with an opportunity to position itself at the epicentre of a new network of public health.

"The Bitter Cry of Helpless Childhood"

The rise of laboratory training for young medical practitioners from the late 1880s onwards[29] had sensitized a new generation of doctors and nurses to the variable quality of water and milk. These transformative changes in the way that health practitioners saw (literally and figuratively) disease have often been associated with the pioneering work not only of the French chemist, Louis Pasteur, but also the German scientist Robert Koch. It was Koch who created a protocol for cell culturing – later known as Koch's postulates – which provided scientists with the consistent empirical approach to isolate the most deadly bacteria of the time. From the middle of the 1870s, Koch and his laboratory team identified the bacterium for anthrax, and several years later, cholera. These discoveries underpinned a new theory of infectious transmission – known by medical historians as the "germ theory of disease." Put simply, it posited a radical new understanding of the origins and spread of pestilence – specific diseases were caused by specific germs (be they bacteria or viruses). Destroy the germ, and one could eradicate the potential for infection.

Of all the bacteria identified by Koch, perhaps none was as cardinal as his identification of the tuberculosis bacillus in 1884. Tuberculosis constituted the single most important killer in the Western world in the nineteenth century, striking down far more people than the shocking, but more transient, epidemics of smallpox and cholera. Although tuberculosis could be spread by a number of means – most notably by coughing and spittle – it was also becoming clear by the beginning of the twentieth century that tuberculosis could also be conveyed through milk. In early twentieth-century Ontario, an estimated 30 to 50 per cent of milk cows carried a particular type of bovine tuberculosis that was harmful and, at times, fatal to humans. Indeed, it was estimated that up to a quarter of tuberculosis cases and fully half of the abdominal and glandular tuberculosis cases at The Hospital for Sick Children were caused by contaminated milk.[30] A retrospective study by staff at The Hospital for Sick Children revealed that in the late 1880s and early 1990s, "from one-quarter to one-third" of patients were actively suffering from tuberculosis.[31] As a consequence, the campaign for clean milk emerged as a major public health controversy in the years leading up to the First World War, one that intersected directly with urban poverty and child health. As one Toronto physician lamented, "our babies, our sick ones in the hospitals, our invalids generally, are drinking 'milk sewage.'"[32]

The first decades of the twentieth century were thus an exciting time of scientific discovery and urban public health. Toronto had established its first permanent Board of Health in 1883. The board reflected a long-standing tradition of urban sanitary reform, with responsibilities for establishing clean water supplies, inspecting tainted food, restricting the presence of farm animals (and their detritus) in the city limits, as well as removing waste and cleaning up cesspools. Among the many challenges, milk became a focal point illustrating the challenges, and potential, of public health. The vested interests of dairy farmers, the limits of Toronto's jurisdiction (which did not extend beyond the city), confusion within the general public about the nature of bacteriology, and the cost of inspection and regulation all stymied comprehensive action. As milk became identified by medical reformers as a major source of illness and disability, dairies and farmers blamed each other, and for that matter, the consumers, for the unsanitary condition of milk consumed in homes. Public health advocates called for the city to establish a municipal pasteurization plant and licensing and inspection system, but others opposed the compulsory pasteurization of market milk as either unpractical or undesirable. Popular serials took up the rallying cry in the first decade of the twentieth century, such as the *Home Journal*, which alerted readers to the "Bitter Cry of Helpless Childhood Against the Cruel Ignorance and Murderous Greed of those that Destroy it with Filthy Milk," to invoke just one rather subtle headline.[33]

Toronto was hardly alone in its challenges of addressing childhood poverty and illness. Indeed, many of its public health reformers were cognizant of the other urban public health campaigns in other North American cities. Urban centres across North America and Europe witnessed active and controversial "pure milk" campaigns to regulate the quality and distribution of milk. One was commonly known as the "Certified Milk" movement. In 1893, the New Jersey physician Henry Coit designed a process to produce raw milk that was "certified" to contain fewer than 10,000 bacteria per cubic centimetre. The milk was produced under strict sanitary conditions supervised and inspected by a voluntary medical commission. Coit's process was complex and expensive, and certified milk only ever comprised a tiny portion (1 per cent) of the milk sold in most major North American cities.[34] Certified milk cost up to three times as much as regular milk in Toronto, and yet was often considered of unsatisfactory taste. By contrast, the Toronto City Dairy sold what it termed "pure," sterilized milk produced by tuberculin-tested cows, but it too was unaffordable to the poor.[35]

Much of the debate over the quality, transportation and consumption of milk centred on the evolving process of what became known, over time, as pasteurization. Louis Pasteur had demonstrated in his personal laboratory that one could destroy the microscopic "germs" in milk and water by heating the liquid for a minimum period of time. Pasteurization thus encompassed a simple (if time consuming and expensive) technique. Given the nature of milk production and distribution, different techniques of sterilization emerged. Commercial dairies that engaged in what they termed pasteurization might well heat the milk for too short a time, at insufficient temperatures, or use unsanitary equipment. Companies often adopted pasteurization for purposes of the preservation of milk as it was transported to market, rather than for the goal of eradicating pathogens. Milk may or may not have been tested to ensure that bacterial counts were low, nor would cows be routinely examined to ensure they were free of bovine tuberculosis.

Some contemporaries called attention to the difference between "scientific" and "commercial" pasteurization. Scientific pasteurization often involved sterilization of milk "intended chiefly for infants and supplying a food with few bacteria and no living pathogenic bacteria."[36] The milk was heated (ideally in the bottle) to a point below boiling (140 to 157 degrees Fahrenheit) for 20 to 30 minutes and then rapidly cooled. Commercial pasteurization, by contrast, brought milk to a high temperature (160 to 180 degrees Fahrenheit) for 20 to 30 seconds, killing the lactic acid bacteria and preventing the milk from souring before it reached the market and the home. This quicker method spared pathogenic bacteria such as the tubercle bacilli. Many advocates argued that scientific pasteurization was the only method that prevented the transmission of tuberculosis and other milk-borne diseases. By contrast, some physicians and public health officials opposed universal scientific pasteurization, claiming that it reduced the nutritional content of all milk and "not only encouraged carelessness in the handling of the milk supply, but also discouraged efforts to create a sanitary source for the production of a clean and safe milk."[37]

Debates over the quality, inspection, and distribution of milk intersected with urban poverty in ways that particularly affected young children. Inadequate milk supply due to poor diet or the need to re-enter the workforce often forced working-class mothers to cut short breastfeeding, placing their children in situations where they sought out inexpensive substitutes, including cheap, untested milk. In response to this problem, physicians in Paris had pioneered the *goutte de lait*, or milk depot, where poor women who were no longer able to nurse their infants could secure clean, safe, and inexpensive cow's milk. In Toronto, the Toronto Pure Milk League built upon this tradition by establishing its own milk depots in 1908.[38] Sensitive to the high rates of mortality in the summer months from intestinal afflictions, the Canadian Household Economic Association (CHEA) raised funds and organized a Milk Committee to provide "certified" milk for poor children during the warmer months, with a separate organization being in charge of supplying free ice.[39] In 1911, the CHEA reported that it had distributed 12,000 bottles of milk in an eighteen-month period.[40]

Professional bodies also joined the campaign for clean milk. An appeal at the 1908 Canadian Medical Association annual meeting triggered the creation of "milk commissions" in conjunction with the Ontario Legislature and the Toronto Academy of Medicine.[41] The Provincial Commission reported that approximately 40 to 50 per cent of Toronto's milk was pasteurized commercially, while only two firms used a more comprehensive scientific pasteurization.[42] The Academy commission, which included several physicians from The Hospital for Sick Children, pushed for government action. Their report detailed the difficulty of obtaining clean milk in Toronto and recommended the creation of a medical "dairy commission" to oversee the production of all milk.[43]

One of the factors inhibiting a comprehensive regulation of Toronto's milk supply was that its then medical officer of health, Dr. Charles Sheard, was not a strong supporter of mandatory municipal pasteurization. However, in the wake of a 1910 typhoid epidemic spread by inadequate municipal sewage and water treatment, Sheard ultimately resigned. His replacement, Dr. Charles Hastings, was known as a leader of the clean milk campaign. Hastings used his position to push hard for municipal pasteurization, employing the Toronto Board of Health's *Health Bulletin* as a bully pulpit in favour of compulsory sterilization. He erected exhibits at the Canadian National Exhibition illustrating to the public what tainted milk contained. His campaign against "germs" and for the cleanliness of the domestic environment even employed that popular competition of the time — the fly-swatting contest. Microscopic slides from the city's "diagnostic laboratory" presented a visual comparison of the bacteria count of regular, certified, and pasteurized milk.[44] Provincial Board of Health tests showed that much of the milk sold in the city had millions of bacteria per cubic centimetre, far more than the limit of 50,000 set by most experts for the designation of "clean" milk.[45] Meanwhile, between 1910 and 1912 Dr. Helen MacMurchy published three reports on infant mortality for the Ontario provincial government. MacMurchy condemned irregular feeding, unregulated patent foods (which she referred to bluntly as "Baby Exterminators"), soothing syrups, and unclean milk, emphasizing the importance of breastfeeding as long as possible.[46] It was due to Hastings's efforts that Toronto became the first municipality in the province of Ontario to pass a by-law under the 1911 Ontario Milk Act, a permissive piece of provincial legislation which gave the green light to municipalities "to enforce standards of cleanliness and quality" for milk products.[47]

"Pure Milk Means Life for Babies"

Amidst the push for municipal pasteurization, John Ross Robertson reacted in a manner that characterized so many of his actions as paterfamilias to the institution. Robertson had taken a personal interest in the urban reform movement that was emerging across North America, something of which, as a proprietor of a major North American newspaper, he must have been well aware. In 1908, he attended the Toronto Academy of Medicine symposium on milk, which resulted in a petition, signed by six hundred doctors, condemning the quality of the city's milk.[48] A few months later, Robertson joined Toronto public health officials, and a committee from the Toronto Academy of Medicine, to tour the much-publicized Nathan Straus plant in New York City and interview experts on milk and child nutrition. Upon his return, Robertson personally purchased and supervised the construction of a state-of-the-art pasteurization plant on the premises of The Hospital for Sick Children. The plant, modelled on the Nathan Straus facility, was installed in October 1909 and opened in November. Robertson appointed his sister-in-law, Miss Jean Holland, who had trained at the Straus operation, as superintendent. The plant was temporarily located in an adjoining property before it was moved behind the hospital three years later. As the importance of the plant grew, a new facility was completed in 1914, just months before the outbreak of the Great War. The two-story red-brick building included a

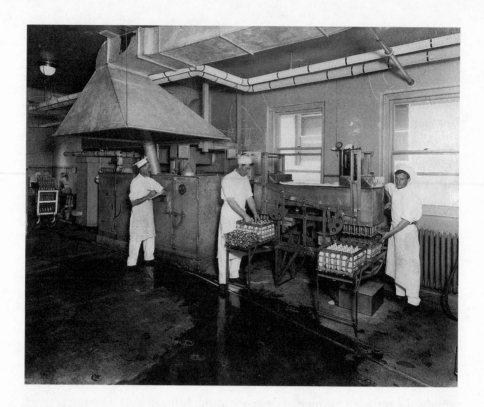

business and office area, receiving room, order room, modification room, pasteurization room, private entrance to the superintendent's apartment, and a runway connecting it to the hospital.[49] This new "milk modification laboratory" could pasteurize up to 200 gallons of milk per day. It was proclaimed the first of its kind in Canada.[50]

Over time, the pasteurization plant became as symbolically important to the outpatient department of the hospital as the new surgical wards were for the inpatients. It represented scientific technology and modern medical science, situating the hospital at the centre of a new push for public health reform. From then onward, the hospital trumpeted that it pasteurized certified milk of "exceptional purity and keeping quality."[51] Each day, milk was delivered at 8:00 a.m. and nearly 3,000 bottles were returned and cleaned in an automatic washer, steamed, and then baked overnight in an oven at 260 degrees. The hospital's bacteriological department tested the milk before and after pasteurization daily. Meanwhile, the city health department independently evaluated the milk weekly, with the city medical officer of health and laboratory director declaring it "the best milk in Toronto."[52] The hospital advertised the benefits of bacteria-free pasteurized milk as "As Good As Mothers" [sic], publishing testimonials of grateful women, before-and-after photographs, and bacteriological evidence to demonstrate the link between pasteurized milk and healthy babies.[53] "Pure milk means life for the babies," the hospital proclaimed in 1911.[54]

The pasteurization department performed multiple functions for both outpatients and inpatients. It pasteurized milk and prepared special feedings for inpatients. In addition, it provided milk and prescribed feedings for outpatients and the general public, with instructions to mothers, nurses, and medical students in pasteurization, milk modification, and infant feeding. As the popularity and fame of the plant grew, the department extended its reach even further, shipping milk and instructions to city clinic patients, and private patients of physicians. Circulars sent to Toronto physicians advertised the pasteurization plant and its products. Although there was no delivery to individual offices, physicians could prescribe milk and mixtures for their own patients. Individual prescriptions were made up and identified with small tokens such as ivory rings, steel weights, buttons, and pins.[55] In practice, The Hospital for Sick Children was sponsoring its own extensive milk depot, serving hundreds of families within Toronto. It famously posted signs in three languages — English, Yiddish, and Italian — reflecting the principal communities of its outpatient department. As one reporter wrote in a semi-edited draft for the *Telegram*:

> ... mothers from all parts of Toronto — of almost every nationality — the Russian Italian — the Pole [the Russian] — the Hebrew — [the Dutch] the Galician — the Finlander — the Swede find their way to the Milk Depot, for Baby is as precious in the home of the foreigner as in that of our own race ... Anyone who has seen the listless — blue-veined — sickly little babies daily at the Out-Patient Department, growing round and rosy and happy on the pure milk and feedings supplied at the Hospital's Milk Plant, can only express wonder at the broadening field of work at the Children's Hospital. From the suburban shack to the congested tenement in the heart of the City, the crowds daily appear ... [56]

The dairy sold milk for 4 cents less per quart than it paid the farmer, as well as "a certain amount of surplus skim and whole milk, and cream."[57] By the 1920s, an average of seventy-five children per day whose parents could not make their own feedings were "supplied regularly with a 24-hour set of bottled feedings, prepared on doctors' orders."[58] The department also began to produce quarts of lactic acid milk for those who made feedings at home, and sent cultures of lactic acid milk to homes throughout the province for home preparation (see table 5.1). Even after pasteurization was made mandatory in Toronto in 1914, "the pasteurization plant of the Hospital for Sick Children was the only source of pure milk for infant formulas."[59] By this time, all of the hospital – patients and staff – drank its pasteurized milk. [60]

Table 5.1 Pasteurization plant daily output

Year	Gallons	Outside milk bottles distributed	Bottles of baby feeding prepared
1910	54	512	
1911	72	602	n/a
1912	100	1,500	475
1913	150	1,700	755
1914	160	2,000	925
1916*	110	700	875
1917	110	700	900
1918	100	700	1,000
1919	n/a	n/a	2,000

Sources: AR 1910, 10; AR 1911, 9; AR 1912, 10; AR 1913, 10; AR 1914, 10; 1916, 10; AR 1917, 7; AR 1918, 12; AR 1919, 5; AR 1925, 17.

* Statistics were not listed in the 1915 annual report.

The pasteurization department became a self-described "clearing house for the Baby Welfare Work of the city."[61] But the chain of production and distribution was not without weak links. Working with the city's Health Department, the hospital supplied milk, feedings, and prescriptions to the Infant Home and Settlement House depots among others. The Health Department inspected depots and institutions receiving the hospital's milk, uncovering problems of swapping and inadequate milk storage.[62] Public health nurses and physicians referred "difficult and troublesome cases found at the various clinics scattered throughout the city [...] to the Hospital,"[63] and visiting nurses followed up cases receiving "Baby Feedings made from the Hospital Formulas."[64] In 1912, the Health Department, CHEA, and HSC coordinated and jointly distributed milk to depots partnered with the city health department.[65] In 1914, the Health Department of Toronto reorganized, and public health nurses employed by the city took over

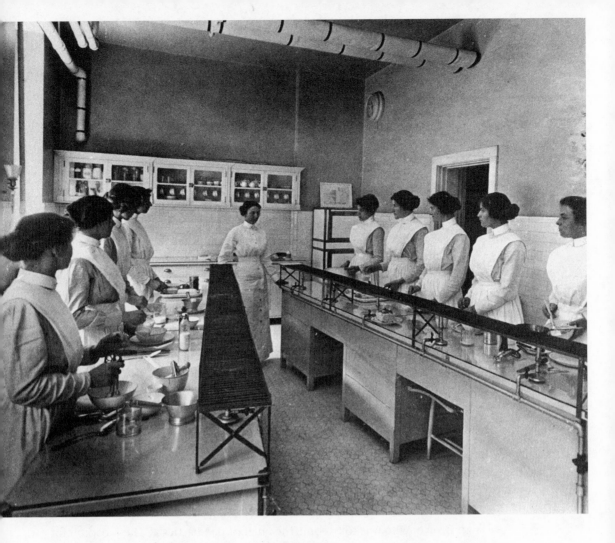

management of the volunteer-run milk depots and "soon organized the most elaborate and systematic infant health system in Canada."[66] In time, a public health nurse supervised every neighbourhood, visiting families, teaching hygiene, and running child hygiene and baby care clinics.[67]

5.4 Although Toronto had created its own Women's Medical College in the 1880s, there were many barriers to the entry of women into medicine. By contrast, other more culturally acceptable opportunities arose, including nursing and dietetics (pictured here).

This realm was staffed by a new type of trained medical subordinate armed with a diploma from a domestic science training school: the dietitian. *Maclean's* magazine heralded dietetics as "A Progressive Profession for Girls," emphasizing the scientific basis of artificial infant feeding.[68] The dietician's work was vaunted as curative and preventative: "the scientific feeding of the sick has in many cases taken the place of drugs in the treatment of disease, and the doctors' prescriptions in the matter of diet must be carried out."[69] As the hospital explained,

[T]he feeding of the sick is now an important and special branch of modern therapy. Diet is relied upon in many cases almost exclusively for the cure of a patient. The Hospital is particularly equipped in its kitchens, diet kitchens, and baby feeding laboratories for a satisfactory and up-to-date service. Scientific diets are furnished on prescriptions, that is, diets having a definite chemical composition or caloric value.[70]

In the milk laboratory, students and dietitians concocted formulae and feeding preparations using oatmeal, barley flour, cane sugar, and malt sugar. Symbolizing the growing importance of diet, a resident dietitian was added to the staff in 1912 to "superintend[...] the culinary department."[71] A significant portion of the dietitian's work was instructional. Dietitians, who lived in an apartment above the dairy, taught nursing students, nurses from affiliated schools, student dietitians, medical students, postgraduate nurses, and mothers the principles of milk modification and the preparation of special feedings. University of Toronto household science students completed three-month training rotations in the "diet kitchen" and "dairy" (as the pasteurization unit was informally known), and often joined the staff as dietitians, provided, of course, they were unmarried.[72]

Conclusions

Alan Brown, who was to become the chief of paediatrics at The Hospital for Sick Children during these formative years, considered milk depots, when medically supervised, to be "one of the most effective agencies known for the reduction of infant mortality."[73] The hospital credited pasteurization, as well as cattle inspection, with contributing to the near-disappearance of bovine forms of tuberculosis among Toronto-born children by 1921. Near the end of his career, in 1943, Brown even boasted in the *British Medical Journal* that "We have not had a case of milk-borne infection (including bovine tuberculosis) enter the Hospital for Sick Children – having lived in the city of Toronto and used nothing but pasteurized milk – since 1915."[74] His views are substantiated by considerable historical evidence. The infant mortality rate in Toronto declined by 50 per cent between the two world wars,[75] and continued its downward trend for the rest of the twentieth century. Within a generation, infant mortality would evolve into something relatively rare.

It would be too easy to attribute this dramatic decline in infant mortality (and subsequent rise in life expectancy from birth) singularly to the hospital's pasteurization efforts; the downward trend in infant mortality occurred throughout North American and European cities. Rather, it is more reasonable to conclude that the pasteurization plant figured among a host of important social and public health changes at the time. Clearly, general improvements in public health sanitation – such as the public health initiatives of the City of Toronto – must have had a significant impact. Indeed, some historians have argued that the preoccupation with clean milk campaigns in the years leading up to the First World War has overshadowed the contribution of water chlorination, which began at almost the same time. Trash removal, the more comprehensive inspection of abattoirs, and sewage improvements all played a role in improving health. In addition, one can assume that home visits of public health nurses and public education campaigns that increasingly worked cooperatively through schools and well-baby clinics also contributed to a new sense of personal and domestic hygiene. Increased standards of living intersected with enhanced transportation and refrigeration of foods to enhance better nutrition for mothers and young children.[76]

In 1914, a Toronto city bylaw mandated the pasteurization of milk sold in the city. Pasteurization at The Hospital for Sick Children would continue until 1929, when a quality supply was available locally. The Milk Modification Department's work within the hospital was reoriented to "the preparation of special milk mixtures for babies."[77] The department continued selling lactic acid milk, cultures, and emergency feedings, collecting breast milk, and making sugar solutions for sick babies. And yet, pasteurization was not made compulsory in the entire province of Ontario until 1938. Legend has it that in October 1937, following a dinner at the home of J.P. Bickell, president of McIntyre Porcupine Gold Mine, Drs. Alan Brown, D.E. Robertson, and John L. McDonald invited Premier Hepburn to see the hospital's iron lungs. The doctors then brought Hepburn to the girls' surgical ward to witness those afflicted with tubercular conditions. This experience is said to have convinced Hepburn to sponsor pasteurization legislation.[78]

If the near disappearance of bovine tuberculosis was a feat, something else also disappeared from this remarkable period in public health. The Ward itself – long targeted as the source of infection for the city – became slowly reconfigured. The Hospital for Sick Children itself had expanded southward to build its nurses' residence, something that only occurred through bitter negotiations between Robertson and the landowners. When the impressive new Toronto General Hospital was constructed on College

Street (moving from its previous location on Gerrard Street in the eastern part of the city), the city permitted the demolition of 232 row house dwellings, one of which, ironically, was the site of the first rental home of The Hospital for Sick Children. Meanwhile, the expansion of the Eaton complex of warehouses and factories accompanying the store at Queen and Yonge involved the demolition of an additional fifty houses.[79] When the Toronto General Hospital opened a private patients' pavilion in the late 1920s, the construction was contingent on the expropriation of property. By this time, many of the landowners were Jewish: "practically every owner is a member of the Chosen People," Toronto General Board chair Howard Irish confided to fellow trustee and future Chairman Joseph Flavelle, "and, therefore, a bit 'fussy' in his dealings."[80] During the First World War, the garment industry and Jewish community began shifting west to Spadina and Kensington, while the Italian community moved west along College Street. Nevertheless, there persisted a complicated relationship between the Jewish community and the hospital. In the 1920s, editorials in the *Canadian Jewish Review* backed a new fundraising campaign of the hospital to construct a convalescent hospital at Thistletown, northwest of the city, telling readers that

> No group in Toronto more than the Jews should be desirous of seeing carried to success the Sick Children's Hospital Campaign ... For the Jews are greatly in debt to this wonderful institution. To it they owe the lives of thousands of little ones and if not actually the lives, at least the good health and the use of limbs.[81]

The periodical praised the "non-sectarian" nature of the hospital: "Do you realize what would happen to our Jewish kiddies if the Hospital for Sick Children did not exist, or if it were not absolutely non-sectarian? As Jewish citizens of Toronto we appeal to you on behalf of our Jewish children to show your appreciation by sending your contribution ..."[82] Yet, despite the official support, resentment was growing among the Jewish community in Toronto about the unofficial prohibition on the hiring of Jewish doctors and nurses. It would cascade into a very public rebuke by the Chief Rabbi of Toronto in 1925[83] and lead to discussions to expand a Jewish dispensary into a full-blown Jewish hospital modelled on Mount Sinai in New York.

As the Jewish community moved west and northward, The Ward remained a receiving ground for the most recent immigrants, and new developments pushed Toronto's budding Chinese community northwest into the area. Ultimately, during a period of "urban renewal" in the 1950s, many of remaining parts of The Ward and "Chinatown" were demolished to make way for the new City Hall and the adjoining Nathan Philips Square.[84] It is one of the paradoxes of the history of hospitals in Toronto that the expansion of the Toronto General Hospital, the establishment of University Avenue sites for The Hospital for Sick Children as well as Mount Sinai and Princess Margaret Hospitals, and the construction of so many government buildings, from the post-war City Hall to the nearby municipal courthouses, would only be achieved through the expulsion of many of the poorest members of the city whom these public institutions were dedicated to serving.

The pasteurization plant represented one of the last grand projects of John Ross Robertson, who passed away in May of 1918. Sir Edmund Osler was subsequently elected chairman and the composition of the board of trustees underwent significant change. Later that year, a medical advisory board was established, including the chief of the medical staff and the chief of surgery. Within a few months of its creation, Alan Brown, who had only officially joined the hospital in 1915, would accede to the position of chief of the medical staff, a position he would hold for over thirty years, until his retirement in 1951. Brown would dominate paediatrics at the hospital for the next generation, ruling his department with an iron fist. He would fundamentally reconstruct the staffing at the institution and build upon the success that Robertson's pasteurization plant had created. In particular, Brown was drawn to the potential of the new science of infant feeding, which he was dedicated to refining and expanding.[85]

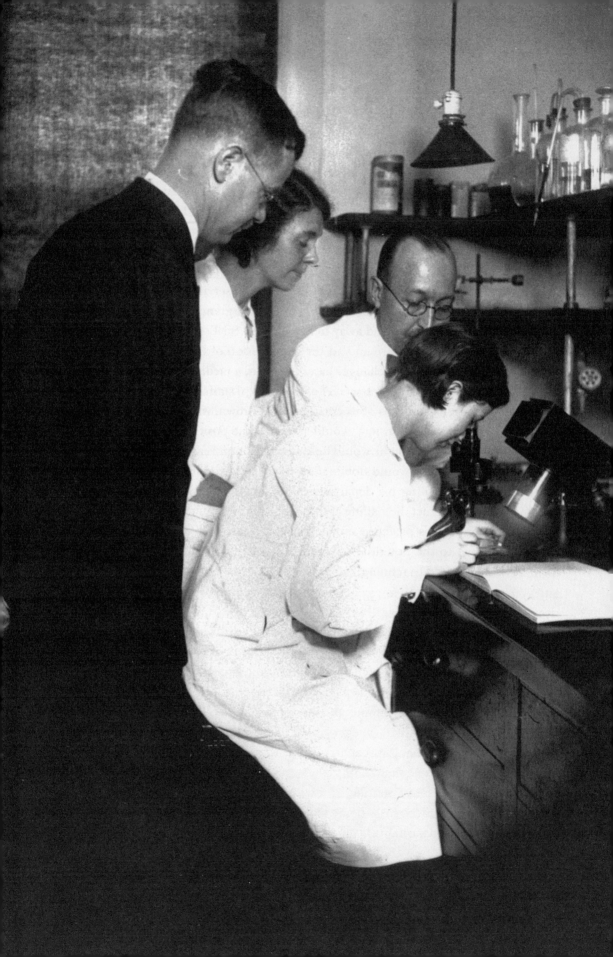

SIX

Irradiation

Alan Brown ... preached, pressured, commanded and brow-beat everybody on the subject. When he found that a mother was weening [sic] her baby, he would lecture her and say, "You are subletting your duty to a cow. Now go home and use what the good Lord gave you."[1]

Dr. Harry Ebbs, remembering Alan Brown, 1975

"Cow's Milk is for Calves"

The pasteurization plant at The Hospital for Sick Children placed it at the heart of an unprecedented network of child and infant welfare work that combined traditional elements of paternalism and social reform with the latest technologies of bacteriology and medical research. Over the next two decades, paediatrics as a discipline would come into formation, revolving around the activities of The Hospital for Sick Children and the imposing figure of Dr. Alan Brown. The hospital is replete with stories of this legendary physician who is often considered the founding father of Canadian paediatrics. One recounts that, when the young medical graduate had difficulty gaining an appointment at the College Street hospital (allegedly due to professional jealousies), he approached John Ross Robertson through his nephew, a surgeon at the hospital. In 1915, Robertson granted Brown a staff appointment contingent on his promise that he would reduce the infant ward mortality by 50 per cent within

6.1 Scientists in the hospital's Chemical Research Laboratories – such as (from left) Drs. Frederick Tisdall, Pearl Summerfeldt, Theodore Drake, and (laboratory technician) Ruth Herbert – devised fortified foods and pursued popular avenues of inquiry, particularly the effects of ultraviolet rays.

the year. As recounted by his successor, A.L. Chute, the resourceful and ambitious Brown reputedly fulfilled his promise, at which point Robertson entrusted him with a major reorganization of the medical and nursing staff.[2] Ultimately, Brown would become physician-in-chief and rise to prominence as the most influential paediatrician of his generation. His zealous advocacy of breastfeeding and imperious attitudes towards the hospital's expansion into the community would make him one of the most arresting figures in twentieth-century Canadian medicine.

Like many controversial figures in medical history, Alan Brown's ideas about medical care evolved over time and were far from consistent. He began his career as an ardent proponent of breastfeeding and was highly critical of weaning children onto cow's milk. He declared repeatedly that "breast milk is for babies, cow's milk is for calves."[3] He insisted that nearly all women could nurse their children when properly instructed and dismissed complaints of breastfeeding difficulties as largely "fictitious" and the result of commercial enterprises that sought to promote artificial foodstuffs.[4] Brown was well aware that breastfeeding as a cultural practice had begun to decline since 1900 and was less common among the Canadian-born and the well-to-do. Indeed, he affirmed in 1920 that breastfeeding had declined by one-third over the previous two decades.[5] What disquieted him most was the belief that middle-class mothers increasingly associated artificial feeding with "modernity," seeing breastfeeding as "old-fashioned." He orchestrated public awareness campaigns to promote breastfeeding, which he conceptualized as an example of "preventive pediatrics."[6] After conducting a study of Toronto mothers in 1917, he concluded that the "intelligent instruction" of mothers could improve breastfeeding rates. He held health-care practitioners ultimately responsible for encouraging mothers to persevere, maintaining that "[i]t is our duty as physicians to remedy this evil."[7]

Brown soon appreciated, however, that he was swimming against the tide. Across North America, breastfeeding was on the decline and there was a limit to what any one person — even someone as powerful as Brown — could do to reverse the long-term trend. Moreover, one must assume that he himself understood that his early criticisms of cow's milk might be misinterpreted as an attack on the pasteurization plant at the hospital, which was widely regarded as a public health triumph in the city. As a consequence, although Brown would continue to prioritize breastfeeding, he soon supported clean milk campaigns, ultimately judging the "milk meant for calves" as preferable over the alternative — proprietary infant foods. As a converted bovine booster, he decried commercial food advertisements: "the exploiting of photographs of crowing, fat, red-cheeked babies which are used to illustrate the supposed virtues of this or that manufacturer's food composed principally of maltose is not a very high-minded procedure on the part of the manufacturer who thus stoops to steal the credit which belongs to a cow."[8] As breastfeeding continued to fall in popularity, Brown searched for something between the ideal of breastfeeding and the dangers of commercial infant foods. In a letter to John Ross Robertson, he acknowledged the compromise that had to be made: "Pediatricians are unanimous concerning the superiority of breast fed babies over that of bottle fed babies," he began by way of emphasis, "but, at the same time, we can rear bottle fed babies who physically and mentally are equal to the most vigorous breast fed infants."[9]

As Alan Brown searched for an alternative to commercial foodstuffs, he turned to the burgeoning science of nutrition. He was greatly aided by the existing infrastructure of the new laboratories in the College Street hospital. The first labs in the hospital were traditional bacteriological ones, testing water and food for pathological microorganisms such as tuberculosis and cholera. Later, as the pasteurization plant grew in importance, the laboratory facilities were expanded to test daily bottled milk produced at the hospital and in certified dairies. It also took on an important diagnostic role, for blood exams, throat cultures, urinalyses, lumbar punctures, and typhoid tests, as well as the occasional autopsy.[10] With the growing scientific interest in infant nutrition, however, Brown expanded the remit of the laboratories even further. He oversaw the establishment of the Chemical (later, renamed the Nutritional) Research Laboratories, which had a mandate more focused on basis research than testing. The laboratories began scientific research on the contents of breast milk and indigestion in children, including work on carbohydrate intolerance in infants as it related to malnutrition and intestinal intoxication. Inspired by the discovery of insulin in 1922, which had been accomplished in University of Toronto laboratories just down the street, the hospital researched "blood sugar curves [in infants] after treatment with sugar by mouth, interstitial or intravenous injection, with and without insulin."[11] A pathologist studied the bacteriology of the intestinal tract of infants and conducted post-mortems of victims of digestive ailments. The research findings informed modifications in infant feeding formulas.[12]

Over the course of the 1920s, the laboratories began to occupy an increasingly important role in the hospital. Angelia Courtney directed the laboratories from 1919 to 1929, leading investigations into the etiology of infant digestive disorders and infant metabolism.[13] During this time, Frederick Tisdall would rise to national prominence in infant nutrition, succeeding Courtney as Director in 1929 and continuing in that capacity for another two decades. The hospital would also convince Frederick Banting, the 1923 Nobel Laureate in physiology and medicine, to be an affiliated researcher, giving the laboratories enhanced prestige. By the time of Tisdall's accession, the laboratories boasted fourteen full-time staff. Although Tisdall and Banting would become the best-known researchers associated with the hospital during this decade, the daily work was led by women, including the physicians Pearl Summerfeldt, Elizabeth Chant Robertson, and Gladys Boyd alongside technician Ruth Herbert, bacteriologist Marion Johnston, her assistant Mildred Kaake, and Juanita Thomson, a research pathologist.[14] Their presence must have been noteworthy, considering the rarity of regular women doctors on the wards of the hospital in the 1920s.

There may well have been push-and-pull factors involved in the clustering of women in research-oriented hospital positions at this time. Although the Medical Advisory Board, chaired by Brown, recommended a handful of women doctors for internships in the 1920s, they were most often overruled by the hospital trustees on the grounds that there were no residential accommodations for women at the hospital. Summerfeldt was one of the few exceptions, completing an internship at the hospital; but even she decided to pursue a research career. After she completed her two-year internship in medicine in December 1925, she underwent a fellowship in the United States with the renowned nutritional expert Emmett Holt. She returned to Toronto and was appointed Clinical Assistant 1929–34 and, later, Assistant Physician 1935–7. Aware that this issue would likely reoccur, the trustees sought to resist the incorporation of women doctors and exert their authority over the medical staff. They were not, however, always successful. The trustees had initially denied Doris Monypenny's appointment as an externe, but in March the trustees relented and approved Monypenny's appointment to a three-and-a-half-month externship. That fall, the hospital reversed its decision again, appointing her to a two-year internship when an unexpected vacancy arose and a change in the housing of nurses provided vacant space for accommodation.[15] Given this environment, it is perhaps not surprising that many highly educated women doctors drifted towards research, where there was some degree of freedom from the existing hierarchy and where they might find mutual support of other women doctors and scientists. Other graduates of the now coeducational medical programs of the University of Toronto and the University of Western Ontario may well have voted with their feet and simply not applied to the children's hospital, or became affiliated to Women's College Hospital.

Rats on the Rooftop

Pearl Summerfeldt's fellowship in nutrition reflected the scientific trends of the 1920s. As Aleck Ostry has demonstrated, that decade was a period where vitamins captured the public imagination in Canada. Scientific studies garnered much publicity, and vitamins were promoted both scientifically and commercially as near-magical "protective" elements. American historian Rima Apple captured the obsession of the time by entitling her book on the era *Vitamania*.[16] The public health fad, however, had profound scientific implications, as it ushered in a new, complementary understanding of disease. Until the 1920s, medical theorizing about disease had been largely focused on the new "germ theory of disease," whereby the presence of specific germs (bacteria like cholera or viruses like influenza) led to specific diseases. The nutritional research that emerged across North America in the 1920s added a new dimension — a rethinking of certain conditions as the longer-term developmental result of specific deficiencies. Studies (often based on feeding experiments with laboratory animals) demonstrated that diseases such as scurvy, pellagra, beriberi, and tetany were induced by vitamin and mineral deficiencies.[17]

Of particular importance for paediatrics as a discipline was the identification of vitamin D, the so-called "sunshine vitamin," and its role in preventing rickets. Rickets had long come to epitomize poverty and malnutrition in industrializing societies, and was by far the most lethal of the "deficiency diseases," affecting thousands of children and killing at least one child per 1,000 live births in the 1920s.[18] Sunlight and cod liver oil had traditionally been used to prevent or cure rickets and bolster general health, but the cause of their efficacy was hitherto unknown.[19] However, in 1919, the British researcher Edward Mellanby demonstrated that "foods rich in fat-soluble vitamin A (cod-liver oil, butter, and whole milk) were able to prevent rickets." In 1922, researchers at Johns Hopkins "concluded that the anti-rachitic substance found in certain fats was distinct from fat-soluble vitamin A[.]"[20] This new entity was named vitamin D. Subsequent studies further proved that both sunlight and cod liver oil prevented and treated rickets in young children. Mellanby's animal research spread quickly, and Canadian child health authorities, including Helen MacMurchy and Alan Brown, began officially recommending cod liver oil and sunbathing for children.[21] Unfortunately, the vitamin was found to be greatly lacking in ordinary foods, and the latitude and atmospheric conditions of Toronto were found to further deprive its citizens of vitamin D–containing ultraviolet light.

Researchers at The Hospital for Sick Children determined that one teaspoon of cod liver oil contained the equivalent amount of vitamin D found in 1,500 servings of spinach and fourteen egg yolks.[22] Yet cod liver oil was widely considered a vile substance. Administering it to children was an unpleasant task for mothers. So hospital researchers pursued other avenues. For example, they studied the effects of heliotherapy, by exposing white rats to solar radiation on the hospital's rooftop,[23] while the effects of donated Vita Glass or Vio-Ray Glass (which did not block ultraviolet rays like regular glass) were observed on actual wards. In the latter case, Colonel Eric Phillips, an Argus Corporation plutocrat and later chairman of the board of governors of the University of Toronto, donated one hundred square feet of Vio Ray Glass for research in the efficacy of this approach. Certain hospital beds were placed under direct light passing through the Vita Glass.[24] Ultimately, they found that in Toronto, winter sunlight was only one-eighth as strong as that of the summer months.[25] Suntanning on rooftops was not a practical therapeutic option for most Toronto families; instead, researchers undertook to discover ways of adding vitamins to nutrient-deficient foods.

As mentioned above, the researchers in Toronto were part of a larger network of biochemists and scientists becoming interested in nutrition. In 1924, Harry Steenbock in Wisconsin and Alfred Hess in New York each had developed, independently, a process of adding vitamin D to food through a process that was called "irradiation," the exposure of foods to ultraviolet rays.[26] It was found that different foods contained trace amounts of a substance called ergosterol, which exhibited the antirachitic (or anti-rickets) properties of vitamin D when it was exposed to the ultraviolet rays of mercury vapour quartz lamps.[27] In 1926, soon after this research was published, the trustees of the hospital authorized the purchase of such lamps, to be used for both clinical and research purposes.[28] With the success of the pasteurization plant no doubt in their minds, the next step was to identify a way to produce and distribute irradiated foods for community consumption. Hospital researchers sought to make vitamin D available through a palatable food commonly eaten by all, particularly the poor, at no extra cost to the consumer. In developing the lab's first product, an enriched biscuit, Frederick Tisdall collaborated with researchers at the Ontario Agricultural College in Guelph, who were researching enhanced chick food.[29] By 1930, the work of the team had yielded publishable results. The biscuit was made of whole wheat flour, irradiated wheat germ, milk, butter, yeast, bone meal, iron, and copper, and contained vitamins A, B_1, B_2, E, and D. They identified the product as "belonging to the essential or protective class of foods," and recommended that it replace regular "nonprotective" breadstuffs.[30]

The production and sale of these laboratory biscuits required the team to obtain a licence from a Wisconsin foundation to use the patented (Steenbock) irradiation protocol. The Wisconsin foundation was a novel compromise in the competitive world of meal-preparation patents. Steenbock had reluctantly patented his process of irradiating wheat germ in order to protect it from commercial exploitation and ensure that it would be used to bring affordable enriched food to the people. There are also suggestions that Wisconsin authorities wished to protect the Wisconsin dairy industry from the oleo-margarine industry. An independent body known as the Wisconsin Alumni Research Foundation (WARF) was formed in 1925 to hold the patent and control licensing, manufacturing, advertising, and royalties, which were used to support research at the University of Wisconsin. This not-for-profit foundation operated as a model for over fifty similar organizations in the United States.[31]

At Toronto's Hospital for Sick Children, three of the four principal researchers – Brown, Drake, and Tisdall, but noticeably not Summerfeldt – used WARF as their impetus to found the Paediatric Research Foundation (PRF) of Toronto, an organization designed solely "to make available and scientifically control" the products developed by the Nutritional Research Laboratory.[32] The PRF oversaw the manufacture, tested the quality, supervised the advertisement, and managed the royalties of commercialized products created in the hospital's labs. The founders emphasized that the PRF's role was "to adequately control the biscuit from the scientific standpoint."[33] They would apply for licences and patents in the name of Tisdall, and then turn them over to the foundation. In the early years, the Paediatric Research Foundation dispensed annuities to Drake and Tisdall, who authorized grants to support research at the hospital. Dr. T.C. Routley volunteered to share his business knowledge, helping Tisdall conduct negotiations regarding patents and licences. As the importance of the foundation grew, two senior physicians, Alexander Primrose and F.N.G. Starr, joined Brown, Tisdall, and Drake as trustees, for "it was felt that it was essential for the Paediatric Research Foundation to have further medical standing and medical advice[.]"[34]

In 1929, the principal researchers struck a deal to commercialize the super-biscuit. They finalized a contract according to which the foundation would maintain responsibility for the "scientific aspect" of this biscuit and receive royalties from the private company to be used for research purposes. The research foundation also completed what would ultimately become a short-lived contract with the United Biscuit Company of America to release the product in the United States. A London, Ontario–based subsidiary, McCormick Manufacturing Company, produced and distributed "McCormick's Sun Wheat Biscuit."[35] In January 1930, the biscuits were available for 21 to 25 cents per 10-ounce package, a price comparable to similar products.[36] Demand greatly exceeded expectations; grocery stores in Toronto, such as Loblaws, ran out of stock within the first week, publicly apologizing to consumers and promising to meet future demand. In response to the market success, McCormick acquired more equipment to increase production by 100 per cent, and expanded distribution to department stores, general stores, and druggists. In 1931, McCormick's ran ads promoting the biscuits' new and improved flavour, and claimed to have sent a coupon worth 5 cents to every home in the city, redeemable at any grocery store.[37] Newspaper advertisements promoted Sunwheat Biscuits as a doctor-approved source of nutrition, proclaiming, somewhat modestly, that they constituted "the most important scientific advance ever made in the history of food preparation."[38]

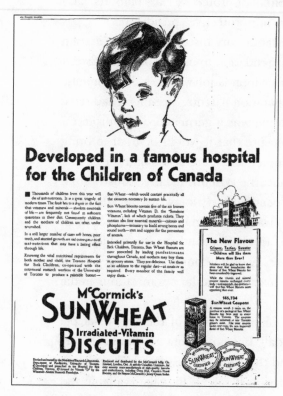

6.2 Fortified foods became all the rage in the interwar period, as child health researchers became emboldened by the decline in infant mortality. The hospital's Chemical Research Laboratories pioneered, and patented, several fortified products that brought fame and fortune to the researchers and the hospital.

The biscuit was only the beginning. From 1929 to 1934, the group published results of their creation of a vitamin- and mineral-enriched irradiated whole wheat biscuit, irradiated loaves of bread, a cereal mixture, and, most famously, the pre-cooked version of this cereal mixture.[39] Although the pre-cooked version would prove to be the greatest success, researchers were initially much more interested in promoting enriched white bread. As they explained:

> Bread is consumed in large amounts by the wage-earning class. In a survey of the consumption of bread in a large city, it was found that about one-eighth of a loaf per person per day was consumed in the well-to-do families, while in the poorer sections of the city the average consumption was from one-half to one loaf per person per day. The reason for this is that bread is the cheapest form of food. It is reasonable to conclude, therefore, that bread is a particularly valuable food in which to make vitamins available, not only on account of its universal distribution but because it is so largely consumed by those who frequently cannot afford to buy the more expensive vitamin-containing foods.[40]

In May 1930 the team began irradiating tons of wheat germ, using "several thousands of dollars [sic] worth" of quartz lamps. At this time Robertson orchestrated the formation of a company to be known as National Foods Limited, which would handle the "business end." In December 1930, he disassociated himself from the project, possibly due to growing concern that the hospital would be seen as profiteering off of the new products, and folded National Foods into the Paediatric Research Foundation. National Foods had acquired the rights through WARF for the Steenbock process, but found that irradiating wheat germ "would increase the price of the bread and would probably be commercially impossible."[41] Discouraged by the high cost of irradiating tons of wheat, the team successfully developed a process for adding vitamin D by irradiating ergosterol in the shortening used in the bread. Immediately following the announcement of the development of irradiated bread early in 1931, newspapers reported that certain American parties were offering as much as $1,000,000 for the right to use the Toronto bread irradiation process.[42]

The bread appears to never have been mass produced or used by The Hospital for Sick Children, but the Paediatric Research Foundation did ultimately license U.S. and Canadian companies to employ the process. The

U.S. General Baking Company of New York, for example, manufactured irradiated bread in Boston.[43] In Toronto and Montreal, irradiated bread was sold as Weston's Bread and Weston's Buttermilk Scone Loaf (George Weston Bread & Cakes Ltd.) and Vitos Bread (Ideal Bread Co.) beginning in August, 1931.[44] The "fraction of a cent on each loaf" was used to meet the expense of ergosterol, product testing, and licensing payments to WARF. The team kept the price as low as possible, applying all net profits to research.[45] By 1933, the bread was being sold in fifteen Canadian and sixty-eight U.S. cities.[46] During the Second World War, hospital researchers worked with the Dominion (federal) Department of Agriculture, Dominion Department of Pensions and National Health, and milling companies to develop a "Canada Approved Vitamin B white flour or bread" containing nearly as much vitamin B and iron as whole wheat bread.[47] The sale of this bread nationwide according to standards set by a new Food and Drug Act increased the availability of government-certified vitaminized breads and flours throughout the country.[48]

The invisibility of both vitamins and vitamin deficiency posed challenges to the verification of products. As Rima Apple observes, American advertisements for vitamin products often used subtle if somewhat coercive tactics, suggesting that seemingly healthy children could be secretly suffering from deficiency diseases due to dietary neglect.[49] Vitamin D had, within a decade, become a "vital food ingredient" that was "essential" for child health. Vitos Bread, distributed in Toronto, was advertised as a "priceless health source" for the whole family, the daily consumption of which would "probably" enable the consumer to "enjoy better health and develop a greater resistance to sickness."[50] Licensed North American bakers promoted their product as containing "the sunshine vitamin D" and displayed letters and seals from WARF and the PRF certifying the truth of their nutritional claims. Products in the United States sometimes listed the approval of the American Medical Association.[51] Such certification was felt to be essential to fostering trust in the brand, for "false claims for vitamins – particularly for vitamins added to breakfast cereals – emerged as a major issue in 1929 as manufacturers began to add vitamins to their products and to make unrealistic health claims for them[.]"[52]

This potential for fraudulent or unsubstantiated claims was the grounds on which the hospital's team defended the decision to patent their product. Pointing out that irradiation was invisible and undetectable by the consumer, they argued that patenting was necessary to guarantee to the public that the bread contained the promised nutrients. As the hospital researchers announced, somewhat defensively, "Our whole object in this project is to make available to the public an additional source of Vitamin D ... we want to emphasize again that our object in doing this work is to put into practical effect measures which have been shown from a scientific standpoint to be of value in the prevention of disease."[53] In PRF certification included in advertisements, Drake stated,

> We have bestowed upon the General Baking Company the exclusive right to make available to the American public through Bond Bread and other bread, that vital food element known as the "sunshine" vitamin, or vitamin "D."
>
> We assume the responsibility continuously to analyze the product to insure and guarantee that all such loaves made shall supply said vital food element to the degree that our research has proved to be adequate and efficacious.
>
> Since ours in a non-profit institution, our paramount interest is public service.[54]

Mead's Cereal

Energized by the success of the irradiated foods, the research team undertook to develop a children's cereal rich in vitamins, proteins, and minerals that would retain whole and part grains without inducing constipation or other digestive trouble. Observing that cereals provided 30 to 60 per cent of average daily caloric intake, the team sought to develop one that would resemble "widely used products."[55] In 1930, the NRL introduced "A New Cereal Mixture Containing Vitamins and Mineral Elements," containing irradiated wheat germ and yeast. In partnership with Mead Johnson Company, "Mead's Cereal" was made commercially available. Like many other available cereals, it required tedious hours of cooking to be rendered digestible for infants. It was tested and then used exclusively on the wards of the children's hospital. Recognizing the burdens posed by such lengthy cooking times, the hospital lab team endeavoured to develop a process of pre-cooking the cereal so that it would be ready in minutes.[56]

In 1934, in the midst of the Great Depression, Pablum was introduced to the market. Fortified with minerals (calcium phosphorus, iron, and copper) and five of six known vitamins, Pablum was made with nearly the same recipe as its predecessor: wheat meal/farina (52 per cent), oatmeal (18 per cent), corn meal (10 per cent), wheat germ (15 per cent), dried bone meal (2 per cent), dried brewers' yeast (1 per cent), alfalfa (1 per cent), sodium chloride (1 per cent), and iron salts. The mixture "was cooked in large steam kettles under pressure with air excluded ... then dried on heated rolls and scraped off in the form of fine flakes."[57] Parents could prepare a meal in minutes through the addition of hot milk or water. The same process of commercialization followed: the product was patented by Tisdall on behalf of the PRF, and a contract formed between the PRF and a private manufacturer, Mead Johnson and Co., which had offices in Evansville, Indiana, and Belleville, Ontario. The contract granted royalties to support the hospital's research for the next quarter-century.[58] Mead Johnson was a well-respected producer and distributor of infant foods, complimented as "foremost among manufacturers of infant dietary and medicinal specialties" by the *Wall Street Journal*, who also observed that it "painstakingly developed and retained" the good graces of physicians.[59] It was one of the first companies to develop artificial infant foods, and, after 1915, had operated its own paediatric nutrition research facility and manufacturing plant. The company was also a long-time producer of the standardized cod liver oil often recommended by Alan Brown and Frederick Tisdall.[60]

Mead Johnson introduced Pablum to the North American public as a product that was unique due to its "medically approved" status. Pablum was initially sold through drug stores, a step that, though it limited the first wave of sales, also reinforced its "scientific" standing among the public. Newspaper advertisements from the 1930s indicate that in Toronto, Pablum was sold at I.D.A. Drug Stores and G. Tamblyn, Ltd. Drug Stores.[61] Mead Johnson advertised the cereal in medical and nursing journals, aggressively presenting itself as a steadfast ally to physicians. In ads decrying the "Exploitation of the Medical Profession" through false advertising and the distribution of free baby food samples to laypersons, the company positioned itself as one that respected physicians' authority:

> It has been said that ten more years of the present trend of interference in medical practice will do away with the need for private practice of infant feeding and other branches of medicine.
>
> Mead Johnson & Company have always believed that the feeding and care of babies and growing children is an individual problem that can best be controlled by the individual physician ...
>
> When more physicians specify MEAD'S Products* when indicated, more babies will be fed by physicians because Mead Johnson & Company

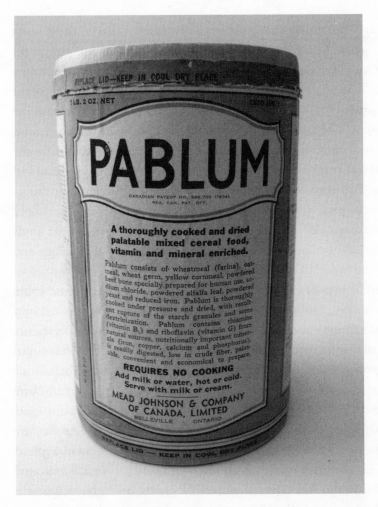

REPLACE LID—KEEP IN COOL DRY PLACE

1 LB. 2 OZ. NET

PABLUM

CANADIAN PATENT NO. 346.700 (1934)
REG. CAN. PAT. OFF.

**A thoroughly cooked and dried
palatable mixed cereal food,
vitamin and mineral enriched.**

Pablum consists of wheatmeal (farina), oatmeal, wheat germ, yellow cornmeal, powdered beef bone specially prepared for human use, sodium chloride, powdered alfalfa leaf, powdered yeast and reduced iron. Pablum is thoroughly cooked under pressure and dried, with resultant rupture of the starch granules and some dextrinization. Pablum contains thiamine (vitamin B₁) and riboflavin (vitamin G) from natural sources, nutritionally important minerals (iron, copper, calcium and phosphorus), is readily digested, low in crude fiber, palatable, convenient and economical to prepare.

REQUIRES NO COOKING
Add milk or water, hot or cold.
Serve with milk or cream.

**MEAD JOHNSON & COMPANY
OF CANADA, LIMITED**
BELLEVILLE · ONTARIO

REPLACE LID — KEEP IN COOL DRY PLACE

6.3 A whole generation of Canadians was raised on this fortified breakfast food. The royalties from Pablum flowed back into the hospital's Research Institute, providing it with unparalleled funding in an era when government support for research was still rather meagre.

earnestly cooperate with the medical profession along strictly ethical lines and never exploit the medical profession....

Please enclose professional card when requesting samples of Mead Johnson products to cooperate in preventing their reaching unauthorized persons.[62]

Pablum was met with international applause and publicity, adding to the growing reputation of The Hospital for Sick Children and the University of Toronto, the latter of which had been basking in the reflected glory of the discovery of insulin.[63] Tisdall was contacted by British physicians and Glaxo Laboratories, which, like Mead Johnson, was experimenting with the production of "a vitamin-fortified farinaceous food." Glaxo adapted and released a different version of Mead's Cereal in Britain, paying royalties to

Tisdall through National Foods, under an agreement "that in those parts of the world where Mead Johnson were unable to handle marketing, and the Nathan Company was more appropriate, sole rights would be reserved to the latter."[64] Upon the development of Pablum, Glaxo took out a patent for its own "process of preparing a cereal food in soluble form," released in Britain as Farex.[65] Mead Johnson modified the Pablum recipe over time, and by 1951 four different versions of the cereal – Pablum Mixed Cereal, Pablum Oatmeal (previously called Pabena), Pablum Barley Cereal, and Pablum Rice Cereal – were commercially available.[66] These newer "tasty" versions were, in part, to reverse the popular perception of "Pablum" as "a synonym for blandness." As one journalist put it, "It tasted (to the adult palate, at least) like boiled Kleenex. It had the consistency of mucilage and smelled like the inside of an old cardboard box."[67]

The scientific uses of fortified cereals did not cease with the remarkable commercial success. Pablum continued to be used within hospital research. It was fed to various species of living creatures in scientific experiments through the 1930s and 1950s, including the *Aëdes aegypti* and the book louse, and to *Xiphophorus hellerii* fish to assess its impact on their mating behaviour. It was also fed to exotic creatures in the public eye: in 1945, the *Toronto Daily Star* reported that "Pablum, Milk and formula, regular scientific baby food, are fed Barbara, 4 ½-month-old gibbon at Washington zoo."[68] As the *New York Times* reported, Pablum was a core part of the diet of two pandas gifted to the Bronx Zoo by China in 1941.[69] Throughout the 1930s, Tisdall indicated ongoing research into "the effect of diet on the condition and development of teeth in children" and "the effects of diet on the mental development of children."[70] Pablum had entered popular culture and carried with it the name and reputation of Toronto's Hospital for Sick Children, although the vitamin-D chewing gum never proved to be a success.

"The Mush that Made SickKids Rich"

Despite, or more likely, because of, the self-evident success and prestige associated with Pablum, some principal supporters of the hospital felt decidedly uncomfortable about what they feared was the commercialization of the Nutritional Research Laboratory. The hospital trustees, for example, expressed discomfort and unwillingness to enter into indirect or direct relationships with the Paediatric Research Foundation and National Foods due to their "very definite commercial aspects." Reflecting their uneasiness with the royalties that were being accrued, and the potential danger of the appearance of profiteering, the board appointed representatives to the PRF, and decided that medical staff members should not "have any direct or indirect contact with the above-named organizations." As a consequence, Drake and Tisdall were told in 1931 that they would have to resign from either the hospital staff or from the boards of the PRF and National Foods.[71] That year, a memorandum of agreement specified that the PRF would undertake major research, keep their own accounts and records, and dispense funds only with the trustees' knowledge and consent. Furthermore, the trustees insisted that they have authority over "any arrangement in the Province of Ontario connected with the announcement of, or sale of any discovery or process"; that the PRF and trustees would cooperate to create a formal research endowment fund; and that the trustees would "direct that any discovery or process made by the Paediatric Research Foundation which may be considered as of benefit to humanity at large shall, in the Province of Ontario, be made available to all and sundry who care to take advantage of it on a fair and equitable basis."[72] All research funds were to be henceforth managed by the trustees. Trustees minutes indicate that, thereafter, Tisdall sent proposals for major research projects to the board and superintendent for approval.[73]

In the decades before organized governmental support (the Medical Research Council of Canada being established in 1948), research funding was acquired piecemeal from private organizations with overhead costs and salaries absorbed by the hospital. In the early years, the research department operated on a shoestring, haphazard budget. Alan Brown obtained funding from private sources to initiate research from circa 1917 to 1923, during which time the hospital held the funds in trust. The hospital provided the facilities necessary for the work: "space, equipment, heat, light and power, cleaning service, telephone and all other sundry and general overhead expenses."[74] Facilities were often makeshift: there were even plans approved to convert the chapel into a temporary laboratory.[75] In 1930 the trustees funded the renovation of three rooms for nutritional studies for the department, which had annual operating expenses of $30,000. Brown reported that these funds were raised "through the efforts of the individual members of the Department. It is earnestly hoped that, at an early date, it will be possible to arrange for an adequate permanent budget, so that the members of the Staff of the Laboratories, unhampered by financial worries, will be able to devote all their energies to the work of the Hospital."[76]

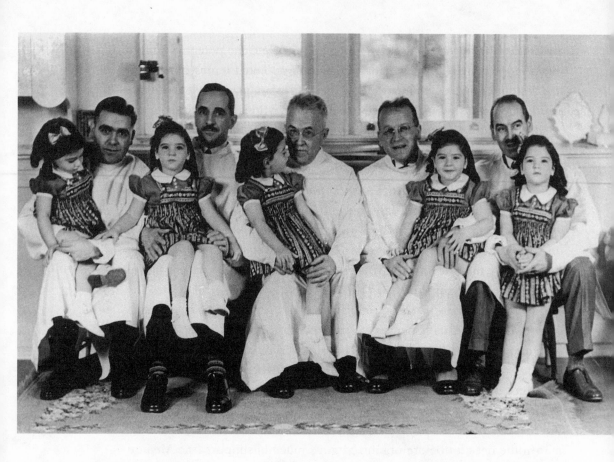

6.4 The powerful incentive of discovery led to research activities and protocols that would today be considered ethically problematic. Here, senior medical staff including Alan Brown (second from right) pose with the most famous (and studied) sisters of their generation – the Dionne quintuplets.

The patenting and commercialization of products developed in the research laboratories ended this shaky, ad hoc financial situation, providing researchers with the stable financing that they craved and forming the basis of hospital's research endowment fund. The foundation gave the research laboratories about $79,000 from royalties by 1932,[77] and by 1935 had given an additional $500,000 in cash and bonds to the hospital.[78] Despite the desperate economic conditions of the 1930s, royalties continued to flood in. Superintendent Bower reported that in 1953 the PRF had received about $1.6 million, nearly all from nutritional products.[79] The PRF was to dissolve and transfer its funds to HSC upon the death of the last members of the Pablum-Sunwheat team. Executive Director Douglas E. Snedden recalled that upon Drake's death in 1959, "assets of over one million dollars came to the Hospital and were set up under the Research Endowment Trust Section of our General Ledger Accounts."[80] Drake himself, director of research from 1949 to 1953, left the hospital another \$300,000 posthumously.[81] By 1978, Pablum had brought the hospital's research foundation an estimated \$7 million. Perhaps, unsurprisingly, local media identified and celebrated Pablum as a gold mine for the hospital. One writer described it as "the mush that made SickKids [...] rich."[82]

Research Experimentation

The research into fortified foods also reflected an ambiguous and fluid research environment involving patients. By the 1920s, it was common to employ animals in the first round of experimentation, as reflected in the horses used to develop the diphtheria toxin, the dogs used by Banting and Best to refine their research into insulin, and indeed the rats suntanning on the roof of the children's hospital. But research and clinical practice were seldom so easily distinguishable. Much of clinical practice was, by necessity, experimental and involved professional and ethical choices that may appear, in retrospect, vague and undefined to researchers today. An eclectic approach of auto-experimentation, research on animals, and (involuntary) trials on captive populations was extremely common for the period. In the case of the nutritional research at The Hospital for Sick Children, food products were tested first on laboratory animals (mainly rats) and then on many different groups of children: patients in the hospital itself, preventorium residents, the students of the St. George Nursery School, unspecified groups of "normal children," and infants attending well-baby clinics. In some cases, such as those in which mothers administered vitamin D–fortified substances to their children, a degree of parental consent was assumed; in others, such as those involving institutionalized children, the terms of the subjects' participation were decided by the researchers themselves.[83]

The new "cereal mixture" was tested in the laboratories and the wards of the hospital. In 1930 it was "used almost exclusively" for several months, during which time it was observed that

> [i]n the infant wards, from the standpoint of a laxative or constipating effect, no difference was noted from the results obtained with the refined and finely milled cereals ordinarily used. The palatability of the product was evidenced by its being eaten with the same avidity as the ordinary cereal, not only by the infants, but also by the older children.
>
> Further laboratory and clinical observations are being conducted on this product.[84]

Experiments were carried out to ascertain the effects of adding vitamins and minerals to the diets of women and children. Studies involving institutionalized children compared the effects of regular diets with those supplemented by the "special cereal mixture" on the health and hemoglobin levels of children from orphanages, other institutions, and more privileged class backgrounds and even children of fellow researchers.[85] In 1932, Pearl Summerfeldt led a twenty-week study on "The Value of an Increased Supply of Vitamin B_1 and Iron in the Diet of Children" by feeding a "special cereal mixture" (nearly identical to Mead's Cereal/Pablum) to twenty-one "normal" children, most of whom had recently resided in an unnamed preventorium. In 1932, a scientific article stated categorically that "nearly all" hospital patients were fed the cereal.[86] Sometimes the research was conducted concurrently on animals and children concurrently, like a study on "the curative effects of cereals and biscuits on experimental anaemias," wherein different products were added to the diets of rats, "a group of normal children," and two infants (with little success with the last group).[87] In a similar study, 350 Toronto children in four institutions participated in a study of the effects of diets supplemented with vitamin D and phosphorus.[88] In the late 1930s, Doris Monypenny investigated "The Early Introduction of Solid Foods in the Infant Diet," studying the effects of adding eggs, Pablum, and vegetables to the diets of month-old infants in foster care. She observed the greatest success in the introduction of Pablum at one month of age.[89]

By 1934, irradiated milk was available commercially in Toronto.[90] With the approval of the Medical Advisory Board (MAB) and trustees, researchers conducted a five-month study comparing the vitamin D potency of cod liver oil, viosterol, and irradiated milk with 529 "well babies" from comfortable households.[91] Several five-month observational studies of the antirachitic value of irradiated yeast and other sources of Vitamin D were conducted with a total of 1,228 infants representing "a cross-section of the infant population of Toronto."[92] Nutritional studies were also carried out with mothers, mainly those of the poorer classes. In the 1920s, Angelia Courtney had studied the effects of "defective diets" on the breast milk of several nursing patients' mothers.[93] Elizabeth Chant Robertson carried out further observational work on the effect of prenatal nutrition on the health of women attending obstetrical outpatient clinics at Toronto General Hospital.[94] It would be tempting to assume that all of the children caught up in the dragnet of these early decades of paediatric research hailed from poorer households. But this does not appear to have always been the case. Indeed, as the reputation of the hospital grew rapidly in the 1920s and 1930s, researchers often commented on the involvement of children from comfortable households volunteered by parents eager to assist the research activities of the hospital.

Conclusions

Royalties from Pablum and the other signature enriched products jump-started the endowment fund for the postwar research institute of the hospital. These laboratory-developed food products stood at the forefront of a new generation of food production. By the end of the Second World War, it was common for food manufacturers to add vitamins "to flour, bread and rolls, cornmeal and grits, macaroni and spaghetti, breakfast cereals, oleomargarine, and milk."[95] As Cynthia Comacchio puts it, "not only the feeding process but food itself became 'scientific.'"[96] Brown himself came to see the Nutritional Research Laboratories as the defining aspect of the institution, stating that the hospital itself was now " ... regarded practically everywhere as the centre, not only for the treatment of the sick child who is brought to its doors, but also for the dissemination of the newer knowledge regarding both the treatment and prevention of diseases of infants and children."[97] Brown and the hospital medical staff could not be accused of hypocrisy: Sunwheat biscuits were fed to children at the hospital for over fifty years.[98]

Some of the individual clinician-researchers received national and international attention. Alan Brown, of course, was, by the 1930s, the leading paediatrician in the country, ruling the hospital with an iron fist and publishing widely on the nutrition of children. His 1926 textbook — *The Normal Child* — and his dozens of peer-reviewed scientific articles on nutritional research would bring him international attention. He used his scientific stature and his position as "autocrat-in-chief" of the hospital — as one unsympathetic observer referred to him — to promote nutritional foods. Pearl Summerfeldt, by contrast, in a fate besetting many women researchers of the era, was quietly marginalized in terms of her own contribution. In an unusual personal twist, she married Abraham L. Rose, the vice-president of the company commercializing Pablum, and moved to Indiana. At the wedding, Frederick Tisdall was a groomsman. Her obituary suggests that she "gave up medicine" when the couple moved to the United States, because she didn't have a licence to practise south of the border.[99]

Frederick Tisdall, by contrast, would be catapulted to the national scene. His close association with Pablum enabled him to appeal to diverse groups for ongoing research support. Under his directorship, the Research Laboratories' annual budget increased a remarkable ten-fold.[100] During the Second World War, he was appointed chairman of the Canadian Medical Association Committee on Nutrition and advised the government on the nutritional content of army rations. Later, he became chief scientific officer of the federal Department of Nutrition, part of the Ministry of Health and Welfare. His passion for nutritional research, however, would manifest itself in a multitude of research projects, some of which would prove ethically controversial. For example, he is now well known as the principal author of a federal study involving the Department of Indian Affairs, comparing the nutritional implications of fortified foods by withholding foodstuffs from near-starving Aboriginal communities (including children) during and immediately after the Second World War. In effect, he took the opportunity of using isolated Aboriginal communities suffering from severe malnutrition to conduct a controlled study, with certain communities receiving nutritional foods, and others not.[101]

The health impact of the new craze in nutritional foods is more difficult to assess historically. Certainly the principal players in the drama of Pablum trumpeted the beneficial effects, as witnessed most dramatically in the decline of rickets and scurvy in the 1930s. During the Second World War, Alan Brown and Elizabeth Chant Robertson observed that these deficiency diseases were becoming part of the past of medical practice: "It is with the greatest difficulty we obtain sufficient cases of rickets and scurvy for demonstration to our students" – a pseudo-complaint laden with a great deal of professional satisfaction.[102] Cause of death data clearly indicate a significant drop in the mortality rate from nutritional deficiency diseases in 1930s Canada, though the decline was nationwide and indeed most pronounced in Quebec.[103]

On an occupational level, the growth of the laboratories also encouraged the proliferation of a new type of hospital worker – the laboratory technician, who began to populate modern research hospitals by the hundreds. From the beginning these workers were predominantly women who operated in a quasi-domestic sphere of a hospital-based domestic science. Food preparation (considered a women's sphere of knowledge) combined with the new scientific practices of bacteriology to usher in a new locus for female science. As described in chapter 5, *Maclean's* heralded the new occupation of dietetics in the 1920s as "A Progressive Profession for Girls."[104]

These dietitians, central to the new science of hospital feeding, concocted formulas and feeding preparations using oatmeal, barley flour, cane sugar, malt sugar and created such enticing formulas as Barley Gruel, Groats Gruel, and Granum Gruel.[105] The dietitian straddled several worlds – the domestic and the institutional, the familial and the scientific.

The success of Pablum also introduced an interdependent, if awkward relationship between laboratory research and clinical care. On an instrumental level, research required ultimately its application to patients, a protocol that was not clearly defined in the era before the Nuremberg Code and other codified protocols of consent. In addition, the enormous and somewhat unanticipated profits posed particular issues for individual researchers and for hospital trustees. Should researchers benefit financially from their discoveries? And to whom do the patents belong, the hospital or the laboratories? The Steenbock protocol clearly provided a useful mechanism by which the hospital could support research, but in a transparent manner that would deflect any suspicions of individual profiteering. In the context of the economic privation of the 1930s and war years, these perceptions were first and foremost in the minds of hospital trustees. Indeed, although patenting would become widespread in the post–Second World War era, in the 1930s it was considered, in the words of one legal historian "indecent," particularly in the British medical context.[106] In 1943, a San Francisco court invalidated Steenbock's patent, arguing that irradiation was a natural process that could not be patented. Ultimately, the research at the hospital cascaded into a larger cultural phenomenon of health additives. Scientific and popular accounts identified the urban environment as "unnatural"; indoor desk jobs, full-time schooling, overly refined foods, smoke, dust, glass windows, and clothing – as contributors to widespread vitamin D deficiency. Vitamin enrichment thus became one of the more popular ways of addressing the deleterious effects of "modern civilized life."[107]

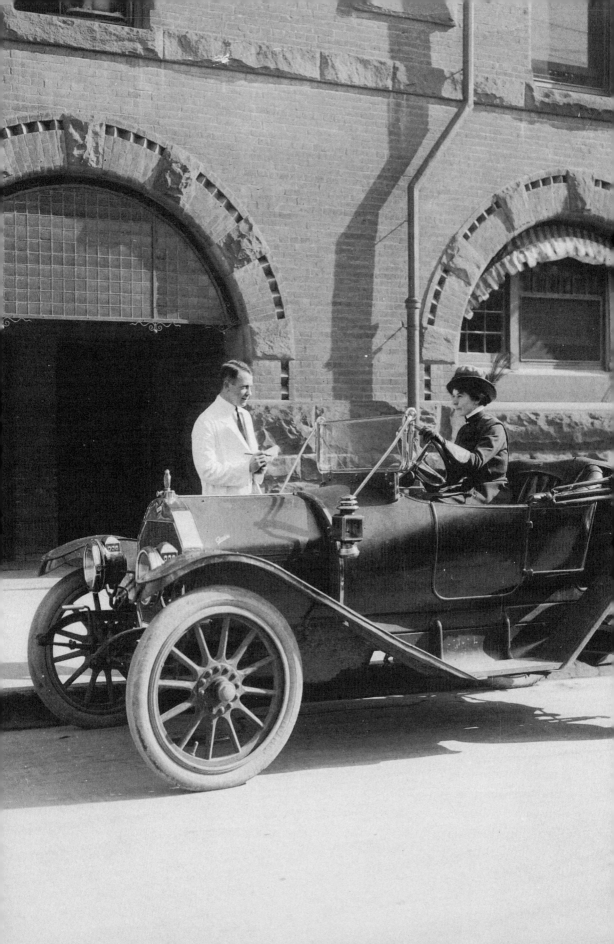

SEVEN

Iron Lungs

> It might be said, and I think correctly so, that paediatrics has been
> the pioneer specialty in preventive medicine.[1]
>
> Dr. Alan Brown, "Preventive Paediatrics," 1931

Forty-three Errands of Mercy

In July 1912, the elderly John Ross Robertson gave a motor car to Florence Charters, the hospital's first social service nurse. Charters had begun visiting the homes of outpatients and discharged inpatients in 1908. Initially, she travelled by foot or streetcar, averaging a dozen visits per day. The motorized vehicle, still unusual in the streets of pre-war Toronto, enabled her to double her weekly visits to 150.[2] Her routine was, to say the least, challenging. Each morning she received orders from staff physicians and a list of names and addresses of her target patients for the day from the hospital secretary. As she called upon house after house, she instructed mothers in hygiene practices, sometimes reapplied dressings, and, upon her return, advised the hospital of the need for admission for those "that are not thriving at home."[3] To ensure the continued success of the pasteurization plant, she also supervised the feeding of children whose parents had applied to the hospital for pasteurized milk. Her criss-crossing of the city was, of course, well documented by Robertson's own *Evening Telegram*, where a special reporter followed Charters and recounted to readers, "One Day with the District Nurse in her whizzing motor car. Forty-three Errands of Mercy Between Sunrise and

7.1 With the growing importance of outpatient treatment, the hospital devised innovative ways to reach out to the community. Here, Florence Charters embarks on her daily follow-up with former patients in one of Robertson's "Motor Cars."

Sunset, from far East to farther West forty-two miles on the Streets of Toronto and its Suburbs ... from Suburban Shacks among the trees to Swarming Tenements in the Heart of the City the Soother of Suffering Speeds."[4]

As delightful as the image of this "soother of suffering" was, the urban adventures of Florence Charters reflected the end of one era and the flowering of another. In the years leading up to the First World War, a remarkable transformation was afoot. The City of Toronto Health Department was reorganizing its activities and centralizing its operations. Rather than having concurrent or overlapping systems of visiting nurses – one managed by The Hospital for Sick Children, another by the City – Alan Brown and the medical officer of health for the City of Toronto, Charles Hastings, agreed to a novel arrangement – to have all child welfare nurses under Brown's authority. Brown was subsequently appointment as "part-time Medical Director" of the city's Division of Child Hygiene in 1915. In this symbiotic relationship, Toronto's Health Department opened a centre in the outpatient department of The Hospital for Sick Children, and a Health Department clerk and two child welfare nurses were present each day to perform the recording and follow-up work. The nurse supervisor of child welfare, Nora Moore, attended the outpatient department of the hospital to "receiv[e] physicians' orders which were delivered to the nurses in the field through her district superintendent."[5] These nurses, in turn, reported back on the home conditions of the patients, sometimes recommending admission to the hospital or attendance at one of the hospital's outpatient clinics. By 1929, the hospital was directing thirty-one "Child Health Centres," a situation which, Brown proclaimed, had "no parallel in any other city in the world."[6] In this way, Charters was superseded by an entire army of child health workers, paid by the city but under the direction of The Hospital for Sick Children. Much of the expansion of the hospital throughout the city had its roots in the vision of the young, soon-to-be chief of medical services, Alan Brown.

Alan Brown's views on the role of the paediatric hospital reflected a new generation of medical thinking. Many childhood disease specialists had formed the opinion that a small hospital for the sick poor augmented by a single dispensary had become hopelessly outdated. Brown envisioned an expansive role for the modern paediatric hospital as a community institution and centre of medical education, stating, with a certain rhetorical flare, that "a children's hospital should not be just an institution for treating sick children."[7] Rather, in his opinion, the hospital was a "clearing house" for infant and child welfare work.[8] By the end of his career, which lasted a remarkable three decades, the list of activities he envisaged for the hospital appeared limitless. As he preached to the American Hospital Association in 1939, the paediatric hospital ought to

> embrace all children's activities beginning with cooperation with obstetricians in the prenatal and antenatal care of the infant ; supervise all children's homes and insti[t]utions ; cooperate with all governmental departments of health ; be a centre for education of medical students, nurses and postgraduates; be called upon for public addresses on problems relative to the child ; cooperate with all service clubs ; embrace all problems of psychological medicine relative to children's work, which means cooperation with the Juvenile Courts and all other organizations having to do with children ; cooperate with all nursery schools ; and have a well organized research laboratory.[9]

The realization of his vision, however, was neither straightforward nor without opposition. The early twentieth century witnessed the advent of public health departments in urban areas across North America. Sometimes these municipal units clashed with pre-existing hospital power structures, causing tension between public health and institutional medicine. Brown's genius was to respond to, and in many instances co-opt, this public health movement so that it revolved around the hospital and operated under his personal authority. In this way The Hospital for Sick Children became the centre of a hub-and-spoke structure of child health throughout the city, coordinating public health nurses responsible for child welfare and home visits, arranging follow-ups after discharge, and building on the network of well-baby clinics that had proved so useful in the distribution of pasteurized milk. As Superintendent Joseph Bower explained, "The Hospital is in fact largely an adjunct to the City Health Department ... some time ago, it was found that approximately 85% of the children attending our Out Patient Department, many of them subsequently becoming in-patients, were referred here by the visiting nurse of the City Health Department, either directly from the home or following the periodic inspection made by the nurses and doctors at the schools."[10]

In this ever-expanding system of child health services, attendance at outpatient clinics soared, and new specialist clinics were added, including those that dealt with nutrition, venereal disease, neurology, dermatology, child welfare, cardiology, and diabetes. In 1923 alone, over three thousand massage therapy interventions for conditions such as paralysis, rickets, malnutrition, and torticollis (twisted neck) were given, half of which were for outpatients.[11] Central to the mindset of the interventionist public health movement was the emphasis on preventive paediatrics and reforming the household environments of poor families. As one hospital report reminded friends of the hospital, "In the Out-Patients' Department ... efforts are concentrated not only on the cure and prevention of disease, but also on the education of parents along lines to be followed in order to minimize sickness and otherwise to help in raising healthy families."[12] Clinic reports highlighted the instruction of mothers – who were encouraged to observe the treatment in the clinic – as a primary focus.[13] Brown oversaw this expansion, including the selection of physicians for the clinics; he was also personally involved in the direction of nurseries in not only every hospital maternity ward in the city but also relevant units run by Children's Aid Societies, children's homes, and other paramedical institutions.[14]

Although the rapid expansion of specialist clinics and the referral practices of public health nurses were, from the hospital and city's perspectives, unmitigated successes, community paediatricians and general practitioners took umbrage with the imperial agenda of Brown and the army of public health nurses under his command. In October 1921, two side-by-side editorials in the *Canadian Practitioner and Review* claimed that outdoor clinics "overstepped" the institution's role and cheated physicians out of their "proper revenue."[15] The charge was clear: community medical practitioners feared that Toronto Public Health nurses were directing potential paying patients to the hospitals' free services, thus undermining the viability of their individual clinical practices. Charles Hastings, the city's medical officer of health, called the article "a malicious misrepresentation of the facts" and defended his nurses, insisting that they referred parents first to family doctors and to clinics only if they lacked a physician or money. Furthermore, he attested to the hospital's practice of investigating each family's ability to pay for private care.[16] For his part, Brown insisted that the well-baby clinics "came into being to fill a want created by the great numbers among the poor who, because of overcrowding and ignorance, require advice relating to health, hygiene and manner of living."[17] In a revealing turn of phrase, Hastings affirmed that the principal function of these nurses was to "keep the community well, never to treat the sick."[18]

General practitioners in Toronto were not persuaded by what they saw as a disingenuous sleight of hand. Children were considered an integral part of building a thriving practice, and community practitioners unattached to the hospital were alarmed by the intrusion of the hospital and the expansion of free public health clinics administered by the city. General practitioners had few qualms with the hospital treating the poorest children in the city, whose parents were not able to pay for private care anyway, but suspected that many families of middling incomes were making use of free clinics and community nurses in lieu of paying for private care. The editorials in the *Canadian Practitioner and Review* criticized, in particular, the practice of city nurses sending patients to "some so-called children's specialists conducting baby clinics" rather than family physicians. One doctor bitterly attacked the aims of the well-baby clinics:

> Once these children are taken to the "Clinic," the mothers are told to bring them back regularly and have the children weighed and cared for. In many instances they are taken into the hospital.
>
> Now, all this is wrong, and is bound to give rise to severe criticism. The medical profession of Toronto is not going to stand [for] this sort of thing.[19]

This criticism echoed other contemporary concerns about the rise of school medical doctors and nurses who, it was alleged, were using their privileged access to children to steer cases to the hands of certain medical practitioners.[20] As one "East End Practitioner" wrote in response to the editorial, "I have frequently found that the school doctors follow the case to their homes and have recommended the employment of certain specialists for the removal of enlarged tonsils. They, of course, get the anaesthetic fee."[21] It should be remembered that, at this time, no physician at The Hospital for Sick Children, not even Alan Brown, received a full-time salary from the hospital. All ran private practices in the community, thus opening them up to accusations that the hospital staff, or the city's public health nurses, were guiding potential paying patients to their own practices or to those of friends or colleagues.

The anxiety of private practitioners that doctors affiliated with the hospital were "stealing patients" was understandable, given the popularity of the well-baby clinics and the explosion in the numbers of patients attending the outpatient department. Publications proclaimed that it had become

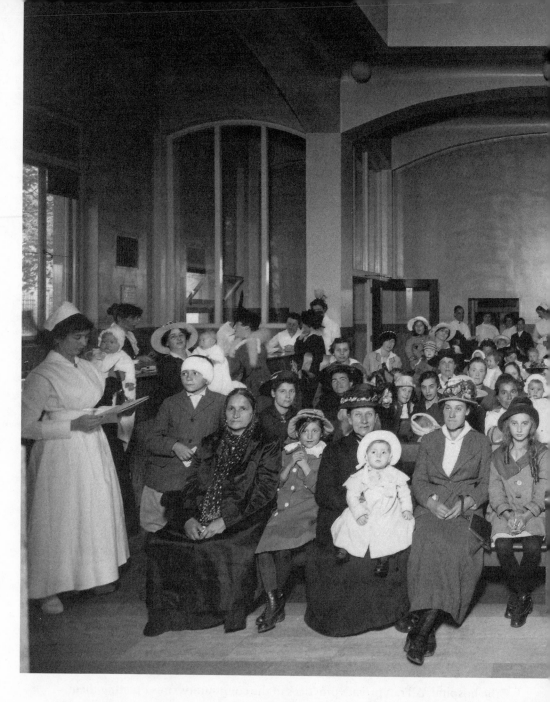

"the largest out-patient clinic, in connection with hospitals for children, in the world."[22] A few statistics, drawn from annual reports, quantify its growing popularity. In 1911, a daily average of forty-one patients attended the outpatient department. By 1920, this had more than tripled to a daily average of 132; in 1921, it climbed to a daily average of 188. In 1933, an all-time high of 98,351 patient visits were recorded, with a daily average of 323. One particularly busy day topped 500 children. Baby carriages lined up outside

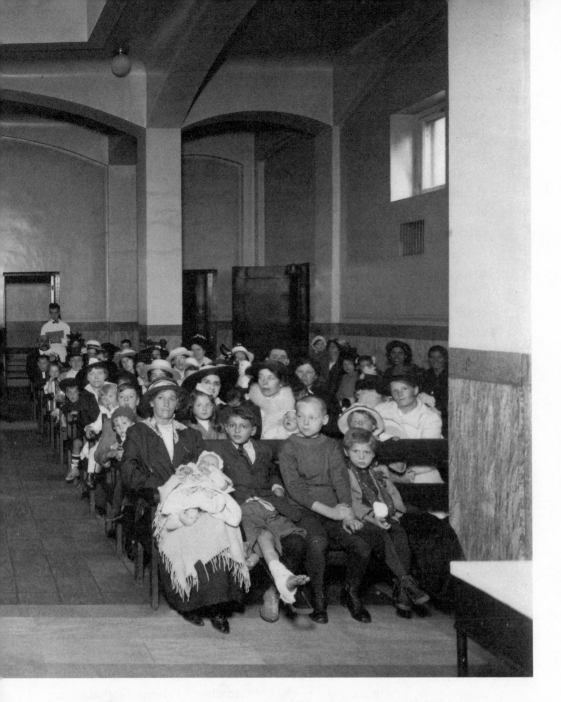

7.2 Local families – many immigrant and working-class – filled the outpatient department of The Hospital for Sick Children in the decades before Medicare.

the Elizabeth Street door of the hospital had become a familiar sight to those taking the College Street street-car in the morning.[23] Contemporary photographs capture rows of mothers and children, dressed in something approximating their Sunday best, lined up on long wooden benches awaiting their turn (see image 7.2). The influence of this new emphasis on outreach was not limited to Toronto. Brown and

W.E. Gallie encouraged hospital medical staff to occasionally organize clinics throughout the province of Ontario and to send "crippled children" to The Hospital for Sick Children for treatment. Surgical clinics, for example, were held in Kitchener, Sault Ste. Marie, Sudbury, Chatham, Woodstock, Welland, Port Colborne, and Oshawa.[24] The provincial Department of Health and service organizations such as the Red Cross and Rotary Clubs also organized "popular lectures, baby clinics, and so on, with the result that unusual surgical conditions occurring in children [were] discovered."[25] Indeed, the demand was becoming so great that calls were repeatedly issued to locate other teaching centres in outlying parts of the city.[26]

The suggestion that the hospital and city sponsor teaching centres in other parts of Toronto, however logical, was resisted by university authorities. The hospital's physical location on College Street – situated right beside the newly constructed Toronto General Hospital and within walking distance of the main University of Toronto campus – made it the ideal location for training physicians, nurses, child welfare workers, and, later, dieticians. As chapter 3 illustrated, The Hospital for Sick Children also constituted an important locus of training in the early years of orthopaedic surgery. The interwar period built upon this foundation, which was mutually beneficial to the hospital and the university. Stakeholders argued that the hospital's "educational value ... would be decreased were any portion of its work removed to a considerable distance from the Medical Lecture Rooms of the University."[27]

The growing importance of The Hospital for Sick Children to the University of Toronto was reflected in a fundamental reorganization of clinical and teaching staff in the university's Faculty of Medicine, one that prompted a similar administrative reconfiguration in both Toronto General Hospital and The Hospital for Sick Children itself. The reorganization was propelled, in part, by a substantial endowment in 1919 from the powerful Eaton Family, which provided a remarkable $500,000 over twenty years to fund, among other things, a full-time chair in clinical medicine.[28] Duncan Graham, the recipient of the endowed chair, presided over the Department of Medicine from July 1919 until 1947. Graham removed 40 per cent of the staff positions, and appointed Alan Brown (by now the head of Medical Services at The Hospital for Sick Children) as associate professor of medicine in charge of paediatrics. Brown was to devote half his time to what was then the sub-department of paediatrics. He rearranged clinical staff into a hierarchy mirroring that of academic faculty at the university, from clinical assistants as the most junior rank, to assistant physicians, associate physicians, and full physicians. The same structure was imposed on the surgeons. Concurrently, Brown organized the "specialties," medicine, surgery, laryngology, ophthalmology, pathology and bacteriology, chemistry, radiology, and anesthetics, into administrative departments within the hospital.[29]

As if the Eaton endowment was not enough of a windfall, the same year, 1919, the Rockefeller Foundation announced that it would grant $5 million in support of Canadian medical education, $1 million of which was earmarked for the University of Toronto. This generous subvention provided financial space for redefining the relationship between the medical school and medical staff at its affiliated hospitals. For example, in 1921, the university elevated Clarence Starr, formerly surgical chief at The Hospital for Sick Children, to full-time professor of surgery in the medical school, with his own resources to appoint other full-time faculty.[30] As for the remaining physicians at The Hospital for Sick Children, almost all would henceforth hold joint appointments, most of which were largely nominal, with the sub-department of paediatrics. In return for these university affiliations, the clinicians would be responsible for part-time clinical instruction of undergraduate medical students, medical clerks, nurses, and dieticians. None would receive salaried payments from the hospital, though honoraria were paid by the university for teaching sessions. Sensitive that the public might be confused about the entangled relationship between the hospital and the university, the hospital trustees, while praising the philanthropy of the Eaton family and the "close co-operation" between the hospital and the medical school of the University of Toronto, also emphasized that the hospital "retains its full independence from any measure of outside control."[31] Apparently Robertson's bequest was predicated upon the independence of the hospital; as a consequence, University of Toronto representation on the board may well have jeopardized his substantial posthumous gift.[32]

As the hospital enhanced its relationship with the University of Toronto's medical school, its own teaching facilities were augmented through the addition of a lecture theatre and the expansion of an existing one. Most of the training, however, was clinical, as the outpatient clinics described above would be "more than ever thronged with students eager to learn the last word in pediatric science."[33] In time, undergraduate medical education leading to an MD would be supplemented by postgraduate specialization. Brown, for example, began a summertime graduate course in paediatrics in 1921. Ten years later, the surgeon W.E. Gallie began his own "Gallie Course," the first dedicated postgraduate course of surgical training in the country. In 1920, the Medical Advisory Board voted to open residencies to individuals other than students enrolled at the University of Toronto, suggesting that they were limited to them previously. Graduates, initially two at a time, could also pursue full-time fellowships involving clinical work and laboratory investigation.[34]

The Faculty of Medicine reimbursed these part-time instructors for their teaching work, and also paid the salaries of the research assistants, technicians, and secretarial assistants in the laboratories. Instructors of postgraduate courses received honoraria. In the 1935–6 academic year, for example, $700 was split among thirty-five individuals in the department, including medical and surgical staff and the heads of the milk and radiology departments. Brown himself received nominal remuneration through the department ($350 in 1935, plus a $50 honorarium and $160 from the School of Nursing), in contrast to Duncan Graham's annual full-time take-home salary of $9,690, and the $500–$2,440 paid to other assistant and associate professors in the Department of Medicine. Brown's successor, A.L. Chute, claimed that Brown never received more than $800 from the University of Toronto in any given year. It is important to note that the new, closer relationship to the University of Toronto also directly benefited the hospital financially: receipts from student fees more than doubled from $773.35 between 1917 and 1918 to $1,703.31 in 1921.[35]

Faculty of Medicine calendars describe the course of lectures and clinical instruction in paediatrics offered to fourth- and fifth-year medical students. As of 1920, fourth-year students received thirty-two clinical lectures in paediatrics and would rotate through the hospital for approximately six weeks. They were also required to take a course on orthopaedic surgery at the hospital. Fifth-year students gained clinical experience in the wards, dispensary, milk modifying laboratory, outpatient department, and child welfare clinics. They also wrote specific examinations in paediatrics. Some students might accompany other hospital medical staff and nurses on home visits. Postgraduate residents could also supplement their meagre stipends of $25 per month with clinical work paid for by the city and by giving blood. At a 1919 conference on medical education, Assistant Physician G.S. Strathy commented insightfully that The Hospital for Sick Children was "practically a university hospital."[36] By the 1930s, the relationship between the hospital and the university had fully formed.[37]

"Too Poor to Collect"

The sudden wealth bestowed upon the University of Toronto's medical school masks a harsher financial reality of its affiliated hospitals during the 1920s and 1930s. The financing of patient care at The Hospital for Sick Children in its first fifty years had been a constantly changing mixture of annual grants from the city and the province, charitable donations from ordinary citizens, private fees, and the occasional remarkable intervention of a few extraordinarily wealthy Torontonians. The guiding principle had always been that the hospital was there to provide medical care for the respectable sick poor. Charitable donations were there so that "no child knocked in vain," to invoke the mantra of the institution. But these lingering Victorian conceptions of relieving the "respectable poor" were breaking down in the face of twentieth-century public health initiatives.

For better or worse, from the 1880s the hospital relied on municipal and provincial grants. These included block operating grants as well as per diem grants for specific patients under the Charity Aid Act. In return, hospitals in receipt of public monies were required by law to accept all needy poor patients. These "indigent" patients, as they were still called in the 1920s, were supposed to apply for a municipal grant that would partially offset their maintenance and medical treatment. Although these grants rarely covered the entire cost of a patient's inpatient care, they gave the impression, to the general public, that the hospital was a public hospital open to, and supported by, the entire community. In addition, the growing interest of the middle class for access to the latest in medical technology led to a demand for hospital care among wealthier clientele. No longer did the middle class shun medical institutions as little more than glorified poorhouses; they increasingly sought hospital care and scientific medicine for their household members, although in a manner that was commensurate with, and reflective of, their social standing. In these cases, public ward patients were charged a base fee of $1.50 per day (or $10.50 per week); semi-private patients, by contrast were charged $3.00 per day (or $21 per week). At this time, there were no private wards. As the 1928 regulations of the hospital warned, these base fees excluded "X-Ray costs, Operating Room charges, or any other expenses that may arise out of the treatment of the ... semi-private patient."[38]

Hospital administrators found themselves in the challenging situation of accepting all poor patients demanding admission and, at the same time, trying to squeeze as much money as possible out of paying patients. The difference was made up by charitable donations from friends of the hospital. Such a balancing act was manageable, although barely, in the prosperous 1920s, but it fell apart in the depths of the Great Depression. Indeed, it was this crisis in the financing of the hospital that, according to the historian David Gagan, constituted a key structural problem leading to provincially run hospitalization insurance programs in the 1950s.[39]

Paediatric care constituted the first wave of a new belief in free hospital care in Canada. By the 1920s, the balance of public and political feeling was beginning to swing to the opinion that all children's medical care should be covered by public funds. This contention combined a lingering Victorian sentiment about the innocence of childhood with more hard-hearted and quasi-eugenic beliefs in raising fit children for national military preparedness. Precedents had also been established, in the creation of free school nurses and medical officers and in the free milk depots discussed earlier in the book. But even if there was growing support for free paediatric care, such a principle became difficult to put into practice. What constituted "medical care"? Should this be restricted to hospital care? Did it include pharmaceutical prescriptions? Should the remarkable work constructed in the orthopaedic workshop – the artificial limbs, the braces, the devices of numerous types – be given free of charge? What about the milk and the bottles in which it was given? Even the grant from the City of Toronto became a source of debate, since as many as one-half of the patients being treated at the hospital came from other municipalities. Should these cities – London, Hamilton, and Ottawa – reimburse the hospital, and indirectly the city, for the care they received?

This debate would wax and wane throughout the interwar period. Meanwhile, the trustees of the hospital found themselves confronting the issue of both private and public patients' unpaid hospital fees. Within the confines of the administrative offices, these bills represented a financial and public relations headache. Although most "bad debts" related to the daily maintenance charges for public patients who had not received a provincial or municipal grant, there were also scores of unpaid debts owed by private patients. In one list from 1922 to 1924, a period of relative prosperity compared to the next decade, over 100 patients, almost all of whom were from Toronto, owed a total of $1,042.50, including one "Municipality Account" from Oshawa for $43.50. The fees on this list were in addition to those included on a separate list of over fifty "untraceable" patients who collectively owed $795.[40] In October 1926, the board wrote off the not-inconsiderable amount of $1,334.50 for maintenance accounts ranging from $25.50 to $365.[41] Smaller amounts were regularly in arrears for orthopaedic appliances and X-ray services. In 1926, the board wrote off X-ray accounts totalling $654.50 for the years 1922–5.[42] In all areas, particularly orthopaedic and X-ray services, the hospital was in a no-win situation. "If the work is not done," lamented one trustee, "the Hospital has to take the blame of the consequences."[43]

The Hospital was limited in its ability to enforce payment of the individual accounts of paying patients. Engaging collectors and solicitors was costly and could result in negative publicity, which any medical institution dependent upon charitable support was anxious to avoid. Nevertheless, in 1922, the secretary did contact the city solicitor "to ascertain if it would be possible to get some assistance in the way of extra pressure on delinquent parents and guardians."[44] Five years later the secretary spoke to the trustees about

> the desirability of enforcing payment in cases where the Hospital has reason to consider that a reasonable amount can be paid by the parents for maintenance. This applies particularly to such cases as have not been protected by a City Order, by reason of its having been refused, owing to neglect to apply etc., etc. Unless the public are educated to realize they must make payment when able to do so, the whole problem becomes very serious to the Hospital.[45]

The hospital first tried to obtain payment from families by sending bills and letters reminding them of hospital charges that were in arrears. Less often, the hospital's own solicitors were brought in to resolve certain cases. If necessary, the hospital haggled and accepted partial payment to settle accounts. By July 1925, the trustees authorized the secretary "to engage a man to handle the collection of accounts for the Hospital."[46] In light of the large Jewish clientele being served by the hospital, one trustee "agreed to enquire into the possibility of obtaining the services of a Jewish girl to assist the clerical staff of [the outpatient] Department in dealing with Jewish families."[47] Records indicate that in August 1925, before the trustees wrote off fifty-two maintenance, orthopaedic, and X-ray accounts, different collectors were sent to nineteen Toronto homes, usually multiple times.[48] The hospital's monthly trustee minutes, dry as they are, convey the self-evident frustration of the members with individual families deemed financially solvent, but who simply refused to pay the hospital. To settle a $36 account, members of the medical staff met with a patient's father, who was connected with the Canadian Business College of Toronto, and reported back to the Trustees that "this man was able to pay, and had no right to withhold settlement from the Hospital." The trustees directed their solicitors, Messrs. Tilley, Johnston & Co., "to take the necessary proceedings to collect."[49]

In 1921, the executive committee of the board of trustees advised the trustees that it would be "bad policy for the Hospital to sue [individuals] in the Courts,"[50] yet the threat of legal proceedings was employed from time to time, in particular with patients from the private Cottage Hospital. Several years later, when dealing with outstanding accounts for two such siblings, the secretary "reported having written Mr. G.T. Clarkson [a trustee from 1921–46] who is reported to be in charge of the liquidation of the Company with which Mr. Thomas is employed, regarding his ability to pay this account. Authority was given to take such legal proceedings as were necessary to recover payment."[51] One month later, for a separate debt, the trustees authorized the secretary "to instruct the Hospital's solicitors to enter suit and obtain judgment against this debtor in the event of his neglect to liquidate his account amounting at present to $90.00."[52] Writing off bad debts was hardly a phenomenon limited to The Hospital for Sick Children; at this time, "hospitals large and small were forced to resort to the services of collection agencies to recover unpaid maintenance fees, a task made all the more difficult by the transient nature of city and town populations."[53]

In many cases, mail was returned and families had disappeared: "Removed and cannot be found," "Bootleggers – moved, when coll'r. called," and "Dutchman. Gone back to Holland" were some of the conclusions reported to the hospital by collection agents.[54] When families were located, they most commonly cited poverty as a reason for non-payment: "Very poor – no chance of collecting [$4.50]" [sic];[55] "father out of work – 7 children"; "Out of work";[56] "Father drowned. Mother cannot pay"; "Illegitimate child – Father not working – shiftless";[57] "Foreigners – no money."[58] In some cases, parental reluctance to apply for a city relief order deprived the hospital of reimbursement: "Mother in Hospital – father out of work. Would not apply for C. Order"[59]

Although it might be tempting to conclude that some parents were simply stiffing the hospital with bills that were rightly theirs to pay, one also senses an older tradition of paying according to an assessment of culpability. For example, parents at times refused payment for accident cases, presumably holding other parties liable for their children's injuries. The secretary of the trustees complained of "the difficulties of, and the injustices to the hospital in respect to some accident cases. When money is obtained from the party causing the accident, the charges due the hospital are not paid, and a bad debt is incurred."[60] Some parents also refused to pay when their children died in the hospital, when they were dissatisfied with treatment, or when the cost increased because a patient's discharge was delayed due to certain institutional measures, such as quarantine.[61] For example, in 1903, a Simcoe farmer refused to settle the outstanding maintenance charges incurred by his daughter, who was hospitalized for six months and then discharged and treated at home when the family was unable to afford hospital fees. The family also owed a Dr. Bingham sums for private treatment. When the Medical Agency of Canada acted as a third party to collect the debt, the father wrote to John Ross Robertson, complaining that "As for a cure, [my daughter] has been much worse since she left the hospital than she ever was before going to the hospital, that I doubt that she received any benefit whatever from the treatment already paid for." The trustees investigated the family's circumstances, and in the end the father paid $37 to avoid going to trial, enclosing the funds with the following message: "You can give the money to Dr. Bingham if he still thinks he is entitled to it after being informed of these facts, and I hope it will do him the good that it is depriving my family of."[62]

Municipalities, including the City of Toronto, were responsible for paying for the maintenance, treatment, and burial of indigent patients by means of a city order, often referred to as a "C.O." or "C. Order" in the sources. Yet municipalities often failed to fulfil this responsibility, and hospital solicitors had difficulty extracting payment. The secretary appears to have occasionally clashed with the City of Toronto relief officer, a Mr. Skippen, over reimbursement for the treatment of city order patients. In 1924, the board of the hospital complained that he had even refused to "take any cognizance of accounts of patients, who died on the day of admission."[63] There was occasionally debate about liability for fees. In one complicated case, there was disagreement over whether the patient's family, the City of Toronto, or the Children's Aid Society was responsible for maintenance charges. An exasperated staff surgeon expressed a desire to sue in his own name for the outstanding charges. To make matters worse, some families who were too poor to pay for care refused to cooperate in applying for a city order, presumably because of the shame attached to receiving relief.[64]

Unsurprisingly, the hospital repeatedly sought larger grants from the city to cover city patients' accounts. In February 1912, trustees petitioned for a nearly 50 per cent increase in the base grant, from $18,000 to $25,000.[65]

In addition to the haggling over the terms and application of municipal grants, such wrangling could not even address those who fell outside the regulations of provincial subsidies, such as the cost of care for non-residents, of very recent immigrants with no fixed address, and of residents of the province of Ontario who resided in "unorganized districts," that is, areas of the province not under direct municipal governance. With regard to the last group of patients, the provincial government finally agreed to "stand in the place of a municipality, in a district where no municipal organization exists," assuming a $2,000 debt accumulated by the hospital.[66] Payment, however, was nearly impossible to obtain for non-residents, such as in one case involving outstanding fees of $99.50 for the "Child of [a] British Jamaican, living in New York, whose wife was visiting her mother in Toronto. No money, and City refused to acknowledge."[67] In 1930, the board contended with an outstanding maintenance account for $503.50 for an immigrant child who did not meet the residency requirement for municipal relief. The secretary wrangled with the Department of Immigration and was instructed by the trustees to "insist on receiving a satisfactory explanation covering the admission of this child to Canada, when, according to the opinion of the members of the Hospital Staff, the child was decidedly a tubercular case at the time of entry to Canada."[68] By the 1920s, immigration officials were supposed to ensure that all new immigrants to Canada had no detectable physical or mental impairment before being granted entry to the country. If they were mentally or physically disabled they were to be returned to their country of origin.[69] In this case, the hospital contacted the Cheerio Club for assistance. Six months later, when the patient's account had risen to $800 and it was determined that "the child will require to remain in hospital for possibly another year," the trustees decided to continue treatment regardless of the impossibility of reimbursement. Other service organizations, such as the Junior Red Cross, supplied funds to settle uncollectable accounts (in this case, to cover the cost of orthopaedic appliances).[70]

As if these multiple categories of non-paying patients were not challenging enough, the hospital also had to contend with negotiating the financial support of Aboriginal paediatric cases. Aboriginal children, under the Indian Act of 1876, were considered the responsibility of the federal government, regardless of their province of residence. Indigenous children were, in a legal sense, wards of the federal government under this controversial piece of legislation and, although there were some so-called "Indian hospitals" in the Prairies, there were none in Ontario until after the Second World War.[71] This situation led the provincial government to inform the hospital secretary in 1929 that "no claim would be accepted with respect to the per diem allowance for Indian patients in the Public Wards. It was decided, therefore, since these patients are wards of the Federal government under the Department of Indian Affairs, that the Hospital's account be sent to that Department, at the rate of $4.00 per day (representing the average per diem cost of maintenance) instead of at the public ward rate of $1.75 per day, as heretofore."[72] First Nations children would figure increasingly prominently among long-stay patients in The Hospital for Sick Children from the 1940s onwards.

With the stock market crash in 1929 and the Great Depression of the 1930s, hospital finances became an increasingly pressing concern. The number of paying patients declined, as did donations, at a time of rising medical costs, though the decline in the numbers of paying patients had less of an impact than it did at adult hospitals of the time, since only about 5 per cent of the beds at the children's hospital were private ones.[73] In response to the financial crisis, the province slashed the public ward per diem from 60 cents to 10 cents for any patients staying over 120 days. In 1933, the province also reduced the provincial grant by 15 per cent.[74] Hospital trustees were considering a new hospital building before the Depression and the outbreak of the Second World War forced them to shelve the plans until the mid-1940s. Meanwhile, the city, which had previously met the annual operating deficits of Toronto's hospitals, ceased this practice in 1931. After this time, annual losses accumulated steadily.[75] The hospital responded by reducing salaries for nurses and non-medical staff, among other measures. The trustees followed the lead of other city hospitals by reducing the salaries and wages of its employees by 5 to 6 per cent in April 1932.[76] By February 1933, the net expenditure on salaries and wages had been reduced 12 per cent from the previous summer.[77] In the midst of this worsening financial crisis, The Hospital for Sick Children would be confronted by an epidemic, which produced consequences that would catalyze not only technological innovation, but also a rethinking of the very financing of public hospitals.

The New Epidemic[78]

Poliomyelitis constituted a relatively unimportant disease over the course of the nineteenth century, dwarfed as it was by the major infant and childhood infectious killers of the era, such as measles or diphtheria. In its most basic form, polio was a relatively benign viral infection, with low morbidity and mortality rates. As a disease, it typically presented with symptoms that were often indistinguishable from the seasonal flu virus, such as fever, headache, stiff neck, loss of appetite, general fatigue, and gastrointestinal distress. In most cases, poliomyelitis would run its course in a manner not unlike a case of the seasonal flu. Paralytic poliomyelitis, by contrast, was an uncommon variation of this self-limiting childhood infection, where the virus infected the central nervous system, attacking the motor neurons of the brain and spinal cord. Indeed, the disease was first termed "poliomyelitis" in the 1870s in reference to the "inflammation of the grey matter of the spinal cord."[79] This more severe, if hitherto uncommon, variation often left sufferers with paralysis of the limbs, among other disabilities. As a consequence, even though the paralytic form of the disease had previously been quite rare, the disease was also commonly referred to in the medical community as "infantile paralysis," or, among the general public, simply as "polio."[80]

Polio constitutes a case study in the paradox of public health reform; it was a disease that flourished because of the success of sanitary reform measures a generation earlier. Medical historians have hypothesized that many of the public health effects of the late-Victorian sanitary reform, such as better hygiene, may well have lowered the immunity of specific social groups. Dr. Helen MacMurchy, who had become a nationally recognized champion of child health, observed the paradox that "[o]ften the vigorous and healthy are attacked and those who have comfortable homes and good care."[81] What was once an endemic, unremarkable gastrointestinal ailment surfaced in increasingly severe epidemics "due to a growing population of immunologically susceptible individuals of increasingly older ages."[82] This, and the fact that middle-class women had begun to breastfeed for shorter periods of time, made children more vulnerable to what would be dubbed a "middle class plague."[83]

As a consequence of these social and immunological factors, polio appeared to increase in virulence over time, with serious outbreaks erupting in Europe beginning in the 1880s. The first major North American epidemic occurred in Vermont in 1894, followed by more widespread epidemics throughout the Northeast and Midwest. In each wave, poliomyelitis seemed to return with increasing severity, attaining "pan-global status" by 1910, the year it became a reportable disease in Ontario.[84] As MacMurchy put it, that year was, "in a terrible sense, a 'wonder year' for epidemic poliomyelitis" in Canada and globally.[85] Reports of medical officers of health and provincial authorities showed a succession of Canadian outbreaks through the 1910s, including in British Columbia (1912); Ontario (1913, 1914, and 1916); Quebec (1914); and Nova Scotia (1915).[86] In 1916, New York City was struck by "one of the largest and most intense outbreaks of the disease ever globally recorded," which involved over 23,000 documented cases. As a result, polio had come of age as a major public health problem.[87]

Placed in the context of interwar period, one can understand the anxiety of parents and medical professionals. The First World War had taken a terrible toll on families and communities, claiming the lives of some 50,000 Canadian troops and support staff. As medical historians have also demonstrated, however, another 50,000 Canadians perished of influenza in the twelve months following demobilization because infected soldiers and medical personnel returned to their hometowns and unwittingly brought diseases and further heartbreak with them.[88] Like the Spanish flu of 1918, polio was a disease without any known effective medical response. As it began to gain traction in its outbreaks in 1916, 1922, and 1929, politicians and the medical elite scrambled to understand the origins of the disease and respond in a timely manner. Their job was not easy, considering the mild and ambiguous early symptoms. Indeed, only the onset of paralysis itself, or the results of a painful and intrusive spinal tap, could confirm diagnosis. Thus, while statistically fewer individuals were stricken or killed by polio than by other infectious diseases of the early twentieth century, polio's highly visible and long-lasting effects, tendency to strike healthy middle-class kids, and unknown etiology maximized the panic it raised among the public.[89]

The first interwar epidemics took place in Alberta, Manitoba, Saskatchewan, and Ontario between 1927 and 1928, shadowed by Ontario's first serious epidemic in 1929, which was followed by an even more serious outbreak in 1930. Outbreaks flowed from west to east, arising in the summer months and often peaking in September. The medical reaction combined traditional public health responses with the new medical science of the 1920s and 1930s. With the experience of the Spanish flu epidemic of 1918 in the minds of political and public health officials, provincial and municipal governments imposed controversial health measures, including isolation, quarantine, travel restrictions, and school closures. However, with the success of the diphtheria toxin during the first two decades of the twentieth century, it was inevitable that medical authorities would turn to the laboratory for a possible "serum" for polio. Polio's infectious nature was shown during a Swedish epidemic in 1905 and confirmed in 1909 by Simon Flexner's laboratory experiments at the Rockefeller Institute for Medical Research in New York. Flexner promoted the theory that the disease entered the body through the nasal passages, while other researchers suggested that it entered via the alimentary tract. Flexner's nasal-neurotropic model, while not universally accepted, dominated prophylaxis until it was disproved in the 1930s, after which the oral-fecal route became gradually more accepted.[90]

During the polio outbreak in 1929, Ontario replicated the strategy used to distribute diphtheria toxoid: funding and coordinating blood collection, preparing (at the Connaught laboratories) and distributing the serum through public health departments, and training physicians to diagnose and administer serum. Potency, dosages, and modes of administration varied, however, and there had been no controlled trials of the serum's efficacy because it was unthinkable to withhold it from active cases. In 1931, controlled trials in New York City failed to prove the serum's efficacy. Doubts over the serum renewed public and professional inquiry into polio's epidemiology, etiology, diagnosis, and provisions for aftercare. By 1932, there were increasing calls for a vaccine and for the provinces to do more for victims. In the mid-1930s, outbreaks in the U.S. incited vaccine research. In 1935, trials of the Brodie and Kolmer vaccines were undertaken in the U.S. The trials were premature, with inadequate controls, lack of oversight, and tragic results. As a result, experimental vaccine research paused for nearly two decades.[91]

The second wave of polio epidemics occurred in several Canadian provinces, including Alberta in 1935, spreading eastward to Ontario in 1937, then to Alberta and Manitoba in 1938, before a reprieve between 1939 and 1940.[92] Toronto had weathered outbreaks in 1929, 1930, and 1934. The 1937 epidemic, however, was shaping up to be unlike the ones before it. In 1937, cases emerged slowly in June, increased towards the end of August, and peaked in the second week of September. In total, Toronto suffered 786 cases, with 40 deaths, as part of a provincial death toll of approximately 100 children and 2,500 cases.[93] Children aged three to six were most vulnerable, followed by

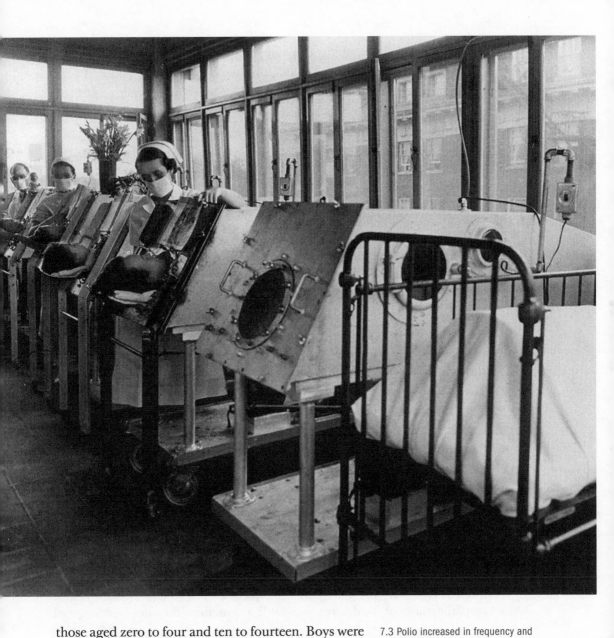

those aged zero to four and ten to fourteen. Boys were slightly more susceptible than girls. The likelihood of fatality increased with the age of patients, although mortality rates varied for different outbreaks.[94]

7.3 Polio increased in frequency and severity in the first half of the twentieth century. During the 1937 epidemic, The Hospital for Sick Children scrambled to construct a new, futuristic apparatus: the iron lung.

As Chris Rutty has demonstrated, the 1937 epidemic catalyzed action in Toronto. Chastened by the public criticism of public health authorities' ineffective responses to previous outbreaks, the province supported new technologies and treatments during 1937, including the now-iconic iron lungs, as well as a pioneering controlled study of the ability of a zinc sulphate nasal spray to prevent polio. The spray acted as a chemical block on the olfactory nerve and had been tested on laboratory monkeys. The spray was based on Flexner's nasal and neurotropic models of polio, according to which the disease entered through the nose and then affected the nervous system. The trial involved 5,000 children and was a coordinated effort between the provincial health department, Toronto's Department of Health, the University of Toronto School of Hygiene, and The Hospital for Sick Children. The study turned out to be an unconditional failure: not only did the spray fail to prevent polio, it permanently damaged the sense of smell of one-quarter of those who received it.[95]

As the 1937 polio epidemic took shape, North American clinicians noticed a higher than usual incidence of "bulbar" cases of polio, ones in which the virus ascended the brain stem and compromised the victim's ability to breathe and swallow. By this time, half of Ontario's 2,500 reported cases were identified as "paralytic;" of these, 80.2 per cent were spinal, and the remainder, 19.8 per cent, were bulbar.[96] In previous decades almost all severe bulbar cases perished. However, with the invention in 1928 of an electric tank respirator by Boston's Philip Drinker, there was at least one, very expensive and visually remarkable, attempt to prolong life. Quite literally, the suffering child was placed in an imposing metal tank, the head alone exposed, which artificially contracted and expanded, respiring for the depleted body. The machine was named the "iron lung." The Hospital for Sick Children obtained a Drinker machine in 1930, which remained the only model in Canada in the early 1930s (see image 7.3).[97]

Since it was clear that new machines would be hard to obtain during the pan-North American outbreak in 1937, the superintendent of the hospital, a civil engineer named Joseph Bower, led the in-house mission to construct more of the devices as quickly as possible. Toronto, London, and Hamilton had machines on order, but it was to take ten to fourteen days for them to arrive. Superintendent Bower determined that The Hospital for Sick Children had to construct their own before those on order arrived; when a four-year-old with chest paralysis was admitted on August 26, "an experimental respirator for premature infants was modified and coupled with a quickly built wooden box in which the little boy was placed and stabilized." His mother appealed to the city's wealthy through the papers, and an anonymous donor provided money for the construction of two additional machines. From August 27, the basement of the hospital was

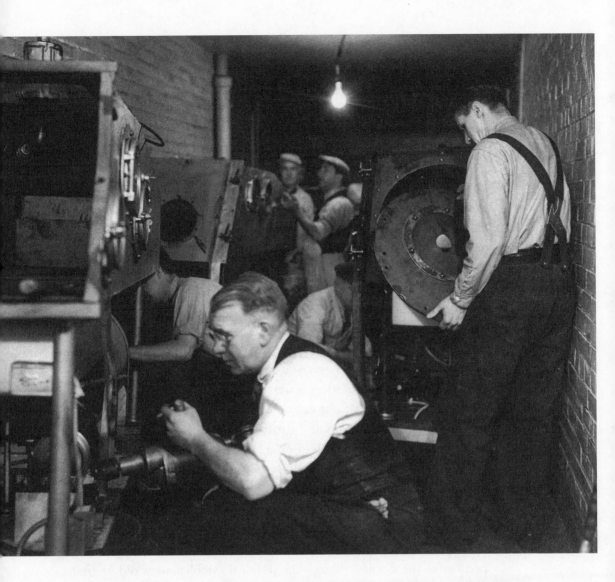

overtaken with the construction of iron lungs. By August 31, the first four lungs had been built, and by the end of the epidemic, skilled technicians had constructed twenty-seven machines.[98] Their much-publicized efforts helped assuage a general public that witnessed over a hundred children die of polio during that summer.

7.4 Workers toiled around the clock in the basement of the hospital during the 1937 polio outbreak. The iron lungs became an iconic aspect of the hospital's history, though there is good reason to believe that, in retrospect, they had relatively little impact on the epidemic.

For the other 2,500 cases of childhood polio in the province of Ontario in 1937, treatment and aftercare was long-lasting, expensive, and potentially ruinous, even for better-off families. As a consequence, the disability of children led to unrelenting pressure for government subsidies. Provinces gradually assumed more responsibility for ensuring access to hospitalization and aftercare services. Before the 1937 outbreak, the provincial response to polio had involved an average annual outlay of only $4,000 for an experimental convalescent serum. By contrast, in 1937, the government spent an extraordinary $197,000 on patient care, including over $150,000 for treatment.[99] The province funded three weeks of free hospitalization, serum, and aftercare. Aftercare consisted of three weeks in the hospital following the acute stage of the illness, which was spent in isolation, the provision of orthopaedic supplies, and free home school instruction for several months. The province also funded some of the iron lungs constructed at the hospital, and standardized specialized splints – "Toronto splints" as they became known – as well as other specialized equipment for all paralysis victims. In September, a 150-bed Ontario Orthopaedic Hospital opened in the former Grace Hospital to function as the centre of hospitalized aftercare. It was supervised by Alan Brown and D.E. Robertson, the chief of surgery. By Christmas 1937, the orthopaedic hospital had treated and released 238 patients.[100]

The response of Ontario was replicated in other provinces and in the United States. In Alberta, for example, the Poliomyelitis Sufferers Act guaranteed free hospitalization and treatment for sufferers.[101] In the United States, long considered the bastion of private medical care, the National Foundation for Infantile Paralysis (NFIP) was created in 1938 to "provid[e] adequate care to all polio victims who needed treatment."[102] Of course, in the United States, the unusual intervention of the federal government in Washington was underpinned by one important fact: the president, Franklin Roosevelt, was himself a polio survivor who suffered lifelong disability because of the disease, though the political establishment did its best to disguise the degree of his disability and suffering during his time in office.[103] By the end of the 1937–8 epidemic, over 750 children in Toronto, and over 2,500 children in the province, had been infected.[104] While the iron lungs generated a great deal of publicity, there was little, in fact, that the medical authorities could do, short of focus on rehabilitation.

Conclusions

By the end of the 1930s, Alan Brown had successfully modernized The Hospital for Sick Children, placing it at the epicentre of welfare in the city of Toronto. His success was greatly aided by the lack of competitors: The

Hospital for Sick Children was the only children's hospital in Toronto for most of the twentieth century, a situation zealously guarded by hospital administrators whenever rumours circulated about the provincial government's intention to establish a second paediatric centre. With Montreal's paediatric community split between the anglophone Children's Memorial Hospital and francophone Sainte-Justine hospital (not to mention further complicated by the presence of Canada's first Shriners hospital for children) Brown had few rivals in the country who could pretend to match the power and influence of Toronto's Hospital for Sick Children. By the time his textbook, *The Normal Child* (1926), was published, the bow tie–wearing "autocrat" was also the pre-eminent Canadian paediatrician of his generation. In the 1935–6 academic year, paediatrics became a full department at the University of Toronto and Brown became the first professor of paediatrics, although he retained the title physician-in-chief at The Hospital for Sick Children.[105] He had promoted the development of paediatrics by entrenching the field in the public health movement and the organizing a professional society, the Canadian Society for the Study of Diseases of Children (later the Canadian Paediatrics Society), which was established in 1922 at a conference at The Hospital for Sick Children itself. McGill's professor of paediatrics, Alexander Blackader, was the first president of the society and Alan Brown was vice-president. Of thirteen founding members, six were from Toronto, five from Montreal, and one each from Ottawa and Hamilton.[106] In 1937, paediatrics was one of nine new specialties recognized by the Royal College of Physicians and Surgeons of Canada, which had previously been limited to internal medicine and general surgery. The first qualifying certificate examinations were held in 1946 by the Royal College of Physicians and Surgeons of Canada.[107]

Brown's Depression-era Hospital for Sick Children reveals multiple dimensions of the nature of hospital care, the growing responsibility of the state, and a new fascination with medical technology. From a strictly therapeutic standpoint the medical responses to the poliomyelitis outbreaks were characterized by the well-meaning pursuit of research and clinical avenues that proved largely ineffective. The technology may have been life-extending, but it could not work miracles. Of the 63 children treated with iron lungs during Ontario's 1937–8 epidemic, 20 months after the end of the epidemic, 40 had perished, only 12 had recovered, and 11 lingered in respirators. In retrospect, one wonders, as Chris Rutty has carefully argued, whether the publicity surrounding the iron lungs became more about reassuring an anxious public that "something, anything"[108] was being done. Ultimately, a vaccine discovered in the 1950s would finally put an end to the terror of polio, rendering it a chapter in the complicated history of medicine and a chronic condition afflicting an adult generation of survivors in the West, while persisting in some developing countries.

The political legacy of polio, however, resulted in important changes. In the depth of the Great Depression, the 1937 polio epidemic and its successors fuelled a growing debate about the role of the state in the organization of hospital care and medical services. Canadians were well aware that, in Britain, a national health insurance system had been introduced in 1911, whereby the state, employers, and employees each contributed to provide basic medical coverage. Universal health insurance would form the framework of the famous Beveridge report (1942) which seeded the National Health Service in post-war Britain.[109] The declaration of hospital care as a provincial jurisdiction in Canada, from Confederation onwards, undermined the creation of a pan-Canadian consensus on the issue. And yet, the financial pressures of the hospital system in Ontario, and elsewhere in the country, proved unsustainable. The older system of public subsidies for "public" (that is, non-paying) patients, and a dwindling number of individuals who were able or willing to pay privately, put the squeeze on hospitals. Such pressures gave rise to a growing chorus demanding comprehensive provincially run hospitalization insurance that would relieve the middle classes.

Of course, there were many groups in society who were deeply suspicious of state-run health insurance, even if it was limited to hospitalization. Yet, paediatric care, in some respects, was the thin end of the wedge. Public health advocates argued effectively that children should be exempted from the moral responsibility of answering for their own ill-health. Children could not be held responsible, even if commentators did not shy away from criticizing their parents. Moreover, immunization programs, school doctors and nurses, and milk depots had legitimized the state, at various levels, as a provider of free medical services. Seen in this light, the public subsidies for hospitalization and aftercare for child polio sufferers merely extended this principle. In 1946, Ontario's worst polio year since 1937, 88.4 per cent of polio cases received provincial hospitalization benefits.[110] Some of the western provinces, Alberta in particular, "developed the most sophisticated and generous polio policies," underwriting free services for prevention, treatment, and hospitalization.[111] As Canadian provinces entered the world of free hospital care for children, a concurrent debate would inevitably emerge over free hospital care for all.

More subtly, there was also a cultural and psychological shift occasioned by the iron lung. As the disappointing results of iron lungs became apparent, and the 1937–8 epidemic subsided, people began to question the psychological impact of immobilizing children for weeks or months at a time. When a new wave of polio epidemics emerged between 1941 and 1946, the hospital responded by becoming more receptive to non-technological interventions. Researchers began to reflect on the emotional state of the children not only as polio victims, but as hospitalized children more generally. Not just diseases, but psychological suffering, came under the microscope.

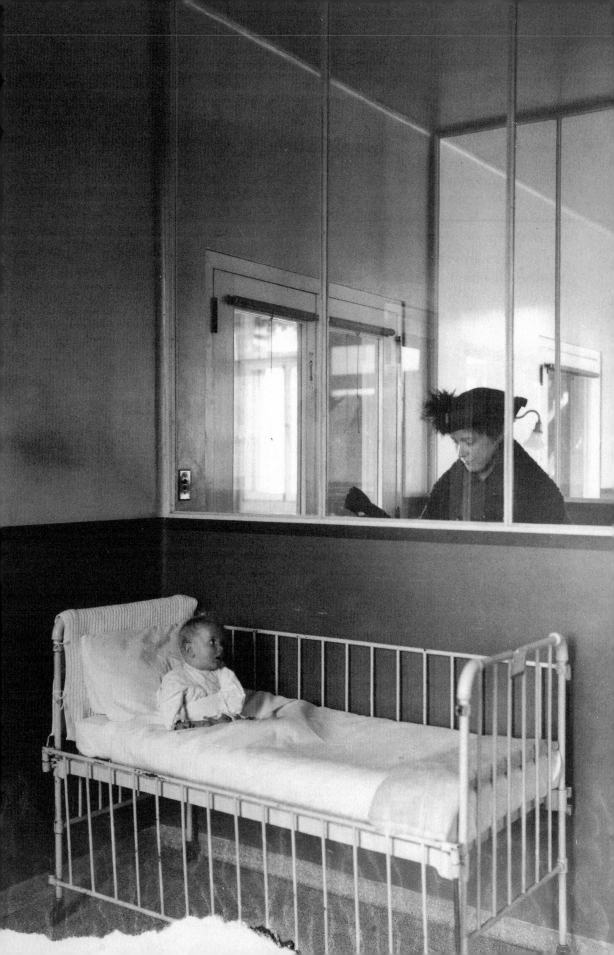

EIGHT

Visiting Hours

> When the doors were finally opened it was like a herd stampeding;
> all the parents hurrying down the halls to have every available min-
> ute with their children.[1]
>
> A mother recollects Sunday visiting hours at
> Thistletown Country Hospital, 1952

During the height of the 1937 polio epidemic, Susannah C. was admitted to The Hospital for Sick Children. The thirteen-year-old appeared to have caught a cold in early September, but within a mere twenty-four hours her four limbs were "completely paralyzed." On the third day of her sickness she was rushed to the hospital with the expectation that she would be placed in an iron lung if one was available. However, she survived the acute stage without the famous apparatus. Instead, after two weeks of hospitalization and monitoring, she was strapped to a Bradford frame, a canvas-and-iron apparatus that, in effect, immobilized her limbs. Over time, the nurses observed that she had become "very depressed and homesick ... demanding to be allowed to go home." Susannah complained that "she knew the doctors had lied to her." They had promised her that she would go home in two weeks and three had already passed. She feared they had also misled her about the reversibility of her paralysis. She was convinced that she would never be able to walk again. After five weeks, however, Susannah was released "a radiantly happy and cheerful girl." Six months later she returned to Toronto for re-examination. She showed marked improvement in all limbs

8.1 As hospitals became preoccupied with isolating diseases, visitors were increasingly seen as dangerous vectors of filth. This photograph from 1916 depicts not only the anxiety of a mother but also, symbolically, the physical separation from her child.

except the left leg. Her chances of being able to walk with the aid of some sort of brace were considered "excellent."[2]

Susannah's story was recounted as a published clinical case study authored by three staff doctors at The Hospital for Sick Children. The article describes in detail the transformation of the patient, the onset of paralysis, the stabilization of her condition with the aid of the Bradford frame (see image 8.2), and then the slow road to recovery. However, the principal purpose of the scholarly contribution was not to recount a dry factual description of what was ultimately a non-fatal case of polio. Rather, the narrative of the girl's hospitalization was really a study of child psychology, an early contribution from the hospital's new Department of Psychological Medicine and a success story for the temporary orthopaedic hospital. The staff writing the article documented Susannah's emotional progression from suspicion, to resignation, to optimism, as she became socialized into the hospital environment with other children who faced similar challenges. The narrative structure detailed her emotional coming-to-terms with her disability, as related by the letters from her mother, who had informed the doctors that Susannah had maintained her "cheerfulness" and "unselfishness" at home. In addition, her mother added, Susannah had been working hard at her studies with the help of one of the teachers from the high school. One of the chief pieces of evidence of her transformation was the fact that she had been responsible for the organization of a troop of Girl Guides among the friends she had originally made at the hospital. Now that Susannah was "optimistic" and "not afraid," the doctors concluded their paper confident that her illness would not leave her with "psychologic and emotional distortions."[3]

The case study of Susannah was authored by Drs. Griffin, Hawke, and Barraclough, three prominent figures in the early history of child and adolescent psychiatry in Canada. Their interest in this case and others like it reflected changing attitudes that were occurring more broadly among paediatric hospitals in the world, but had been dismissed by Alan Brown and other senior staff in the main hospital: namely, a greater openness to studying the effects of prolonged hospitalization on the emotional health of children. And it was not just polio that occupied the attention of these younger medical men interested in psychological medicine; chronic and debilitating tuberculosis and severe burn victims also continued to pose a significant challenge to hospital medical staff and administrators. It was feared that the months of enforced bed rest might damage children mentally. The Department of Psychological Medicine in the hospital was thus part of a growing recognition of the importance of treating children by tending to their *mental,* as well as their physical, health. Indeed, the predominant term in the interwar period for emotional and psychological health was "mental hygiene," implying the conceptual overlap between advances in hygienic practices of the body and those of the mind. As Jean Masten, the head of nursing at the hospital, explained at the time to the journal *Canadian Nurse,*

> One of the chief purposes of the hospitalization period should be to teach these children through educational, recreational and social supervision to face the future with equanimity. They must learn to profit from their long period of idleness by learning healthy mental attitudes as well as useful educational and creative skills. In short, the duty of the hospital should not be only to reduce physical crippling to a minimum, but to prevent the development of any mental crippling.[4]

The new psychological program of The Hospital for Sick Children was central to this psychological rehabilitation of those who were commonly called "crippled children." A neurologist, psychiatrist, and psychiatric social worker directly employed by the institution oversaw the services provided by four occupational therapists and an array of volunteers, including librarians, teachers, artists, and occupational therapy students. The principal strategies were to occupy the interests of the recovering patients with "constructive" activities and to cultivate a "cheerful" and communal atmosphere during long periods of convalescence and rehabilitation. This was done by incorporating a variety of activities, such as music, singing, reading, movies (especially nature and travel films), occupational therapy, and art projects into a carefully scheduled daily routine. As the hospital acknowledged, "the treatment of the mental attitude of the child towards his physical disability is frequently as important as the treatment of the physical disability itself."[5]

A psychiatrist or psychiatric social worker interviewed each child over the age of four upon admission to the temporary orthopaedic hospital to which many disabled patients discharged from The Hospital for Sick Children were sent. The professionals were expected to be frank, yet upbeat, conveying to patients their expected length of stay and realistically discussing their prospects for recovery. Above all, the young patients were encouraged to control their emotions in an environment where they were separated from family and siblings. Unsurprisingly, many children experienced homesickness, which was considered normal. Severe cases, however,

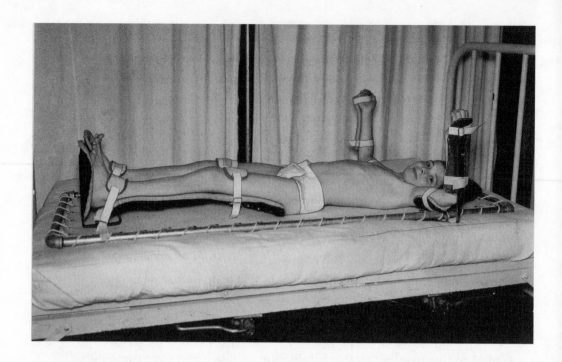

8.2 The after-effects of polio on survivors were significant, including life-long disability. Post-polio patients, as they were called, took months, even years, to recover, with the aid of stabilizing devices, such as the Bradford frame.

were attributed to "an abnormally strong attachment to the mother." Indeed, those who "were emotionally unstable, showing either excessive crying or unusual lability of mood and excitability" were helped "to regain [their] self-control and sense of security" through "reassurance, cheerfulness, and gentle firmness."[6] Ultimately, these social workers and psychiatrists clarified the importance of the ban on parents' and well-wishers' visits. Thus, separating children from their families – a standard three weeks in the temporary orthopaedic hospital – began to be conceived, by some, as a type of psychological imperative. The emotional world of the paediatric patients was being increasingly considered, but it was within the paradigm of reformulating emotions and attitudes within an institutional environment and under medical authority.

Parental Exclusion

The exclusion of family and friends from the hospital environment was a relatively novel phenomenon in the history of medical institutions. For most of the eighteenth and nineteenth centuries, families were encouraged to visit hospitals to provide emotional support and material comforts to kith and kin. Hospital visitors' books of the Georgian and Victorian periods reveal the regular attendance by family members, curious onlookers, benefactors, inspectors, and, of course, medical and nursing students. By the close of the nineteenth century, however, hospitals across the Western world became much more restrictive and formalized in their social regulation and surveillance of non-patients. Medical and nursing students continued to round hospital wards under the watchful eye of senior medical and nursing staff, but by the dawn of the twentieth century, the exclusion of non-medical staff, and family members in particular, was becoming more common. This growing isolation of the hospital was particularly pronounced in the paediatric environment where the rates of infant and child mortality dictated that the regulation of the medical environment was a matter of life and death.[7]

Given the prevalence of infectious diseases circulating in society at the time, the growing conservatism of medical staff and administrators was understandable. As practitioners embraced the so-called germ theory of disease, the ideal hospital environment was a sterile one, isolated from the dirt and disease outside its doors. Photographs from the early twentieth century reflect the culture of the sterile hospital environment. The most extreme exemplar was, as mentioned in an earlier chapter, the new surgical theatres, where complicated rituals emerged involving asepsis and sterilization. These protocols of the surgical theatre became, over time, generalized throughout the hospital environment. Nurses' memoirs and songs commonly referred to the unforgiving standards expected of nurses: "At ten Dr. Brown through the window / Saw six spots of dust on the floor! / She trembled and quaked in a fever / And prayed for deliverance once more!"[8] As doctors and nurses became acculturated to the sterilized environment, there was a creeping sense that the dirt and disease of the outside world needed to be kept at bay, and this could best be achieved by circumscribing the movements of hospital visitors.

The evolution of the infectious ward of the hospital represents an early example of the physical separation of patients and their parents. At the height of the rise in infant mortality in the years leading up to the First World War, the hospital constructed a ward of cubicles, room for twenty-eight acute and twenty-four convalescent patients, separated by glass partitions. Parents were forbidden from entering the rooms containing infectious or vulnerable patients, and thus were required to "talk to their children through the glass"[9] (see image 8.1). As the waves of diphtheria, scarlet fever, measles, typhoid, and, later, influenza swept through Toronto, the need for isolation and quarantine only seemed to grow. The success of Brown and his staff in reducing inpatient mortality in the years immediately after the First World War enhanced the sense that the new controls over parental visitation were working. Thus, if anything, restrictions needed not only to be continued, but to be even more strictly enforced.

Outside of the infectious wards, there was also a growing *psychological* justification for the separation of patients and family members. The presence and departure of parents, in the minds of health-care practitioners, unduly distressed children, disrupted ward routines, and interfered with recovery.[10] Parents, to be blunt, were considered a nuisance; well-meaning, if overzealous, onlookers whose very presence prevented children from adjusting to their medical fate or to their long-term disability. In the hard-hearted reality of psychological theories of the 1920s and 1930s, the isolation of children was believed, by some, to facilitate the needed "mental preparation" and "attitude adjustment" that hospital staff sought to render in their young patients. New researchers in psychological medicine, such as Jack Griffin, feared that anxious, over-attentive parents would spoil a convalescent patient, who might become "a veritable egotistic despot."[11] And the prevailing culture of deference to medical authority – a deference where lack of clinical knowledge was reinforced by social status and, often, by language – facilitated the restriction of visiting.

Some historians have argued that hospital managers of paediatric institutions at the time permitted members of the general public to visit only if they shared the class and cultural background of the institution's professional staff. Genteel visitors played a role in managers' efforts to cultivate an institutional environment that treated patients' "morals and manners" as well as their bodies.[12] At a time when private donations were a substantial source of revenue, wealthy visitors continued to be welcomed as potential sources of future support.[13] As case studies of paediatric hospitals in England have demonstrated, although parents were "effectively excluded" from wards of children's hospitals by the 1930s, private paying families were still permitted entry.[14]

The Hospital for Sick Children in Toronto appears to conform to this general pattern in the Anglo-American world. In the early years, parental visiting at The Hospital for Sick Children was relegated to one or two afternoons per week, usually Wednesdays and Sundays. Only two visitors per patient were permitted, and they were not allowed to stay more than one hour. Some poor mothers were indirectly granted a way around this by volunteering as scrubwomen at one of the homes.[15] The general public, upon whose charity the success of the institution depended, was granted access to the hospital on two other days: Tuesdays and Saturdays.[16] After the construction of the College Street hospital in 1892, the trustees changed visiting hours to 2 to 4 p.m. daily, and ensured that all visitors expecting to be on the wards check in with the charge nurse first who would politely vet and confiscate any treats and foodstuffs destined for patients.[17] In response to worsening infant and child mortality rates in the years leading up to the First World War, visiting hours appear to have been restricted and nearly rescinded entirely. Indeed, by 1921, the hospital trustees even approved staff requests to close the hospital to *all* visitors, as happened periodically during outbreaks of infection.[18] In 1923, acting on the recommendation of Superintendent Kathleen Panton, the Medical Advisory Board reinstated "the old-time system" of Sunday visiting.[19] Through the 1930s and 1940s, public ward visiting was restricted to this one hour on Sundays,[20] though during the inter-war period, parents of semi-private patients "could purchase the right to see their children" for extra visits.[21]

Internal quarantine was a temporary measure imposed during the frequent outbreaks of contagion. Wards were not only closed to parents, but also to other patients. This worsened overcrowding and had deleterious effects on hospital finances because the hospital received no per diem for empty beds in isolated wards. To make matters worse, parents sometimes refused to pay extra fees for children hospitalized due to quarantine. In January 1911, for example, the wards were in and out of quarantine for scarlet fever. By April of that year, a nurse recorded that "scarlet fever – mumps – Diphtheria Chicken pox, whooping cough, Mumps" were present on the wards. On June 25, a further ward was quarantined for measles.[22] By the 1920s the introduction of preventive measures for diphtheria and scarlet fever, made possible by Connaught Labs, reduced the need for quarantine measures.

At The Hospital for Sick Children, as elsewhere, some exceptions to the visitation restrictions were made for critically ill children. In the earliest years, Elizabeth McMaster had set aside a "quiet room" for mothers to be with their dying children in their final hours.[23] In 1909, a nurse recorded that the parents of a terminally ill child were "here all day + with her until the last."[24] Even this compassionate exception was not without a degree of tension among medical staff. One infant ward nurse remembered an incident forty years after the fact: "I recall that in 1949 one of our babies was dying with leukemia. I was in charge and telephoned the parents to come – much to the shock ... of the supervisor."[25] Another young, foreign-trained doctor, who began at the new University Avenue hospital in 1951, recalled that he had to tread very carefully because of the opposition of more senior colleagues to the presence of family members on the wards, even if they were appropriately gowned and masked and regardless of the state of the child.[26] While there were no printed visiting hours for private wards in the 1930s, by 1948 private ward visiting hours were 2:30 to 8 p.m. daily, private and semi-public patients on public wards were permitted daily visits from 2:30 to 4:30 p.m. and 7 to 8 p.m., and public patients were allowed to have visitors only from 2:30 to 3:30 p.m. on Sundays.[27]

The pain of prolonged separation is a salient aspect of the recollections of staff and patients who were associated with the hospital before the Second World War. Journalists covering the Ontario Orthopaedic Hospital, the temporary sister institution in downtown Toronto, dramatized the reunification of mothers and polio victims after weeks or months of hospitalization. Nevertheless, a booklet for parents of polio patients instructed them not to allow their emotions to prompt them to take a child home early, reminding them that they could not "possibly give him the same treatment and care that he gets in the Hospital and you may impede his progress."[28]

The Country Hospital for Sick Children[29]

Long-term patients represented an enduring source of debate among those connected to the hospital. As early as 1882, the Ladies Committee had expressed their wish to have a "Convalescent Hospital somewhere outside the City limits" for year-round use.[30] Likewise, soon after organizing, the Heather Club, a charitable organization involved in fundraising to support the long-term care of tubercular victims, conveyed a desire for a "preventorium" for children, claiming, somewhat sharply, that it was "suicidal to let some of them go back to the homes we take them from."[31] In the 1920s, after the death of John Ross Robertson, Surgeon-in-Chief W.E. Gallie began actively appealing for public support for a permanent country home. Rebuilding the Lakeside Home, which, after all, was only a seasonal retreat, did not appear to be the preferred option. Rather, a branch hospital in the countryside would enable the hospital staff to carry out prolonged rehabilitation.[32]

The perceived need to establish a convalescent branch reflected an era in which disability emerged as a major public health concern. Tens of thousands of Canadian soldiers had been demobilized in 1918 and 1919, and many were suffering from physical and indeed psychological trauma endured during the Great War. Physical disability became an inescapable social reality of the interwar years, one that was entangled with patriotism and reconfigured as a moral challenge to be overcome. Such physical disability spawned a new awareness of the need for prosthetics which affected many hospitals in Toronto. According to the historian Geoffrey Reaume, "By the end of the war, Toronto had become the artificial limb-fitting centre [for Canadian soldiers]."[33] Some of this new medical and social awareness was transferred to the plight of children suffering from a range of permanent physical disabilities, who would, in the parlance of the time, be commonly referred to as "crippled children." Fraternal organizations, like the Rotary, Lions, Kiwanis, and Shriners clubs, all became involved in the cause, leading to the formation of umbrella organizations, such as the Ontario Society for Crippled Children (OSCC) in 1922. The Ontario society coordinated a range of services, including liaising with individual families and transporting children between different types of medical institutions. After an informal census of disability in the city revealed over a thousand "handicapped" children in Toronto, the city opened two "crippled classes" in Wellesley Street Public School in 1926. Orthopaedic specialists at the hospital would assess children for their suitability for admission to these classes. In addition, "it was these same surgeons who prescribed the number of hours of schooling, physiotherapy, and occupational therapy each child could receive per day."[34]

For three decades after its opening in 1883, the Lakeside Home had operated as a summertime convalescent facility for patients with a range of conditions, but with a high proportion who suffered from tuberculosis and chronic asthma. The belief in the healing power of fresh air and heliotherapy (sunshine and UV light), particularly for non-pulmonary tuberculosis, increased during the interwar period. Surgeon-in-Chief W.E. Gallie argued that a country convalescent hospital could provide fresh air and heliotherapy *year-round*. In addition to the self-evident therapeutic effects of the country surroundings, there were practical considerations: a country branch would provide convalescent care on a more economical basis and ease ever-worsening overcrowding in the principal hospital. Internal documents from the early 1920s predicated that a convalescent facility in the country would free up as many as 100 beds for more "active" cases.[35] Accordingly,

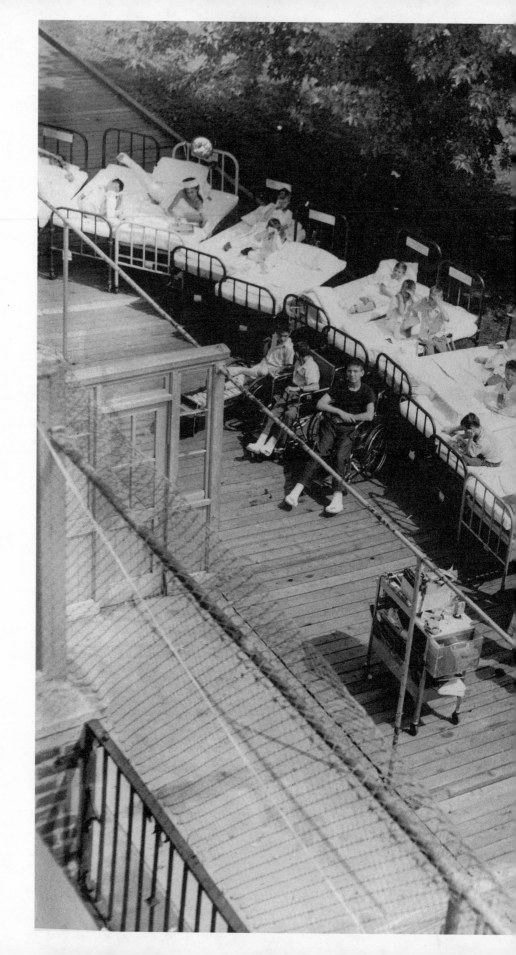

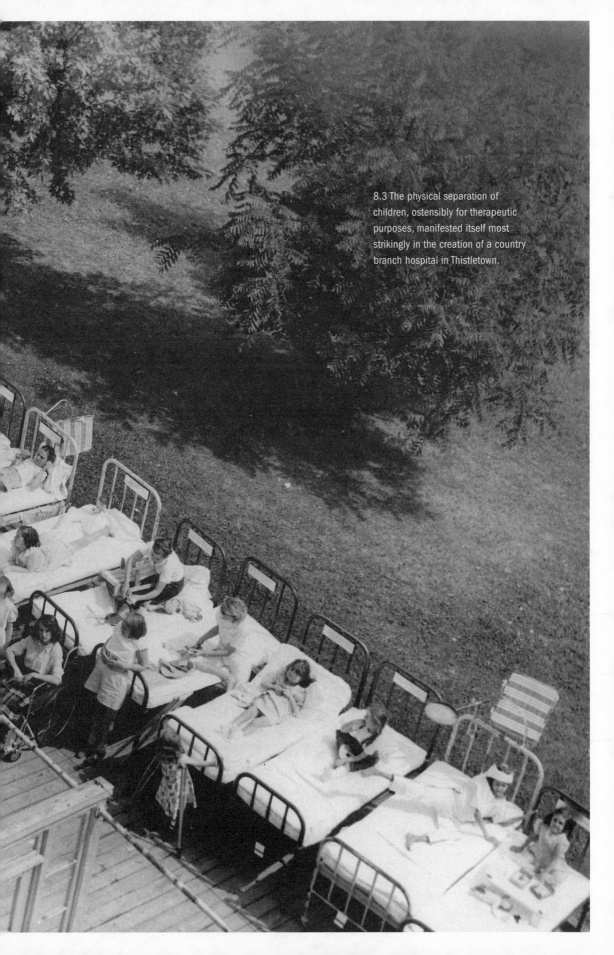

8.3 The physical separation of children, ostensibly for therapeutic purposes, manifested itself most strikingly in the creation of a country branch hospital in Thistletown.

in 1923, Gallie and Chairman H.H. Williams visited three convalescent homes in Boston and New York. In June 1925, confident that they would receive municipal and provincial funding, several trustees were authorized "to negotiate for the purchase of a suitable site" and hire architects to design the new branch institution.[36] The trustees selected Kingdom Farm along the Humber River in Thistletown (in Etobicoke), about thirteen miles northwest of the existing College Street hospital. The property was chosen for the quality of its physical environment. Echoing Victorian preoccupations with getting sick children away from the degrading effects of industrial urban environments, the trustees boasted that, "The ground is high, rolling and fairly well wooded, and from the point where the buildings are to be erected it commands a wide view in every direction."[37]

The fundraising campaign began in early 1926, with the establishment of an appeal committee and an initial goal of $625,000. The capital campaign also raised funds for renovating the old hospital and adding fifth-floor pathological labs in the West Wing. Ultimately, the campaign raised a total of $767,000, including two substantial grants of $100,000 each from the province of Ontario and the City of Toronto.[38] Individual communities within Toronto also provided financial support for the new facility, including $1,000 from the "Chinese citizens" of the city. Senior figures of the hospital's administration also supported the new institution, including the hospital's chairman H.H. Williams, who donated a sum of $50,000 for the campaign, and R.A. Laidlaw, who contributed $9,000. Sir Edward and Lady Kemp added a further $10,000. The Eaton Company employees gave $30,000, along with $25,000 from the *Evening Telegram*, and other trustees and major banks contributed several thousand dollars apiece.[39] Ultimately, the campaign fell $100,000 short of the final cost, which had, like many capital projects, exceeded its original estimate. The trustees withdrew the remaining amount from the hospital's investment funds, enabling the branch to open debt-free.[40] The fundraising campaign was, no doubt, assisted by good timing, since the call for support occurred during the prosperous years of the mid-1920s. And yet, even with the onset of the Depression, Superintendent Bower led a successful initiative to endow cots at Thistletown. It cost a mere $5,000 to endow a cot in perpetuity, $1,000 to name a cot in perpetuity, and $50 to name a cot for a year. These endowments were pegged at half the cost of endowments for the College Street hospital. Despite the hard financial times brought on by the collapse of the North American stock markets only two years earlier, in 1931 Shriners from the Ramses Temple of the Mystic Shrine gave $25,000 to name in perpetuity eleven cots at Thistle-town and a further seven at College Street.[41]

Construction for this "superlatively necessary" country branch began in 1927.[42] The cornerstone was laid by the premier of the province, G. Howard Ferguson, in July.[43] Work at Thistletown ran several weeks behind schedule, and was held up by strikes by workers in the building trades.[44] Ultimately, the facility was fully completed in the fall of 1928. At that time about forty patients returning from the soon-to-be-abandoned Lakeside Home on the Toronto Islands were transferred directly to Thistletown.[45] Members of the Toronto Academy of Medicine visited the "branch hospital,"[46] as it was sometimes called, shortly before the opening ceremony on 24 October 1928 to give their blessing. The Honourable Reverend H.J. Cody, chairman of the board of governors of the University of Toronto, spoke to 500 attendees at the formal opening about the progress of medicine and surgery and the power of open-air treatment. "The discovery of the curative powers of the direct rays of the sun," he opined, "are to be utilized to their fullest extent in the new Country Hospital for Sick Children."[47] Justifying the now geo-graphical separation of the children from their home environments, he inveighed: "Many of those children had known in their homes poverty and sickness, and even harshness and cruelty," but now, "[a]t the Hospital for Sick Children they were given strength to overcome the noxious environment from which they came."[48]

The Country Branch of The Hospital for Sick Children was considerably less ostentatious than the "French chateau"[49] that was the College Street edifice, even if the latter was now showing its age. Thistletown boasted an unadorned principal building, a garage, and a power plant, situated on about 100 acres. The central red-brick building with stone facings, designed in a Georgian style, could accommodate 112 patients in small wards containing eight to ten beds, all of which faced south and opened onto verandas in order to maximize natural light. The primary wing was constructed to allow for two further additions of 100 beds each, bringing the potential bed capac-ity to over 300. In this simple design, a surgical wing with sixty-four beds occupied the ground floor and the forty-eight-bed medical wing the second floor. The building also contained playrooms and a schoolroom. Gallie was effusive as to the potential of the site, and proclaimed the facility "a triumph of science" that "combined efficiency, with a minimum of cost."[50]

At Thistletown, the unassuming architecture of the building contrasted with the attention given to the facility's surrounding environment. The entrance to the hospital was carefully considered and designed.[51] The secretary-treasurer, J. Stuart Crawford, recalled that the road was modified to veer to the left and follow a natural ravine to the highest level, at which point the road swung gracefully around the west side of the building to the north entrance and then to the power plant. "This resulted in a longer and more costly road," he admitted, "but I think everyone who knows the Thistletown Hospital is agreed that the arrangement added much to the beauty of the grounds, particularly when the tree and shrub plantings reached maturity."[52] In order to enhance the rustic locus of rehabilitation, 50,000 saplings were planted before the opening ceremony.[53] After several years, and several thousands of dollars, the landscaping was completed, giving the property a "parklike appearance."[54] The physical environment was intentionally constructed to encourage rehabilitation and ease the long lament of isolation. Such a soothing rustic environment was not lost on nurse Kathleen Symes, who attempted to summarize the co-mingling of suffering and solace by waxing almost poetically that Thistletown "was both a wonderful and horrendous place to have been – a garden planted with lilacs from around the world – the river passing through."[55]

Hazel Elliot, then the night supervisor at 67 College Street, was appointed Supervisor of Thistletown, a position she held for twenty-one years.[56] Once it reached full capacity, the facility was staffed by Elliot, her assistant, a new night supervisor, an assistant night supervisor, five graduate nurses, four ward helpers, two nursery nurses, twelve well-baby nurses-in-training, fourteen maids, five orderlies, three engineers, four laundry workers, two kitchen workers, a chef, and a night watchman.[57] Since they were unable to find specialized "convalescent nurses" in Canada, the trustees hired the hospital's own nursing graduates.[58] A resident house surgeon was in attendance, while one surgical staff member at the downtown hospital visited each patient weekly, and the entire medical staff conducted rounds monthly.[59] All interns spent four weeks of their year-long internship at the country institution. There was always one intern in residence, accompanied by a full-time occupational therapist, and a public school teacher.[60] All provisions were brought from the city hospital, and the Farmers' Dairy Company delivered pasteurized milk on a daily basis.[61]

Although the Thistletown property would slowly become engulfed by the ever-expanding borders of the city after the Second World War, in the 1930s it was very much an isolated location in the countryside. Indeed, it was so far away that the hospital administration was initially concerned that

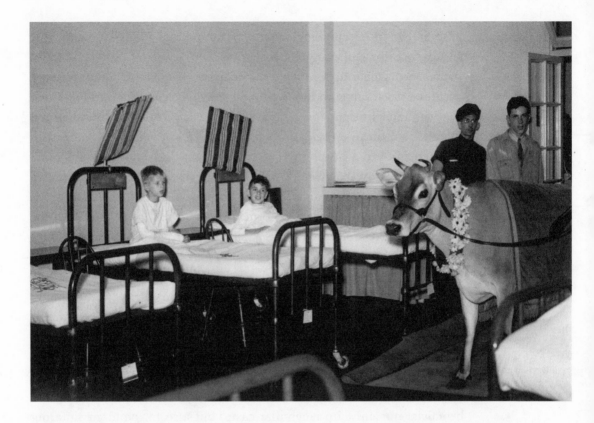

medical staff would voice their discontent with the duration of travel. As a consequence, they arranged for bus service to the city streetcars and then eventually directly between the two hospitals. The trustees also tried to smooth over any possible grumbling by arranging memberships at the Thistletown Golf and Country Club for interns and nurses. They need not have worried. Once at the country hospital, the staff availed themselves of tennis courts, square dancing, bridge parties, afternoon tea in the lounge, and a swimming pool. Service clubs and philanthropic groups regularly provided entertainment for patients and supplied Christmas presents, a pony, puppies, and Saturday afternoon movies. As a site for convalescent children, Thistletown also became a regular locus for contemporary entertainers on tour such as Roy Rogers and Trigger, as well as Elsie the Cow, the world's most famous Jersey.[62]

8.4 Through its three-decade existence, Thistletown was visited by many notable celebrities, including movie stars, politicians, and royalty. Here, Elsie the Cow, the "world's most famous Jersey," pays a visit.

Entertainment provided occasional diversions from the very real suffering of the children transferred to the hospital. Among the first to be moved were tubercular patients with curvature of the spine, tuberculosis of the hip, and osteomyelitis.[63] Nurses led the daily routine of care, which consisted of several hours of schooling, heliotherapy on the verandas, physiotherapy, and occupational therapy.[64] Because of the worsening polio epidemics, polio patients made up a growing percentage of residents. Children received occupational therapy to aid their adjustment to institutionalization and cultivate their independence.[65] On Saturdays, a Protestant minister and (notably) a Roman Catholic priest conducted Sunday schools. For leisure, children enjoyed a wading pool, television sets, a library, a pony and a donkey, walks on the grounds, tobogganing and sleighing, and birthday parties. H. Willenegger organized the Robert Louis Stevenson Boy Scout Troop in July 1930. The scouts formed two patrols: the "beavers" of the medical ward competed with the "stags" of the surgical ward. They held field days and weekly scouts and girl guides programming.[66] Service clubs organized holiday celebrations and more elaborate trips to the annual Canadian National Exhibition and to Maple Leaf Gardens.[67]

Since the late nineteenth century, physicians had identified heliotherapy as a uniquely effective treatment for tuberculosis and other chronic conditions. As discussed earlier in the book, uv ray lamps, or sun lamps as they were sometimes called, were used to supplement natural sunshine. "[P]rolonged rest under ideal conditions of environment" was identified as beneficial not only for tubercular cases, but also for children suffering from rheumatic heart conditions and chronic pulmonary diseases.[68] Convalescence at Thistletown, combined with a carefully controlled diet, was acknowledged to be especially beneficial for coeliac cases, particularly those from homes affected by "poor social conditions."[69] In addition to the therapeutic environment, the hospital emphasized the psychological benefits of institutionalization: "At home these kiddies probably would become cripples, but at the Thistletown annex they are brought into a community where victims are taught to help themselves."[70]

The increasing costs of hospital care and the shrinking length of hospital stays spurred interest in paediatric and adult convalescent institutions in the interwar period. At this time, Thistletown was the country's "largest and best equipped civilian unit" for convalescence.[71] The secretary of the Canadian Medical Association's Department of Hospital Services, Dr. Harvey Agnew, promoted the establishment of convalescent hospitals for all patients "who cannot afford to go away to private health resorts or who cannot enjoy a restful convalescence under ideal conditions at home or among friends." At this time, Toronto also had the Hillcrest Convalescent Home, with thirty-one beds for women.[72] Upon the opening of Thistletown,

Toronto's long-standing medical officer of health, Dr. Charles Hastings, proposed the creation of a public convalescent institution for adults that could be used by the city's hospitals.[73]

Of course, the prioritization of *convalescence* and rehabilitation was a double-edged sword. As previous chapters have illustrated, the province's provision of per diem grants for children was contingent upon residents receiving "active" medical care. In seeming contradiction to many of the publications emphasizing convalescence at a new institution, the secretary-treasurer of the hospital, J. Stuart Crawford, insisted that the Thistletown branch should be considered no more than "another ward of the main Hospital," reminding the public that "[p]atients were transferred daily by bus to the main Hospital for surgery, X-Ray and other services."[74] In 1936, the province, no doubt in response to the difficult fiscal times of the Depression, considered reclassifying Thistletown as a non-acute medical facility with lower provincial per diem subsidies. City, county, and provincial inspectors spent two days visiting the institution and reviewing the records of patients whose treatment was publically funded, people they referred to as "municipal indigents." They concluded that no cases were held beyond the necessary active treatment period, so the facility retained its status as an "active" treatment institution for the purposes of public funding.[75]

The ambiguity of the status of patients at Thistletown spoke to the nature of their treatment and rehabilitation. For the three decades that Thistletown was associated with The Hospital for Sick Children, it was intended to care for the child "who does not require hospitalization with acutely ill children" but who is, by contrast, "not yet ready to return home," a vague description that encompassed both medical and social considerations. Children were transferred directly from 67 College Street when their medical status warranted, freeing up beds for new cases at a time when the main hospital was overflowing.[76] Statistics suggest that the demand clearly existed. During the early years, Thistletown was usually close to maximum occupancy. In 1930, for example, there were 36,876 patient days at Thistletown, with an average patient population of 101.[77] That year, the chief of surgery stated that "On many occasions during the past year, this Branch has been full, and the need for additional space there is practically existing right now."[78] In 1932, there was estimated to be an average of 105 patients. As the facility was overfilled, rooms were temporarily repurposed.[79] Just four years after its opening, the trustees were considering adding a second unit with 100 beds.[80] In 1932, Superintendent Bower reminded the public of the ongoing medical needs of these patients and the short length of stay of many admissions, while also acknowledging that many surgical patients remained for dozens of months. He produced a table (see table 8.1), which gives some sense of the longer-stay children and the conditions from which they suffered.[81]

Table 8.1 Thistletown patients' surgical conditions and approximate length of stay

Type of surgical condition and number of patients now resident		Approximate length of stay
T.B. joints	27	Usually at least a year, up to 2, 3, and sometimes 4 years
Osteomyelitis	17	[ditto]
Congenital dislocation	5	As a rule several months
Stills disease	1	Several months to a year or more.
Poliomyelitis	3	Time variable
T.B. adenitis	2	[ditto]
Patients suffering from Diseases other than those of a chronic nature, but recovering from recent surgical operations.	12	Two or three weeks or more.

Source: Superintendent Bower to Dr. J.L. McDonald, memo, 26 October 1932, Thistletown Subject File, The Hospital for Sick Children Archives.

Parents Personal Service

Despite the long distance from the city, visiting hours at Thistletown were no more generous than those in place at the main hospital, with visits being restricted to 2 to 4 p.m. on Sundays, even during holidays. Only two adults per child were permitted to visit at any one time, with the patient being required to remain in bed during the visits. The emotional intensity of the brief period of regulated visiting was vivid in the memories of those who worked at Thistletown. On the regular wards on Sunday afternoons, "The elevator doors would open, the parents would come pounding down the corridor and the children would all burst into tears."[82] One infant ward nurse who first started working during the 1950s remembered the "terrible situation" that took place during the abbreviated visiting hours at the hospital.[83] Another recalled that "nurses hated working on Sundays. Oh, it was awful. Children pleading and crying on one side, parents weeping on the other."[84]

In a booklet for parents of polio patients sent to Thistletown for convalescence, one physician reassured parents that their absence, and the absence of able-bodied siblings, were ultimately beneficial to their recovering children: "In many ways, it is easier for them to be where they are surrounded by other children in the same situation. They can compare with them and be of help by encouraging those who are more handicapped."[85] One can infer from the documents, however, that the relatives were not always convinced. Hospital publications urged parents to resist the temptation to ask to take their children home early from either hospital against the physician's advice. As nurse Alice Boxill later wrote, Superintendent Bower

> was horrified to discover than many patients were being removed from hospital before the doctor considered the child well enough to leave hospital care. He was determined to try and seek the reason for parents' attitude. He discovered parents were anxious and believed all dreadful tales from all and sundry about the way we treated the children. They could not afford transportation costs or telephone calls and so imagination scared them into a determined decision to take the child "out of that place."[86]

Bower's annual reports mention the fear and apprehension that many parents had about hospitalization. This situation was undoubtedly exacerbated by language barriers and different cultural practices and expectations of Toronto's growing immigrant communities that differed from the expectations of the British and Anglo-Canadian doctors. The hospital also acknowledged the financial hardship that hospitalization could impose, particularly for polio cases, since the province did not cover hospitalization fees for readmissions, surgery, or new braces. While consent was necessary for surgical operations, some parents refused to grant it. In 1930, the Medical Advisory Board passed a resolution that parents who "persisted" in refusing to consent in writing to "any surgical operation which may be found necessary by the attending surgeon ... be asked not to leave the child in the hospital."[87]

In 1930, Bower addressed the problem of premature discharge by further restricting the times during which parents were permitted to remove their children. He found that most cases took place on Saturday afternoon, Sunday, and after 5 p.m. on weekdays, when he and the secretary-treasurer were not on site. New rules, as a consequence, forbade the removal of patients at night and on Sundays. While it was claimed that the intention was "not to deny [parents] the privilege of removal, but to give the superintendent an opportunity to interview these people in the hope that their troubles, whether imaginary or real, may be smoothed out," the restrictions must have imposed a significant obstacle to parents.[88] Of course, seen from another perspective, the removal of a child was one of the few ways that caregivers could exercise agency in a setting in which they may have perceived their parental rights as being suspended.[89] In other cases, it might be in response to a lack of information about the ultimate course of treatment. One woman whose son was hospitalized for five months after contracting bulbar polio in 1948 remembers that "No one could give us any idea as to how long he would be there or what the extent of the recovery of his muscles would be."[90]

The tensions over the rights of parents to remove children against medical advice gave rise to a larger institutional discussion about the relationship of the hospital to the families affected. At the very time that some medical staff were imposing indirect barriers to what they considered the premature discharge of their patients, the Medical Advisory Board adopted a slightly more liberal parental visitation policy for post-operative cases.[91] In addition, the hospital introduced a new program, the Parents Personal Service, in July 1930. Convinced that many parents decided to remove their children from the hospital because of an unfounded fear about the treatment of their children in an isolated hospital environment, the service was an attempt to improve relations between the hospital and parents and "to engender a happier feeling in connection with the word Hospital, and to lessen the fear the word usually conjures up."[92] Bower envisioned the service as a way to follow up not only with parents who withdrew their children, but with those parents he referred to as "the complaining type" – those who were generally dissatisfied, settled their accounts, and "[left] the Hospital in a complaining frame of mind, without registering anything of a definite character." He proposed that nurses, who were already aware of the situation and could identify dissatisfied parents, were best qualified to follow up with the families of discharged patients.[93]

A registered nurse, Patricia Hughes, directed the Parents Personal Service and became the conduit through which parents gained information about their children's conditions, activities, and emotional states. It was her duty "to impress upon the parents the desire of the Hospital to do everything in its power to give the best service possible."[94] She decided which families would be included in the service, prioritizing those who lived far away, but also those who were unduly anxious or whose children were in critical condition. She interviewed parents, personally visited each child in the service, and then wrote letters describing the progress of the child, including the child's remarks, occupations, outfits, and hairstyle.[95] After one year, the service claimed credit for halving the number of children removed by their parents against their physician's advice:

> If the parent is taking the child home against the advice of the doctor, owing to some fancied wrong – not being allowed to visit at any hour, etc., or in many cases, due to lack of funds – this Service is immediately notified, and everything done to satisfactorily adjust matters. Failing that – the majority of foreign [sic] parents are exceedingly nervous and apprehensive – a special effort is made to visit this home within a few days, and usually by then the parents have calmed down and are anxious for Hospital help again.[96]

Although the Parents Personal Service may well be interpreted as a defensive reaction of the hospital to families voting with their feet, it also suggests a more subtle iterative process, through which changing social and cultural views of the relationship between families and their children were being fed back to the medical institution's hierarchy. The 1930s and 1940s were, after all, an era in which new ideas of childhood development were blossoming in North American society. Psychological research amplified concern about the effects of separating parents from children. Researchers in the United States and Britain demonstrated that separation from loved ones harmed children emotionally. They introduced new psychological concepts, such as "hospitalism," "maternal deprivation," and "separation anxiety" which began to enter the lay lexicon.[97] Studies seemed to indicate that visitation and emotional connection were necessary for healthy development. These family experts advocated for the benefits of organized play and daily visitation for hospitalized children. Reformers "promoted the idea of close involvement of the mother in the child's hospital care and the use of play as a therapeutic tool."[98] British reformer James Robertson's 1952 film *A Two-Year-Old Goes to Hospital* compellingly argued that mothers should be admitted with children under the age of five.[99]

The historian Judith Young argues that Toronto's Hospital for Sick Children was especially slow to relax visitation policies.[100] She attributes the reluctance to embrace these newer ideas to the influence of older child rearing theories, espoused notably by Alan Brown himself, that upheld physician authority, discouraged excessive handling of babies, asserted the necessity of independence from mothers, and insisted upon strict feeding, sleeping, and care schedules.[101] Brown, who by the 1940s was entering the twilight of his career, promoted such beliefs in various publications. He insisted that "[t]he environment of the child must be guided by the physician" and that "[h]e [the physician] must give advice concerning the details of early training in obedience, habit formation, temper tantrums, etc."[102] However, it may be that there was a widespread "'theory-practice gap'" during the 1930s and 1940s between hospital visitation policies and new understandings of "the child's need for social interaction and emotional care."[103] A survey of British paediatric hospitals in the early 1950s indicated that less than one-quarter of hospitals permitted daily visiting.[104] Seen in this light, Toronto's Hospital for Sick Children may have been quite representative in terms of the tension between traditional medical authority and a newer family-friendly model of institutional care.

Conclusions

Thistletown embodied many important trends, and indeed contradictions, of early twentieth-century medicine. It reflected a persistent faith in the "nature cure" and a belief in the restorative power of an idyllic retreat from industrial society, particularly for children from working-class families. Media coverage over the decades invariably presented Thistletown as a sort of wonderland for kids. Yet, in many ways, the importance of the country branch faded as quickly as it rose. By the late 1940s, the occupancy at Thistletown declined rapidly as the introduction of province-wide milk pasteurization, sulphanilamides, and penicillin reduced the incidence and impact of pneumonia, empyema, osteomyelitis, and tuberculosis. Ultimately, the vaccine for polio, the great disabler of the early twentieth century, would obviate the need for such a facility. By the mid-1950s, in the wake of the emerging "drug revolution," the country branch held an average of only forty patients. In 1957, the final year of its existence as a branch hospital, the patient population had dropped to eighteen. A 1956 article in the *Toronto Daily Star* referred, somewhat misleadingly, to the "polio hospital" that was now largely "empty" and repeated rumours from city hall that it might be converted to an old age home.[105]

With the opening of the new principal hospital on University Avenue in 1951, the trustees began to consider the future of Thistletown.[106] The board considered closing the branch, but in November 1951 invested $30,000 in necessary repairs and updates.[107] The medical policy committee reviewed the operations of the branch, and determined that it should remain in use and under review for several more years.[108] Ultimately, however, the trustees agreed to sell the facility and use the proceeds to expand the new hospital in the city.[109] In 1957, the province purchased Thistletown for $1,260,000 and repurposed it as a research and treatment facility for a newly identified group in need of specialist services: emotionally disturbed children.[110] From the standpoint of the provincial government, this was consistent with an expanding menu of segregated residential institutions for the developmentally disabled that included huge projects for massive institutions for those then called "the mentally retarded" in rural locations outside of Smiths Falls, Woodstock, and Blenheim. Another former tuberculosis sanatorium, on the outskirts of London, Ontario, was also repurposed as a residential and research institution for "retarded" and autistic children. Thistletown officially "closed" on 31 March 1957.

Following Alan Brown's retirement, the hospital began to slowly liberalize its policy on visiting. Public ward visiting hours were increased to twice weekly by 1955 and then to two hours daily in 1961.[111] During the summer of 1966, visiting hours were extended from 2:30 to 6:30 p.m. to 11 a.m. to 8 p.m. daily.[112] Beyond expanding visiting hours, new services were implemented to support parents of patients. A women's auxiliary unit, begun by Dr. Helen Reid Chute in 1950, liaised with parents of hospitalized children, particularly those in surgery. In 1965, the Parents Personal Service was succeeded by the Parents' Post-Operative Information Centre (also known as the Parents' Post-Operative Service), a service in the main lobby organized by the Women's Auxiliary for parents whose children underwent operations.[113] Although medical paternalism had not perished completely, a new generation of leaders reflected the changing attitude towards the hospitalized child. The physical surroundings of the new postwar hospital framed these relationships in a new era increasingly preoccupied with the psychological state of children. It would be an era dominated by an unprecedented wave of young children — one that, ultimately, became known as the baby boom.

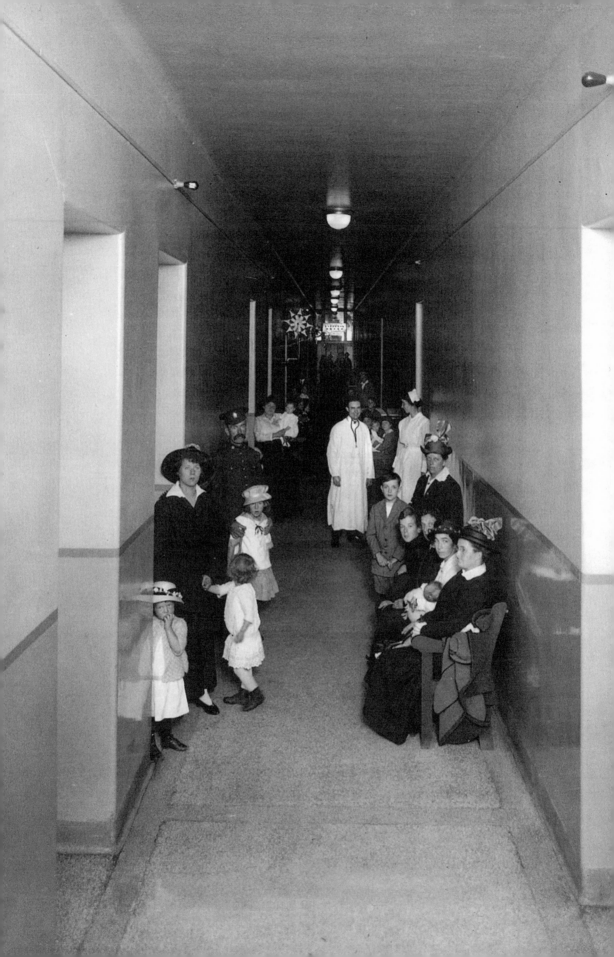

NINE

The Rabbit-Warren

Those who haven't seen the hospital are apt to visualize a gleaming modern building with wide corridors and spacious wards.

Nothing could be further from the truth. The hospital is an ancient mass of discolored brick and stone squeezed into a narrow space on Toronto's busy College Street.

Its corridors are crowded with patients, nurses, laundry trucks and workmen trying to keep the ancient pile together. Surgeons scrub up in a corridor outside the operating rooms. Passageways are crowded with filing cabinets in violation of fire laws.

Doctors across the country wouldn't think of sending patients there except that the hospital, despite all its handicaps, provides the most skilled care to be found in the Dominion. The building is a rabbit-warren[.][1]

"A Worthy Cause," *Rouyn Noranda Press* PQ, 1949

A Pot of Discontent

It may well have been an ant that finally pushed medical staff over the edge. Not just any ant, mind you, but rather an ant infestation in the hospital that was so far reaching that Dr. Nelles Silverthorne reported to Alan Brown that one was observed "walking across the field of operation at the time an operation was being performed."[2] Brown, in turn, recounted the "menace" of vermin that was infecting the hospital to the hospital board, who must have rolled their eyes at yet another complaint from the medical staff. However, this was no idle lament: within

9.1 The College Street hospital seemed to be overflowing soon after it opened its doors, as depicted here in the 1915 photograph of patients (and mothers) lining the hallway.

a few years, Silverthorne, and the rest of the medical staff who had not been seconded to the war, were in open revolt. In 1944, they authored and signed, a scathing six-page report to the trustees outlining the "disgraceful and insanitary conditions" of the College Street hospital that had been accumulating over the past decade. The internal document pulled no punches. It condemned John Ross Robertson's institutional legacy as "a veritable fire-trap" that was not only "antiquated" but more importantly "dirty and infested with vermin." It was self-evident that public wards were "dangerously overcrowded." To borrow a turn of phrase from the manifesto itself, "the pot of discontent [had] boiled over," and no further appeal to patriotism and sacrifice – the twin themes of the war years – could assuage their frustration.[3]

From time to time internal documents can shed much more light on the quotidian reality of a busy hospital than dozens of well-varnished annual reports. And this 1944 manifesto is full of startling insights into the physicality – even the sounds and smells – of the children's hospital by the time of the Second World War. The picture it painted was grim. The sole elevator was hopelessly inadequate, not altogether sound, and packed with "dirty linen, stretcher cases, parents of private patients, cans of garbage and food for the ward patients."[4] There was an overall lack of toilets, utility rooms, linens, and facilities for sterilization and hand washing. Rats were even spotted on the wards from time to time. In the blood bank, the temperature hovered around 80 to 85 degrees Fahrenheit, and there were no waiting rooms, rest rooms, or even cots for blood donors. The outpatient department, in particular, was steadily worsening. The Secretary-Treasurer of the Hospital, J. Stuart Crawford, recalled later in life, that "[w]ithout exaggeration, there were days when it was difficult to get through the corridor due to the number of parents and children awaiting treatment."[5] One "temperature and weighing room" was used for four different clinics *and* as a space for nursing mothers, dressing tonsillectomy patients, undressing larger children, as well as a waiting room for parents and patients during day operations. Overcrowding exacerbated an already-stressful environment: in the physiotherapy and massage room, it was usual to have "2 parents, 2 physiotherapists, 1 patient screaming and crying while other patients wait outside in hall." The din within was considered almost unbearable.[6] The skin and nose and throat clinics were singled out for particular criticism. Patients there were:

> housed in the confined space of a dark and airless dungeon, where
> cases of scabies and impetigo are packed in like sardines with cases of

sinusitis and otorrhoea. Such conditions justify the accusations repeatedly made by Toronto parents and frequently heard by members of the staff, that a child attending the H.S.C. with one disease returns to its home with one or more new ones.[7]

Just a few days prior, the city health department was so disturbed by the conditions that it humiliated hospital staff by informing them that well-baby clinics were to be removed and relocated to another location. As the Medical Advisory Board ominously warned the trustees, "This is the first real official condemnation the Hospital has received but it is an augury of many more to come."[8]

The hospital had celebrated its fiftieth anniversary by 1942 – if one could conceive of such a situation as a celebration – and was clearly showing the strains of events beyond its control. The first problem was obvious: the building, completed in 1892, was by the war years half a century old, and had not received significant structural upgrades during the Great Depression. Indeed, an ongoing nervous joke among staff concerned the elevators that transported patients between floors. One oral interview participant still remembers, sixty years later, the central elevator and the impression that it was literally falling apart. And then there was the physical size of the building itself. The population of Toronto had exploded in the first three decades of the twentieth century, trebling from 208,000 in 1901 to 631,000 in 1931. Nearly all of this growth occurred within the city proper, which had, reputedly, one of the most densely populated urban centres in North America.[9] The population increased by more than 6 per cent annually from 1901 to 1914, roughly twice the annual rates of comparable American cities, such as New York, Boston, Chicago, and Philadelphia.[10] There were simply too many children to be serviced. In addition, the rate of hospitalization had also increased, with new medical interventions spawning more and more admissions. The introduction of new treatments, such as "continuous intravenous," and the increase in active cases as convalescents were moved to Thistletown exacerbated this situation. Of course, a second children's hospital in the city would have resolved some of these issues. Montreal, for example, had two children's hospitals by this time. In Toronto, however, the hospital hierarchy steadfastly countered such suggestions whenever they emerged. This position – that The Hospital for Sick Children should be the only children's hospital in the city – would prove to be both a blessing and a curse.

The pressures of overcrowding were further compounded by the inevitable exodus of doctors, nurses, and non-medical staff to the war front in the early 1940s. Numerous members of the professional staff had left the hospital for active service, including Drs. W.W. Barraclough, A.L. Chute, H. Doney, F.R. Hassard, J.R. Ross, R.M. Wansbrough, and J.B. Whaley. Indeed, by mid-war, 54 per cent of the full-time medical staff was in the service.[11] The number of nurses who had left for the war was considerably smaller, but the drain on non-medical staff resulted in many nurses performing non-nursing duties. For those they could recruit, conditions for teaching, living, and working in the nurses training school became "so poor," in fact, "that for some time it ha[d] seemed questionable whether it is proper or fair to continue bringing in the type of girl we want for [nursing] students."[12] In addition, the College Street hospital hosted rotations of several hundred affiliated students of twenty Ontario hospitals. Medical staff cringed at what these students might retell to their future colleagues when they returned to their home institutions. And yet an even greater problem was non-medical support staff. In 1942, Chairman R.A. Laidlaw acknowledged the obvious when he affirmed that "our greatest difficulty has been in maintaining an adequate lay staff."[13]

Unsurprisingly, the hospital responded to these war-time exigencies with makeshift solutions: the surgical staff admitted fewer patients and, when possible, delayed non-urgent operations until after the war. The shortage of interns forced the hospital to hire two technicians to do blood counts and urinalysis. Student interns were appointed in the place of graduate interns. The newly formed Parents Personal Service was staffed by a nurse who took on the interns' duty of "preparing reports and other data from the histories and records of the Hospital."[14] Supplementary nursing help on the wards was provided by the nurses' aides of the Civil Defence Scheme, the St John's Ambulance Association, the Red Cross Emergency Nursing Reserve, and married graduates working part-time. Between 1941 and 1943, the training school began a nurses' aides program under the Ontario Civilian Defence Committee to teach basic nursing duties and prepare women for work in emergency situations. Nurse shortages were felt most acutely in the summer months, when high school girls aged sixteen to eighteen were brought in to act as nurses' aides on the wards (serving food, reading to and playing with children), and Superintendent Jean Masten issued a public call for trained nurses to work the wards temporarily.[15]

Early Designs

As early as the late 1920s, the trustees had begun to seriously consider a new hospital building, visiting the new Northfield Hospital near Detroit in the spring of 1926 to gather ideas. In 1928, the board hired Joseph Bower as the hospital's superintendent, in part due to his background as an engineer and experience planning military hospitals during the First World War. In the year before the stock market crash, and on the onset of the Depression, Bower began devising preliminary plans for a new building for Toronto's children's hospital. He and senior physicians visited Boston, New York, Philadelphia, Baltimore, Chicago, and Montreal to observe comparable institutions and also complete preliminary studies for a 500-bed hospital.[16] But the Great Depression put on ice any further serious discussion. In October 1929, the Toronto stock market followed New York's "hurricane of selling." A month later, 10,000 men were out of work.[17] In 1933, the city had an unemployment rate of 30 per cent, which marked it as less severely affected than some other parts of the country. Nevertheless, by the following year, 120,000 people were on relief. By the end of the decade, the city had spent $61.3 million on welfare relief, $10 million during 1935 alone.[18] The surrounding suburbs suffered most, where "the numbers on relief ranged anywhere from 33 to 45 per cent of the population."[19] A Toronto "jungle," or transient camp, was located in the east of the city, just north of the Prince Edward viaduct on the Danforth.[20]

Economic depression and the resultant high unemployment rates had multiple effects on hospitals. Poverty and unemployment drove up attendance at the outpatient department and vastly increased the proportion of indigent patients. As a consequence, hospitals throughout the country incurred increasingly large deficits as rising operating costs outstripped stagnant or declining public ward municipal subsidies. As more and more patients arrived on relief orders, The Hospital for Sick Children accumulated an operating deficit of several hundred thousand dollars and began to rely on endowment and investment funds as collateral to increase borrowing.[21] Repeated wage and salary reductions totalling 12 per cent were imposed on all hospital employees and staff by February 1933.[22] Meanwhile, the province attempted repeatedly to reduce per diem grants by 10–15 per cent in response to their own fiscal challenges.[23] "By 1930," Bower confided in a letter to the chairman, R.A. Laidlaw, notwithstanding the deplorable physical conditions on College Street, "it was apparent, however, that probably many years would pass before sufficient money could be raised for such a project [as the new hospital building]."[24] The board even briefly countenanced the idea of enlarging and repurposing the relatively new Thistletown Hospital as the principal institution, while maintaining a smaller city hospital, but dropped the idea in the face of fierce opposition from the Medical Advisory Board who feared isolating paediatric practice in the backwoods of Etobicoke.[25]

In the meantime, the hospital building and property were exploited to their full potential. In 1930, extensions increased the total bed count to a crowded 420. In an effort to expand vastly inadequate private patient accommodation, and thereby increase revenue, the hospital board purchased the small private Wellesley Street Hospital. When this gambit failed to provide sufficient additional revenues, the property was subsequently rented to the Canadian Mothercraft Society. Ultimately, twenty-one semi-private and private beds were added to the main hospital by converting the western half of the fourth floor. The overflowing ranks of nurses and maids were transferred to properties on College, Hayter, and Grenville Streets and University Avenue.[26] The existing site at 67 College Street was expanded east to include the corner of LaPlante and Hayter, "thus completing ownership of the entire [city] block."[27] After that, the hospital could physically expand no further on the existing site. Improvised responses to the "crowded, dilapidated fire trap" were legion:

> The big centre ward was divided into smaller ones; the tiny east elevator was blocked to make a fire escape …; outpatients' department was turned into a laboratory; research went on in a converted potato cellar. The central supply room from where all surgical supplies are issued was developed from an old light well; this meant numerous rooms which are windowless and airless. A suite of tiny offices for doctors was built into an old chimney. A new wing was built, new extensions were added on roofs. But it wasn't enough.[28]

In 1933, annual outpatient department attendances rose to almost 100,000, with a daily average of over 300 treatments. By 1937, average occupancy was 94 per cent, compared to a provincial general hospital average of 65.5 per cent. Indeed, the children's hospital had the highest average occupancy of any general hospital in the province, as well as a waiting list of twenty to fifty patients daily.[29] That year the hospital housed a daily average of 351 inpatients in addition to 101 at Thistletown.[30] By 1945, there was a waiting list of 200 patients, mostly elective surgical cases.[31]

A Modern(ist) Hospital

As the Great Depression dragged on, internal committees continued to dream of a new hospital, even if members were unsure how and when that new hospital might be realized. Superintendent Bower repeatedly revised plans on designs and potential sites throughout the 1930s and during the war years. Perspective drawings made at this time featured a central tower built around banks of elevators, flanked by two lower wings. The designs suggested the long vertical lines of the art deco style would merge into the more starkly modernist features of the 1940s. The base and tower structure of hospital symbolized twentieth-century urbanism, commerce, and efficiency. Studies recommended that the new hospital needed to incorporate some 200,000 square feet, be situated near the University of Toronto (for the convenience of students, nurses, and staff), be easily accessible by streetcar lines (the primary form of transportation for outpatients), yet also be relatively quiet (intersections and playgrounds were a particular concern), and safe from undesirable nearby developments that might obstruct views and sunlight.[32]

Trustees began to comb the downtown Toronto area for potential sites, a challenge that was complicated by the concurrent expansion of municipal offices into the old Ward district, by the multiple proprietors involved, and by conflicting legal opinions as to whether moving the hospital and selling the old building would threaten the legacy of John Ross Robertson. Over time, four sites were considered, all either contiguous to 67 College Street or within two or three city blocks. Ultimately, the board began to seriously consider a site directly south of Toronto General Hospital on the east side of University Avenue, bounded by Gerrard, Chestnut, and Elm. This footprint, known as Site D, was then composed of small, privately owned lots, except for a large parcel at what was then Centre Avenue and Gerrard owned by Inland Investments Limited. Bower considered it desirable because it lay on, or between, several streetcar lines, saving mothers the hassle and danger of transferring lines with multiple children in tow.[33] The trustees had identified this location as their preferred one by 1937 and in November 1938 they obtained a court ruling permitting them to build a new hospital on a new site without "jeopardizing" revenues from the Robertson estate. Ever cautious, the board was loath to assume the financial obligation of purchasing the property with the uncertainty that the European war brought. As the trustees acknowledged, the outlook for the war at the height of the battle for Britain had been "extremely dark."[34]

At approximately the same time, and seemingly to the surprise of the hospital trustees, most of the same parcel of land was purchased or optioned by the organizing committee for the new Mount Sinai Hospital. The existing Mount Sinai had been a modest Yorkville community facility, but the Toronto Jewish community sought to construct a modern hospital with the stature of its namesake in New York. Campaign leader Ben Sadowski, the president of National Motors, was a prominent philanthropist who dreamed of a new downtown hospital affiliated with the University of Toronto. His organizing committee was purportedly unaware that the trustees of the children's hospital had previously expressed an interest in the same site. Lesley Barsky, the historian of Mount Sinai Hospital, recalls that part of the university site was owned by Sinai board member Samuel Lunenfeld, a real estate and steel magnate who was, incidentally, also a well-known donor to The Hospital for Sick Children. Lunenfeld had acquired parcels of land and offered to donate them to the new Jewish hospital, much to the chagrin of some of the downtown tenants. As Barsky tells,

> Considering that Toronto was still in the midst of a sorry era in which both written and unwritten restrictive covenants existed forbidding the sale of certain property to Jews, it wasn't entirely unexpected when some of the occupants along University Avenue were less than delighted with their proposed new neighbours. Those who were involved at the time say the Toronto General was particularly appalled that a Jewish hospital should establish itself next door, and threw up roadblocks to impede such an eventuality.[35]

As the war effort began to turn in early 1944, the board of The Hospital for Sick Children renewed its effort to obtain a new hospital, initiating a campaign that was originally pegged at $5,000,000. When two members of the Sinai committee approached the hospital to name a cot, the board of The Hospital for Sick Children requested a meeting with the intention of discussing Site D. They ultimately reached an agreement that, if the board of The Hospital for Sick Children could find an equally suitable site for the future Mount Sinai, the trustees of the latter would relinquish the property on the east side of University Avenue.[36]

The negotiations, however, were not just about swapping key properties along the prime downtown real estate of University Avenue in Toronto. Discussions suggest a more subtle and unusual quid pro quo. The board members of Mount Sinai were indeed intent on building a new hospital in the city centre. But more important to them than the actual location was that the hospital be affiliated to the University of Toronto as a teaching hospital. It appears that the board saw The Hospital for Sick Children as a sympathetic ally, one which could be strategically useful in the face of the hostile medical staff at the Toronto General Hospital (who occupied many of the senior medical appointments at the University of Toronto Medical School). Yes, the Jewish community had complained bitterly about the lack of Jewish interns and medical staff at The Hospital for Sick Children and elsewhere in the 1920s and 1930s, but things had begun to change in the 1940s, particularly after the death of the Chief-of-Surgery D.E. Robertson (in 1944),[37] whose anti-Semitic views were too seldom kept to himself.[38]

Barsky suggests that Ben Sadowski agreed to cede the property just south of the Toronto General to the board of The Hospital for Sick Children in return for a commitment of support that the future Mount Sinai would be granted status as a University of Toronto teaching hospital. Furthermore, as the full weight of the Nazi atrocities against the Jews came to more public view by the end of 1945, he suggests that the provincial government in Ontario was eager to put the embarrassing years of the interwar period behind it. As a consequence, certain provincial politicians leaned on senior members of the Toronto General Hospital to relent in their opposition of a future Mount Sinai being affiliated to the university's medical school. Ultimately, the gambit worked. The Hospital for Sick Children acquired their target property, Mount Sinai received a lot across the street, and the new Jewish hospital would became affiliated to the University of Toronto.[39] Quite apart from the fascinating political negotiations, this chapter left a remarkable physical legacy to the city, with three of the largest hospitals in the entire country coexisting literally on adjacent blocks.

The Irreducible Minimum

Having secured a good proportion of the property that would be numbered 555 University Avenue, the Board had initiated the first major funding campaign for the new hospital. Between 1938 and 1939 the trustees had made an abortive attempt to rouse public and government support.[40] But with the German invasion of Poland in September 1939, Britain's declaration of war, and then Canada's, a few days later, it was clear that all available monies would be diverted to the war effort and, in particular, to war bonds.

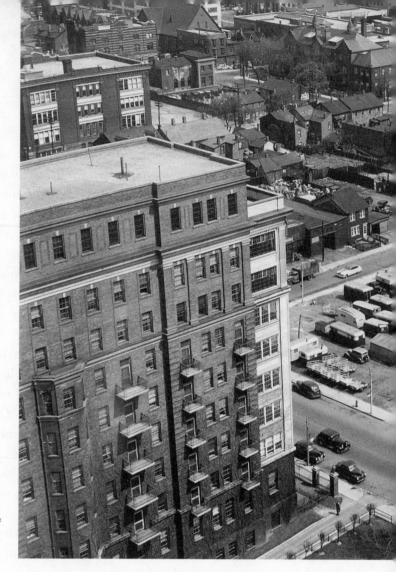

9.2 By 1947, the trustees had identified a location for a new hospital on University Avenue. One problem: it was occupied by a trailer park of families, some of whom were ex-servicemen of the Second World War.

Fundraising was put on hold until after the invasion of Normandy in 1944. Meanwhile, the board strained to successfully woo Norman C. Urquhart to lead the Campaign Executive Committee. The Trustees were adamant in courting Urquhart, who was a mining magnate, former president of the Toronto Stock Exchange, board member of the Royal Bank of Canada, and chairman of the National Executive Council of the Canadian Red Cross. Urquhart was already acting as chairman of the Prisoners of War Parcels Committee of the Red Cross and chair of a Special Mining Commission. After several months of politely declining, he finally relented. Bower stated that he was chosen for his "unusual and outstanding" abilities, qualities, and status in the community, although Urquhart may have been on to something when he asked if he had been chosen for his previous experience as chairman of the hospital's Special Names Committee, through which he

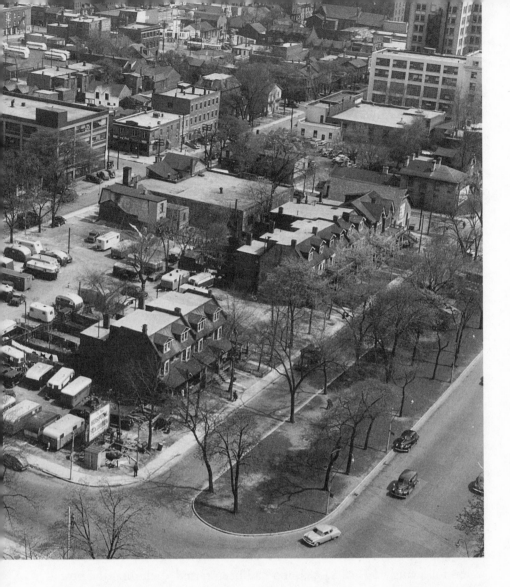

acquired "valuable information as to where the money was and as to who were the most likely prospects for large donations."[41]

The campaign was launched on 18 June 1945, with a revised objective of $6 million. It included several post-war innovations. The principal strategy was to enlist large companies to coordinate their own employee-led fund-raising committees, in effect mobilizing tens of thousands of sympathetic employees in the Greater Toronto Area. The *Globe and Mail* reported that employee committees had formed to canvass for building fund donations "in the business houses, factories and industrial plants in the Greater Toronto area,"[42] and the hospital campaign's employee committee provided firms and companies with literature and materials to coordinate internal canvasses for funds. Support often came from further afield: the International Nickel Company (INCO), based in Sudbury, donated $50,000 raised by its employees.[43] The *Globe and Mail* published the names of corporations undertaking internal canvasses, which included the newest and most important feature of the Toronto economy of the time: Canadian subsidiaries of large American companies, such General Motors and General Electric. The immediate post-war years witnessed a surge in unionization in Canada, so it was little surprise that factory committees of unionized employees were crucial in canvassing fellow factory workers for contributions. Indeed, trade union officials were credited as the "guiding spirits" of these employee committees.[44] Elroy Robinson, president of the Toronto Labour Council, led delegates of the Ontario Federation of Labour on "an inspection tour" of 67 College Street, and encouraged members of the Canadian Congress of Labour to support the building fund. His curious comments began by stating categorically that no "good trade unionist" would put up with the deplorable employment conditions at 67 College Street, but then changed tack by acknowledging that "It is the working man who avails himself of this great institution" and adding, for good measure, that "hospital staff not only put up with, but overcame doing a magnificent job despite ancient facilities and overcrowding."[45]

The initial phase of fundraising was spectacularly successful and efficient, vindicating the hospital's decision to ignore door-to-door canvassing for donations, which had been the common practice for hospital fundraising across North America for the first half of the twentieth century. Rather, individual donors could send cheques via a bank, to the hospital or to participating newspapers. Within ten days of the campaign's launch, just weeks following VE Day, $4,584,660 had been raised, including the promised $1-million grants from the city and from the province.[46] The campaign formally closed during the first week of August with a grand total of $7,010,535 – $1 million more than the objective. It was, to quote a gushing and rather self-congratulatory *Globe and Mail* editorial, "A Magnificent Achievement."[47]

The euphoria of the end of the Second World War and the completion of the campaign, which both occurred in August 1945, raised expectations that the mess that College Street had become would soon be replaced by a gleaming new post-war hospital. But hopes of a rapid and uneventful transition were dashed almost immediately. Assured of the funds for the new hospital, soil testing commenced in February 1946 in the midst of the demobilization of tens of thousands of Canadian soldiers, including medical military personnel.[48] Contrary to the fears of many politicians that the country might plunge into another Depression as thousands of young men returned to Canada and began seeking employment, quite the opposite occurred: the economy took off. Inflation and costs rose as economic production surged, spurred on by unprecedented American investment. Construction costs began rising at a rate of 1.5 per cent per month. Wages for skilled tradesmen increased from $1.15 to $1.70 per hour, and the price of steel rose from $125 to $260 per ton. Initial plans were premised on an estimated cost of 90 cents per cubic foot, which almost doubled in three years to $1.75 per cubic foot.[49] Estimates for the total cost of building ballooned from $7.5 million in 1945 to $12 million by 1948.[50] By December 1946, the hospital realized it no longer had enough money.[51] And to make matters worse, the fundraising campaign had officially ended with the city assuming that the goal had been achieved.

Faced with massive cost overruns, hospital administrators engaged in fifteen months of "intensive replanning, re-estimating and negotiating with the staff for overall reduction."[52] All members of the attending staff had been invited to join the planning process. Through the Medical Advisory Board and heads of services, the total space, apart from that for patient accommodation, was slashed to what Bower termed an "irreducible minimum." Space for auxiliary services, operating rooms, research, and X-rays were cut, while the outpatient admitting and emergency services were combined, and some units were required to consolidate in and outpatient work. Instead of demolishing and rebuilding the Ontario Hydro Commission building, it was to be repurposed.[53] *Star* reporter Jack Brehl somewhat delicately acknowledged the hospital's plight, telling readers that "[n]o effort has been spared to cut costs. Original plans have been revised, number of operating rooms cut down, ceilings lowered in certain floors to shorten walls and save bricks and plaster, doors have even been left off many of the closets and staff offices."[54] New draft plans for a building estimated to cost $10 million were approved in the summer of 1947.[55]

Meanwhile, there was another pressing challenge, one that threatened to prove as embarrassing as the now accepted principle that the hospital would have to engage in a second, supplementary fundraising drive. Even at the turning of the soil, the hospital board did not in fact own *all* of the land upon which it intended to build. In some buildings that it had actually acquired, there lived multiple families who did not want to leave. To add to this, and much to the embarrassment of the board members, there stood a "trailer colony" on a key strip on University Avenue and Gerrard Street.

Early efforts to relocate the trailer park had come to no avail; tenants were unable to find affordable housing for their families, and the proprietor was unsuccessful in his bid to find authorization for other potential trailer park sites. The families had taken up residence in trailers in response to an acute shortage of housing – particularly rental properties – in the post-war years.[56] The hospital board, growing frustrated as the problem dragged on and was picked up by the city newspapers, adopted a technical approach, arguing that the trailer park violated municipal housing bylaws. It attempted to pressure the City's Board of Control to declare the site illegal and move the entire colony of fifty-four to sixty trailers of various sizes including some 125 people. The Board of Control, in turn, refused, insisting that it did not have the authority to do so.[57]

The "trailer trouble," as one newspaper dubbed it, dragged on for months, into 1946, and then into 1947. Newspaper reports, relishing in the irony of a children's hospital that was resulting in the dislodging of an estimated 100 to 125 children, began to pick up on the plight caused by the lack of affordable housing. But the city itself was divided: tens of thousands of Torontonians relied on the hospital and indeed had given to the campaign, only to appear to have their dreams stymied by the trailer camp. The Toronto Labour Council helped organize opposition to their eviction, and helped establish a Trailer Residents' Protection Association among the families. Sensitive to a public backlash, the association emphasized that they were more than willing to move, if only granted the space, and reminded the public that it was their status as families with small children that was a barrier to finding rental housing. The president of the residents' committee himself professed to have donated $10 to the new hospital. Events turned from unusual to tragic as a child from the trailer park was struck and killed by a vehicle on University Avenue in front of where the new entrance was to be built. As the city scrambled to find a way out of the impasse, one solution was to displace the families to an unused military barrack in Long Branch, which the families opposed because they feared they would lose civic aid. Ultimately, in October 1947, the city struck a deal with the provincial government to purchase a property that was abutting Ryding Park and east of Runnymede, between a railroad line and Ryding Avenue. While a delegation of the residents' association was meeting with the mayor's office to plead their case for affordable housing, sheriff's officers moved in and physically evicted the remaining families to the "jeer[s] and taunt[s]" of some local residents.[58]

On 17 November 1947, the premier, the mayor, and roughly four hundred others "braved the bleak November weather" to attend the ceremonial turning of the soil.[59] Work on the foundation began that day. By this time, the entire site had been purchased, expropriated, and razed. Centre Avenue, which had been purchased from the city, ceased to exist. In 1949, additional lots on the north side of Elm Street were purchased and expropriated. Arbitration was used in at least one case. Having awkwardly secured the physical property, the building committee's next challenge was to evaluate the bearing quality of the soil, which had always been somewhat suspect due to the fact that it was located on, and adjacent to, "Taddle" or University Creek. Drilling and sample examinations led the committee to choose a reinforced concrete mat instead of caissons or pilings for the foundation. A structural steel frame with open joist floors was chosen because it could be erected speedily with minimal noise disturbance for the neighbouring Toronto General Hospital.[60] The Hospital for Sick Children would be the first major structure in the city to have a welded steel building frame, a construction technique newly allowed by a revised city bylaw. Steel, however, was unavailable for three months, and a building trade strike lasting one month began the morning of 2 May 1949. The American Federation of Labor Construction Laborers Union Local 506 organized a walkout, and all other members of building trade unions respected their picket lines, halting every major construction project in the city.[61] Despite these setbacks, Chairman Robert A. Laidlaw, amidst incessant rainfall, laid the cornerstone on 22 April 1949, Vice-Chairman J. Grant Glassco spoke, and Elizabeth McMaster's daughter was present for the ceremony to symbolize the historic continuity of the hospital project. The hospital's oldest staff member, storekeeper Mr. Charles P. Fry, an employee of sixty years, passed the trowel to Laidlaw. A reception and tea were held after at Alexandra Palace.[62]

Thus, four years after the apparent success of the first campaign, and with a shortfall that was now estimated at close to $4 million, a second fundraising campaign was launched in 1949. It was spearheaded by Laidlaw and, perhaps unsurprisingly, gained traction more slowly than the first. Chartered banks hosted contribution boxes. Newspaper appeals emphasized that over one-third of patients came from outside of Toronto and that that hospital's research benefited the health of *all* children. The campaign was planned to run from 21 November 1949 until the end of the year, but by the second week of December only half of the objective had materialized.[63] One *Globe and Mail* editorial gently criticized other municipalities in the province by stating that donations lagged "largely because the communities beyond this city have not rallied as expected."[64] As in the earlier campaign, the hospital eschewed door-to-door canvassing, relying on the expansion of post-war media – radio and newspaper – to get the message out. By New Year's, the campaign was still short some $637,926. An additional $100,000 from the T. Eaton Company, $101,000 from the Penny Bank of Ontario, and $50,000 from the Toronto Rotary Club finally put the hospital within reach. By February 1951, the amount had been exceeded, and $4,460,913.32 was raised based on 87,000 charitable receipts.[65] Taken together, and excluding the city and provincial grants, the total non-governmental donations exceeded $9 million. By comparison, a concurrent campaign in Boston for a children's hospital struggled to raise half of its goal. The hospital's success in its second campaign purportedly drew experts to Toronto to study the institution's "magic formula." As one staff doctor smugly quipped, the secret was relatively simple: "Everybody loves us."[66]

Even the Bed Pans

At long last, the new Hospital for Sick Children at 555 University Avenue was officially opened on 15 January 1951. A ribbon-cutting ceremony was presided over by six former and current patients selected to represent geographical and cultural diversity in order to communicate the hospital's commitment to non-discrimination and to "represent the hospital's national character."[67] The children included Robert Westlake (a Toronto polio patient), Dolores St. Germaine (a Regina polio patient), thirteen-year-old David (a black asthma patient in the custody of CAS), seven-year-old Elaine Jackson (a "big-eyed little blonde" and former "blue baby" from St. Stephen, New Brunswick),[68] Dorothy Blackmere (a surgically treated rheumatoid arthritis patient from Freeman, Ontario), and Anna (a ten-year-old Inuit child from Port Harrison, NWT, "who had to undergo months of treatment for a serious congenital eye condition").[69] On its front page, the *Globe and Mail* ran a photograph of Alan Brown with Anna and David, described, respectively, as "a little Eskimo girl" and "a negro boy from Toronto."[70] The publicity committee had agreed to avoid teenagers in favour of "younger children" in the photo ops.[71]

The board endeavoured to make the opening a public event, inviting all Torontonians to the ceremony. The department stores Eaton's and Simp-

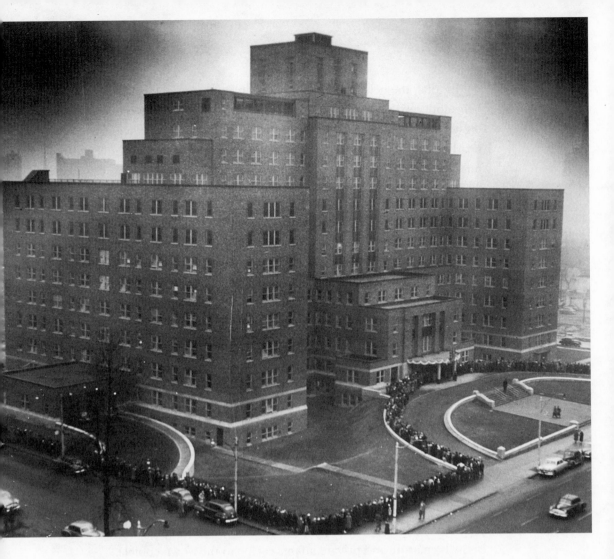

son's featured invitations in their window displays, while newspapers published facsimiles. Board members, who were disquieted by the populist orientation of the opening ceremony, decided that individually addressed invitations to major donors would also be sent out on Laidlaw's personal letterhead.[72] The

9.3 The hospital at 555 University Avenue was opened in 1951 to throngs of well-wishers and the curious. By the time of its completion it was proclaimed to be the largest children's hospital in the world.

opening ceremony was followed by a week-long open house. An estimated 85,000 visitors passed through the building during that week, with huge lines snaking around the building, which were "dramatic testimony of the popular interest. The hope that the people would think of the Hospital for Children as 'theirs' in a real and definite way, has been realized."[73] In what appears to have been a spontaneous gesture, visitors threw $25,000 worth of coins into the new hydrotherapy pool, which then had to be drained to retrieve the largesse.[74]

In total, the new hospital, despite its haircut, was a 495,000-square-foot behemoth capable of accommodating 635 patients. The entire project, including a new nurses' residence, cost a jaw-dropping $13 million.[75] The new facility boasted fourteen operating rooms, twelve X-ray rooms, and a ward for premature babies. Reflecting its central role in paediatrics education for the University of Toronto's medical school, the building incorporated a lecture hall with a capacity of 275 and a smaller room for audiences of up to eighty-five.[76] Construction continued, and the building plans were revised in minor ways to accommodate an expansion of dental facilities and "scientific and technical progress in the fields of Medicine and Nursing" that resulted in UV lights in infant cubicles, as well as piped oxygen, suction, and compressed air in each room. Previously this equipment had had to be transported to individual cots on a portable, rolling apparatus.[77] The service floor at the base held the kitchen, storage, cafeteria, hydrotherapy pool, space for hospital personnel, and records room. On the main floor, one could find admitting, emergency, the outpatient department, including X-ray rooms for outpatients, and the milk laboratory. The first floor contained business offices, heads of services, consulting rooms, and the auditoria. Fourteen operating rooms populated the second floor, as well as the inpatient X-ray department and dentistry, and the third floor was dedicated to laboratory and research space. Patient areas occupied the other seven floors: floors four, five, six, and seven were open to public patients, while floors eight, nine, and ten were reserved for private and semi-private patients. Public wards held two to six patients, with single rooms for serious cases. Premature and private infants each had their own cubicle.[78]

The new facility featured numerous new technologies to augment the comfort and efficiency of patients and staff, such as pneumatic tubes connecting twenty-four departments, intercoms and paging systems for doctors and nurses, as well as air-conditioning in the operating rooms and wards, a therapy pool with a hydraulic lift, a television in one of the operating rooms (for teaching purposes, it was emphasized), three fluoroscopic rooms, and an electroencephalograph. Corridor ceilings, although lowered to cut expenses, were nevertheless sound absorbent. Switches were explosion-proof, floors spark-proof *and* shockproof, and the twelve X-ray rooms lead lined and copper shielded in light of post-war research demonstrating the dangers of repeated radiation exposure.[79] To combat the tendency to render hospitals sparse, white, and sterile, an interior consultant was hired to coordinate a "scientific decorating scheme" that combined a range of soft, complementary colours and colourful murals.[80] The main entrance hall and lobby, however, were designed for adults. The spacious, dignified lobby was praised for "[e]ntirely lacking in the depressing atmosphere of the conventional hospital or institution[;] the impression is one of a modern hotel."[81]

On 4 February 1951, almost 200 patients and nearly all of the equipment from 67 College Street were transported to the new hospital, reportedly in just under three hours. Each child was tagged by a number and moved by doctors, nurses, policemen, and volunteers from the Red Cross and Toronto Hydro using cars, ambulances, and the Thistletown bus. Chairman R.A. Laidlaw carried in the first patient.[82] One interviewee recalls that her husband, a very senior physician, arrived late to the procession and was given a bed pan to carry.[83] The nurses summed up their delight in moving into the new institution with the following doggerel:

> Nineteen fifties, nineteen fifties,
> Now we're moving to a brand new building.
> Everything is the latest
> And what we do is just the greatest.
>
> No cockroaches, no cockroaches,
> Not another one would dare approach us,
> We're insect protected,
> Now they can't come unless selected.
>
> ... Now we're settled, now we're settled,
> There is not a reason to be nettled,
> What! You say it's too small,
> We'll have to build another, that's all.[84]

The Ladies in the Green Smocks[85]

Hospitals are social institutions, reflective of the broader social and cultural trends of the communities in which they reside. Post-war Canada was replete with exhortations for women to "return to the household" and cede the occupational roles they had performed during the war to now-demobilized men. The pressure to return to domesticity was relentless. And yet, at the same time, more and more women were completing university programs and entering the often unwelcoming terrain of the professional middle class. A cadre of educated women were therefore caught up in the tension between women's slow ascendancy within the professions and the cultural pressure to conform to what the historian Veronica Strong-Boag memorably characterized as "suburban dreams."[86] Thousands of post-war voluntary societies, run and staffed by women, occupied this awkward niche of part-time labour within organizations that were still predominantly run by men.

The Women's Auxiliary of The Hospital for Sick Children can best be understood within this context. The original meeting was spearheaded by a remarkable woman medical practitioner, Helen Reid. Reid obtained her medical degree from the University of Alberta in 1935 and joined The Hospital for Sick Children the following year, despite the fact that Alan Brown made little secret of the fact that he "didn't like women doctors." Legend has it that Reid elbowed her way in, sending Brown a telegraph every day for three weeks requesting an appointment until he finally relented. At that time, the Medical Advisory Board, of which Brown was a member, repeatedly cited "space restraints" as the principal justification for allowing only two female interns at a time. It appears, however, that this policy limiting female interns was gradually rescinded; the following year, women were appointed to three of five intern positions. And in 1939, Brown appointed his first female chief resident, Frances Mulligan, the gold medallist in her class, though, as so often happened, she resigned to get married.[87]

Reid worked at the Children's Aid Society Infants Home, at which Brown was a consultant, from 1938 to 1941. During this time she married Andrew Lawrence Chute and had her first child in June 1941. A few days after she gave birth, her husband shipped out to Britain to assist with the war effort. When her "legs gradually turned black as a result of disseminated intravascular clotting," Charles Best, a close friend with whom Chute had worked in diabetes research, brought her heparin daily for several weeks, apparently saving her life.[88] Helen ceased practising for about three years. She then moved to her mother's home in Alberta, arising daily at 4 a.m. to take the train to Edmonton, where she began a part-time private practice and lectured at the University of Alberta medical school. Remembering this time in her life, she later asserted that she "thrived on the work."[89] When her husband returned from war and began practising in Toronto, she "helped out in his office in between looking after her second baby," occupying an unusual position as a mother of young children, the wife of the most senior medical officer of the hospital, and a trained physician in her own right. In an interview late in her career, Reid reflected on her position, declaring that "It's a female dilemma at the age of 45, that is for trained, intelligent women ...

I became concerned about the number of intelligent women whose minds are allowed to decay, whose abilities are not being used."[90]

According to Reid, the idea for the Women's Auxiliary emerged as "pillow talk" with her husband, who was about to succeed Alan Brown as chief of paediatrics. Struggling to raise $2,000 to fund a medical library in the hospital that was then under construction, Chute proposed that Reid lead a group of women to raise the funds. As a consequence, in 1950, eighty-eight women met, somewhat tellingly, in the old nurses residence.[91] At first, they were predominantly wives of medical staff members and trustees, women medical staff members, and members of the previous hospital's sewing group, as well as the head of nursing, Jean Masten. Sensitive to the patronizing elements of women being "put in their place," the charismatic and independent Reid was anxious to foster a women's association that took on what she considered to be "meaningful" tasks within the hospital. She remembered, with evident irritation, the comments of the then vice-chairman, J. Grant Glassco, who attended this first meeting. "Rather condescendingly he said that the Hospital needed a group of women to 'sew and knit and mend.' This made us so mad," Reid scoffed, "that we decided we would show him."[92]

Reid may have been voicing proto-feminist concerns, but the women's auxiliary she envisaged could not be mistaken for being egalitarian and inclusive. Indeed, membership was by "invitation only" and restricted to women of a certain social standing. Wives of professional staff members or trustees and women doctors were eligible. It was also decided that "temporary" or "special" membership could be extended to members of The Hospital for Sick Children's Aid (an existing voluntary sewing group); wives of honorary staff consultants, interns, and fellows; widows of staff members; Miss Hays, the secretary of the building campaign committee; two members of the Junior League; "lady internes and fellows"; and women recommended by permanent members. As the group took shape, the male trustees of the hospital – some of whom, like Chute, were sharing pillow talk with key members of the Women's Auxiliary – offered begrudging support, while seeking, at the same time, to circumscribe the mandate of the organization and ensure its membership would reflect well on the new hospital. Chairman Laidlaw, for example, was chosen to speak with Jean Wansbrough, the wife of the chief of surgery and president of the auxiliary, and "suggest to her that it might be better not to invite members of the employed [non-medical] staff of the hospital to become members."[93]

The executive committee was, perhaps unsurprisingly, composed largely of the wives of senior medical staff. Wansbrough was elected president and Reid herself vice-president. Mrs. Alan Brown was named honorary president and Mrs. D.E. Robertson honorary vice-president. Helen Reid succeeded Wansbrough and became the second president. The secretary and treasurer positions were held by wives of other senior physicians, Drs. Silverthorne, Ebbs, and Jackson. And yet, the leadership was presiding over an ever-expanding guard of women volunteers who were, largely, friends-of-friends. At the end of the first year, the auxiliary had increased to over two hundred members, and after three years, close to three hundred. Reflecting the social void that such a calling filled, a waiting list emerged for the group. Although all members served part-time, again a nod to their concurrent domestic responsibilities, new members nevertheless underwent a three-month training period. They visited every service and each received specialist training in one service.[94]

This small army of Women's Auxiliary members was noticeable from the very opening of the new hospital, when its volunteers led tours for thousands of Torontonians during the open house.[95] Over time, however, their principal tasks would shift towards fundraising and supplementary hospital services. The auxiliary's first coordinated act was to hold a rummage sale that yielded $451.51. These funds were, in turn, used to organize a "monster bazaar" at Casa Loma in November 1950. The bazaar raised $5,772.62, netting $4,738.38. At Bower's request, the auxiliary gave $2,000 of this revenue to set up the new hospital medical library.[96] Encouraged by their success with the bazaar, the auxiliary sought to open a shop to raise funds for the hospital. During a convention in October 1951, they used this space to hold another bazaar, which brought in nearly $3,000, netting $2,400. The auxiliary largely used this money to buy Christmas gifts for the hospital patients. As the main support for the gift fair came not from convention attendees but from the people of Toronto, auxiliary members felt that "[we] had proved that we could run a shop and that our work would sell."[97] The auxiliary was given use of the room for one year pending the board's approval of the equipment and commodities to be sold. The shop was open every day beginning on the first day of October 1952, and featured a myriad of handmade goods, Christmas cards, and a specially made patient booklet, *Billy Goes to the Hospital*, intended to help children understand the process of hospitalization. All of the profits were given over to projects within the hospital.[98]

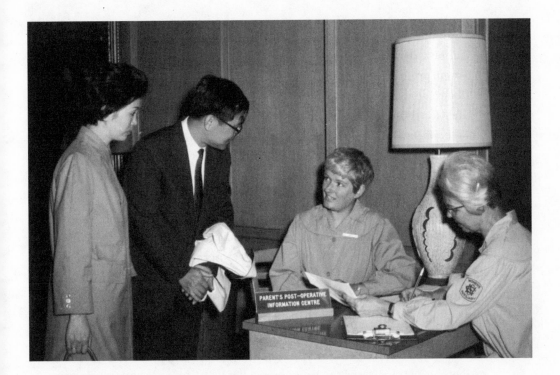

9.4 The hospital was powered by a small army of Women's Auxiliary members. These part-time volunteers were primarily educated middle-class mothers who worked in numerous hospital departments and liaised with parents, particularly those of patients undergoing surgical operations.

Despite the objections of Reid to the tone of Glassco's remarks, sewing and handcrafts had indeed become an important part of the auxiliary's fundraising work. Two of the earliest standing committees were called "Hospital Service" and "Needlework." Sewing groups met twice weekly in the nurses' residence and members prepared innumerable items for sale at bazaars and the gift shop, known as 5Fifty5, including baby clothes, toys, items for use in the occupational therapy department, clothing for post-operative patients who often required specially made clothing to accommodate splints, and the famous "restraint jackets." These special jackets allowed small children to play with their hands but restrained them from touching their face or other post-surgical areas. The production of these "restraint jackets," 135 of which were made in 1953 alone, was both "a service to the hospital and a financing project," for they were also sold widely for outside use.[99] One Women's Auxiliary member recalled:

I had to provide some service and they were looking for someone who would make these restraint jackets in a kind of white canvas material. And they were tricky to make because they were small and the canvas was difficult to manoeuver. I don't know how many I made, I must have made 2 or 3 or 4 dozen until probably they felt that someone with a more professional approach to them should make them, I don't know. I never had the quality of my work criticized, not openly ... but I really felt for those poor little things who were prevented from scratching their faces, because of these restraint jackets.[100]

Within a short time, the Women's Auxiliary had become a fundraising machine. It presented the chairman with annual cheques of ever-increasing value: $9,000 in 1957; $15,000 in 1960; and $20,000 in 1965, a sum roughly equivalent to buying a modest suburban house in Ontario at the time. Within a decade, revenue from these sources permitted the group to make two extraordinary gifts of $15,000 to the hospital. Over time, the auxiliary supported clinical research in the department of surgery, gave grants to the research institute, and established a memorial cot fund. They also provided scholarships for what was thought to be the first bursary program for student nurses and even founded a dental clinic at Thistletown before the property was transferred to the province.[101]

Ultimately, the most significant contribution of the Women's Auxiliary was not the absolute number of dollars raised in the shop and bazaars, but rather the thousands of unpaid hours that the volunteers dedicated to the hospital itself. Women's Auxiliary members began to assist in an ever-increasing array of duties, including helping in the occupational therapy department and even transporting patients during a Toronto Transit Commission (TTC) strike. By 1963, the auxiliary was providing twenty to forty volunteers per day in seventeen different services and clinics, including the medical record library, blood donors' clinic, cleft palate clinic, admitting, X-ray, occupational therapy, cardiac surgery, genetics, and other departments.[102] Volunteers sometimes acted as interpreters for parents and staff, held babies so that genetics researchers could take hand and footprints, helped prepare pre- and post-operative photographs for visual education, and ferried children to and from the X-ray department. Although there was a definite social dimension to the Women's Auxiliary, a *Globe and Mail* reporter warned that this was not a bridge club and that prospective members should be prepared to "work hard."[103]

Volunteers did much to enable the nursing staff to carry out what Jean Masten described as "care of the whole child," an approach to the psychological well-being of the child that had come into vogue in the 1950s. This included school and bedside instruction provided by the board of education; six classes of nondenominational Sunday school taught by medical students; a nursery school run by students from the Institute for Child Study; play therapy and play therapists; Toronto Public Library services and story hours; occupational therapy; and dressing patients "in pretty clothes" to boost their morale.[104] Their initiatives dovetailed with the impetus on the part of nurses and psychologists to reduce the trauma of institutionalization and foster newer theories in child psychology, as discussed in the previous chapter. In 1954, the auxiliary purchased John Robertson's famed *A Two-Year-Old Goes to the Hospital*, a 1952 film documenting the trauma of separating children from parents, along with other films for use in the Toronto hospital. The auxiliary also devoted funds to provide special nursing care for seriously ill children and paid the salary of a social worker for diabetic, psychiatric, and neuro-convulsive patients.[105]

The Women's Auxiliary also helped reshape the interior of the new hospital by planning and funding the creation of numerous play spaces. The auxiliary first discussed providing a rooftop playground in 1951, and realized their vision in October 1957, when the "scaled-down penthouse roof garden" was inaugurated.[106] In 1959, a playroom was opened in the waiting area of the outpatient department, at a cost of $3,000, for children waiting for clinic appointments. In addition to interacting with individual children by visiting their bedsides, reading, showing movies, and throwing birthday parties, the auxiliary supplied amenities and goods to amuse children and encourage play. For example, the auxiliary purchased television sets and record players, paid for the annual Christmas parties, and bought gifts for all patients. In 1962, the auxiliary funded the establishment of the Department of Recreation and Volunteer Services, which coordinated recreational programming for patients and oversaw the distribution of volunteer groups in the hospital. By this time, it included the assistance of 100 retired teachers, students, and housewives. During the evenings these recreation service volunteers may have run into "Uncle Bernie," who had begun entertaining children with balloons and puppet shows in 1948 and, following the opening of the new building, recruited seven friends and his own nephews to regularly visit inpatients. In 1963, two more volunteers groups joined: the Nurses Alumnae Association (identifiable by their yellow smocks) and the "candy stripers," many of whom were teenage girls. Their presence may account for the arrival of a "half-dozen boys" from Upper Canada College who volunteered for two nights per week.[107]

By the early 1960s, the Women's Auxiliary had become entrenched in the hospital, readily visible in their green smocks as they navigated the long corridors of the new hospital. They typed records, numbered and filed documents in patient history folders, and, with the advent of cytogenetics by the early 1960s, helped by counting and classifying human chromosomes in photographs. In the cardiac research department, they performed clerical work for technicians. Director John T. Law acknowledged the auxiliary as the "backbone of our volunteer services," writing that "[a]ll of this volunteer activity helps us tremendously, it permits us to give a level of service that would be impossible on a paid basis, as the cost involved would be astronomical." He added, for good measure, "The volunteer is a better person because of her volunteer activities."[108]

Conclusions

Behind the scenes there was a minor spat between Alan Brown and the trustees over the opening ceremony of the new hospital. The board, who had been discussing the possibility of Princess Margaret, Dr. Ralphe Bunche, or General Dwight Eisenhower cutting the ribbon, apparently feared that the publicity committee was planning an unseemly spectacle resembling a "midway" fair. The publicity committee, by contrast, wanted an opening ceremony that included the general public as much as possible. Somewhat paradoxically, it was Brown, the embodiment of a generation of traditional male medical authority (and now entering retirement), who supported the more populist media blitz. He apparently lectured the trustees and the other medical staff that they "must recognize that it was the public who built the hospital, and that without the publicity committee and the help given by their various media, the campaigns might not have succeeded."[109] The upbraiding of the hospital board may have been one of Brown's final official acts. He resigned as physician-in-chief in October 1951. Brown moved aside to permit a younger generation of medical leaders to take the helm of the new hospital tower. By the time of his retirement, Brown had reputedly helped train three-quarters of all the practising paediatricians in Canada.[110]

The medical men who would take charge of the new hospital – Drs. Chute, Keith, and Salter – represented the medical chiefs of an institution that was, in the wards, teeming with women workers and volunteers. Of the 1,500 employees on its payroll, over four-fifths were women. Women worked in a variety of roles – IBM operators, secretaries, technicians, stenographers, occupational and physical therapists, social services workers, nurses, dietitians, bookkeepers, food services personnel, receptionists, maids, and librarians. Supplementing this paid female workforce was the Women's Auxiliary, part of the estimated 11,000 women in Toronto who participated in twenty-four hospital auxiliaries by 1962. Although volunteers, in the form of lady visitors, date back to the very founding of the hospital, the post-war formalization of volunteerism became a shadow professional group, essential to the smooth functioning of any hospital.[111]

By the spring of 1951, the total space occupied by the new Hospital for Sick Children on University Avenue was almost three times as large as its predecessor. As one reporter somewhat playfully suggested, once the arrows were removed after the open house, "you won't be able to get around the place without a map and a St. Bernard station to bring succour to those lost in the corridors."[112] Unsurprisingly, contemporaries found it impossible not to contrast this gleaming, massive, utilitarian institution with the much loved, if dilapidated, "great red pile" that had been vacated on College Street:

> Whether television, fourteen walk-in refrigerators, deep freeze units, kitchens, dining room and cafeteria second to none, thirteen vast floors, untraviolet [sic] germicidal lights, hearing clinics, allergy sections, diabetic sections, raised bathtubs, giant X-ray equipment and modern lecture auditoriums will make up, sentimentally speaking, for the familiar, homey atmosphere of the old Hospital for Sick Children, we would hesitate to say.[113]

As for the old rabbit-warren itself, the abandoned building at 67 College Street was sold to the province for $375,000, and the main residence and Brent House were leased for a nominal one dollar.[114] As it decayed over the years, 67 College Street began to suffer from lack of attention, a sad legacy to the important role that it played in the history of Canadian health care and the social history of Toronto itself. In 1993, however, it received a new lease on life. It was gutted and beautified, becoming the new Toronto headquarters of Canadian Blood Services. Few hints of its former use still remain, save for the original board room overlooking College Street, some fine china with the insignia of the hospital, and the arched main entrance which still has, blazed in stone, the appellation "Victoria Hospital for Sick Children."

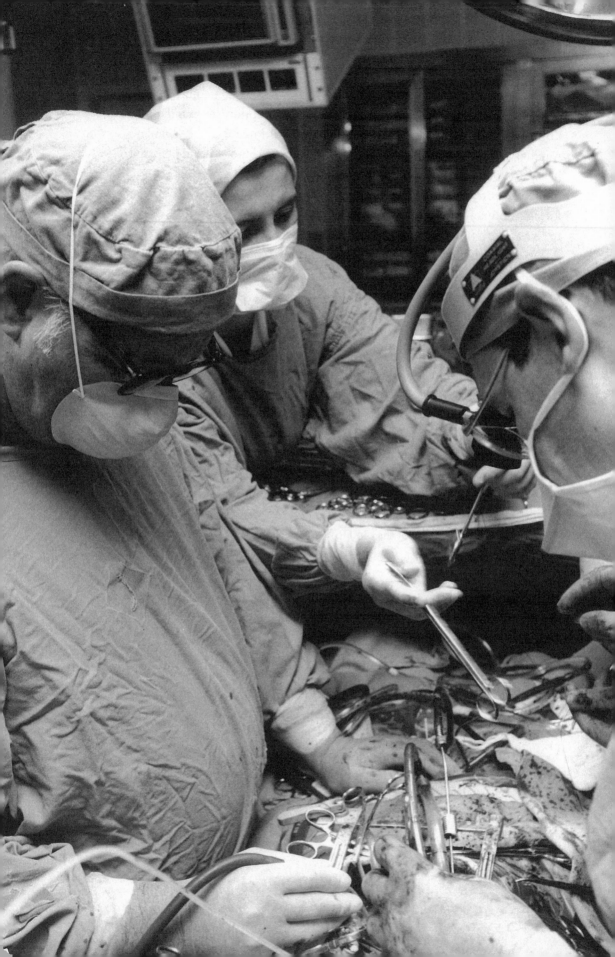

TEN

Blue Babies

The antibiotics, yeah, and ... like today everything's disposable. In
those days it was glass. Glass plungers, and then after there was a dirty
utility room, and you had to wash the stuff out and put it back on the
tray and it went back to central supply where it was sorted, the needles
were sharpened and they set out trays and they sent them up again.
And we had three weeks in central supply, and I was horrendous at it,
I think I had to do an extra week at it. I was so bad. I was bored out
of my skull! Counting these damn syringes and everything, it was
horrible.[1]

Interview with former nurse, participant #12, 2014

The Antibiotic Revolution

The immediate post-war period witnessed the full flowering of advances in
laboratory science, one that would transform the clinical treatment of childhood and adult diseases. A class of new chemicals – known as sulphonamides
or sulfa drugs – had been identified and refined in the 1930s.[2] They were
introduced during the 1938–9 academic year at the University of Toronto
and its affiliated hospitals, revolutionizing the treatment of potentially fatal bacterial infections, most
notably pneumococcal pneumonia.[3] At The Hospital
for Sick Children, Alan Brown and Nelles Silverthorne ran trials of two early agents, sulphapyridine
and sulphanilamide. The results were stunning. They
found that sulphanilamide halved mortality rates for

10.1 As infant mortality declined,
research and clinical attention
began to focus increasingly on
congenital conditions, such as
cardiac abnormalities. It was at the
hospital that William Mustard (front,
left) pioneered his hole-in-the-heart
surgery using the "baffle" technique.

streptococcal infections,[4] which had been almost uniformly fatal in previous decades. They began sulphapyridine therapy for pneumococcal infections in early 1939, which they compared against controls and pneumococcus rabbit serum.[5] Surgeon-in-Chief D.E. Robertson began to routinely administer sulphonamides to patients during the war years, treating eighty-nine patients with acute haematogenous osteomyelitis, a rapidly developing blood-borne bacterial infection of the musculoskeletal system that infected bone and bone marrow. In 1943, he reported to the American Surgical Association a drop in mortality from 22 per cent to 1 per cent, much to the association's delight.[6]

The war front had become an unofficial testing ground for another new antibiotic: penicillin. The compound had first been discovered in 1928 by Alexander Fleming, but had not been further experimented upon until 1940, when pathologist Howard Florey and biochemist Ernst Chain at Oxford University demonstrated its effectiveness on mice, and prompted larger scale production of the antibiotic. Florey and Chain helped refine the powder that would subsequently be used on thousands of Allied soldiers. During the war years it proved decisive in treating a host of bacterial infections affecting troops, including gangrene, pneumonia, and syphilis. It should be remembered that many of the physicians and surgeons of Toronto's postwar Hospital for Sick Children served in Britain or Europe, and would have been familiar with the new antibacterial powders used in the British and Allied armies. Indeed, Major A.L. Chute, the future chief of paediatrics, had overseen a special Royal Canadian Army Medical Corps research unit in Italy involved in the experimental use of penicillin.[7] Back in Toronto, penicillin was first used at the University of Toronto in 1941 at the Toronto General Hospital and the Banting Institute. As early as 1943, the Connaught Laboratories and a number of private firms were producing penicillin, mainly for the Canadian armed forces.[8] A modest stock was used for civilians, funded in part by the National Research Council. For example, a progress report indicated that, by November 1943, "about fifteen patients" had been treated with locally produced penicillin.[9] By the end of the war, a total of over 300 Toronto area patients had received the experimental drug.[10]

While Canadian domestic production of this new wonder drug was being devoted largely to the armed services, staff at The Hospital for Sick Children had resorted to American-produced penicillin in many emergency situations. In the summer of 1942, when faced with a nine-year-old boy dying of a sulpha-resistant staph infection (haemolytic staphylococcal septicaemia),

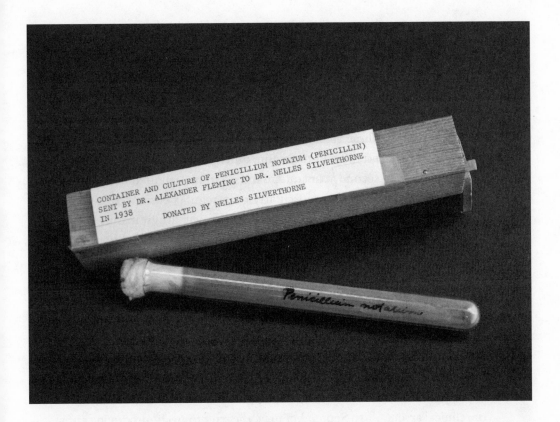

CONTAINER AND CULTURE OF PENICILLIUM NOTATUM (PENICILLIN)
SENT BY DR. ALEXANDER FLEMING TO DR. NELLES SILVERTHORNE
IN 1938   DONATED BY NELLES SILVERTHORNE

Penicillium notatum

Silverthorne obtained penicillin and instructions from Dr. Charles Keefer, Chairman of the (American) National Research Council committee on chemotherapy, who controlled the domestic supply of penicillin in the United States.[11] A technician, Isobel Scott, filtered the penicillin, which was administered every four hours. Silverthorne published the results of two cases

10.2 In the immediate post-war era, penicillin and its sister anti-bacterial agents were employed to near-miraculous effect against staphylococcal septicaemia, pneumonia, pulmonary tuberculosis, osteomyelitis, and rheumatic heart disease.

in the *Canadian Medical Association Journal* the following year, telling of dramatic, if unsteady, recoveries. The first boy spent over two weeks deteriorating in the hospital before penicillin was used: "The night before penicillin was to be administered he was comatose, irrational, and, to all who observed him, obviously dying. Penicillin was administered every 4 hours by continuous intravenous infusion and his temperature for the first time in 16 hospital days became normal." At the time of writing, the boy had returned to "excellent physical condition."[12] Penicillin was similarly obtained and used successfully against haemolytic *Staphylococcus aureus* in a critically ill six-week-old infant hospitalized for pneumonia and intestinal intoxication. Newspapers trumpeted the miraculous effects of penicillin, which in August

1943 was rushed from New York to the Hamilton General Hospital to save the life of a young girl.[13]

In 1944, the Medical Advisory Board appointed a committee to draft regulations concerning the use of penicillin in the hospital, including supplementary fees for its administration, which always occurred on an inpatient basis.[14] These rules were, at first, restrictive, since the drug was still rather novel and difficult to acquire due to limited civilian production. By 1946, however, second-year student nurses were permitted to administer the new class of drugs intramuscularly on a regular basis.[15] This was, in part, a result of the practical application of the new drugs, many of which had to be filtered and administered every four to six hours. Soon, it was important to have a score of syringes at the ready. As the opening quotation illustrates, one student nurse in the early 1950s, recalls the time-consuming routine of cleaning the glass syringes so that a ready supply was always available.

The one-two punch of sulpha drugs and penicillin vastly reduced the fatality rates and recovery times of patients who developed diseases such as pneumonia, empyema,[16] and osteomyelitis.[17] In 1946, streptomycin, an antibiotic particularly effective against pulmonary tuberculosis, was added to the clinical arsenal.[18] In September 1943, the streptomycin-producing strain of *Streptomyces griseus*, which stopped bacterial growth, was first isolated in research laboratories under the supervision of Selman Waksman, a soil biologist at Rutgers University who would ultimately receive a Nobel Prize for his research.[19] Clinical testing followed at the Mayo Clinic, with streptomycin first being administered in September 1944, to a moribund neonate with septicaemia, meningitis, and a *Staphylococcus aureas* infection. That same year, the discovery was made public and the pharmaceutical company Merck and Co. began production.[20] It was found that the drug was uniquely effective against various types of tuberculosis, genito-urinary infections, and influenzal meningitis. It also became the preferred clinical choice for treatment-resistant tuberculosis.[21]

Streptomycin was reportedly used experimentally in Canada in 1945, both in Montreal[22] and at Toronto's Christie Street Veteran's Hospital in May or June.[23] Beginning in 1946 distribution was supervised by the National Research Council of Canada which provided a free supply of the antibiotic to hospital physicians, with some conditions,[24] and then without restrictions to hospitals early in 1947.[25] In 1948, the Federal Health Grants program, a federal initiative in support of public health and under the guidance of the then federal Minister of National Health and Welfare Paul Martin Sr., supported its distribution throughout the country.[26] Early publications, such as that of Gladys Boyd on the results of thirty-four Hospital for Sick Children patients treated with streptomycin since January 1947, demonstrated that it "materially reduced mortality" from "virulent forms of childhood tuberculosis," "permitted cure of all pulmonary cases so far," and also indicated curative effects for tuberculous meningitis.[27] Nelles Silverthorne reported on the successful treatment of meningitis patients with streptomycin during 1946. At the hospital, influenza meningitis had a 98 per cent mortality rate in the pre-antibiotic era. This was lowered to 45 per cent with sulfonamides (with or without penicillin) and serum treatments, and 25 per cent during initial streptomycin treatments.[28] Former nurse Charlotte Burt recalled an overnight race to bring streptomycin from Boston to save a baby dying of influenza meningitis:

> That was one long, lonely night with an infant who refused to do more than indulge in an isolated gasp every now and again. Even the coming of morning didn't improve matters. Eight o'clock, nine o'clock, ten o'clock came and went.
>
> And then it happened. It was our own Dr. [Charles E.] Snelling who was the first to give streptomycin to an infant in Canada. And a few hours later a tiny, pink morsel of humanity slept as though nothing was amiss.[29]

These early results were so promising that Silverthorne boldly concluded "that streptomycin in large enough doses will cure practically all patients with this disease [meningitis] if the patients are admitted in the early stages."[30]

The advent of streptomycin, combined with a generation-long decline in tubercular cases, resulted in a gradual de-emphasis on heliotherapy and the sanatorium aspects of rehabilitation from what had once been dubbed the "White Plague." As mentioned previously, physicians at the hospital boasted that, by the late 1940s, tubercular conditions in Canadian-born children were becoming almost non-existent, though they might have qualified that to exclude Aboriginal children. The tuberculosis death rate was reduced by two-thirds in all provinces from 1947 to 1953, and by 70 per cent in Ontario from 1943 to 1952.[31] In the wake of the chemical revolution, Thistletown, and many tuberculosis sanatoria for adults across the country, were witnessing a steady drop in patients, a phenomenon one social historian referred to cleverly as the "miracle of the empty beds."[32]

Concurrent to the introduction of streptomycin, there was a breakthrough in the treatment of the poliovirus, which continued to terrorize Canadian communities every few years, including the summers of 1952 and 1953. In 1950, the American virologist Jonas Salk announced the creation of a "killed-virus" vaccine for each of the three dominant polio strains. At the request of the National Foundation for Infantile Paralysis (March of Dimes), Connaught Laboratories in Toronto produced all of the polioviruses for the Salk vaccine trials. In 1954, clinical trials were carried out in forty-four U.S. states, two Canadian provinces, and in Finland in one of the largest clinical trials in medical history. National Health Research grants supported crucial polio research at Connaught Laboratories.[33] Led by Andrew J. Rhodes, the director of the University of Toronto School of Hygiene and later director of The Hospital for Sick Children's Research Institute, Connaught researchers developed ways of cultivating poliovirus in test tubes, enabling the large-scale testing of the Salk vaccine.[34] Meanwhile, local health departments coordinated immunizations. In Toronto, the most vulnerable children, identified as those in Grades 1, 2, and 3, were vaccinated with the assistance of local school boards. For example, in 1957, Toronto initiated a polio immunization program in all schools as well as child health centres for those without family doctors. Mothers lined up around the block to have their children vaccinated. Within a generation, polio ceased to be a major public health problem.[35]

The period, then, between the late 1930s and the late 1950s was one of extraordinary success in reducing some of the most feared and intractable childhood killers. Through public health campaigns that emphasized nutrition, comprehensive vaccination programs, and early intervention, common

Table 10.1 Infant mortality table for Canada and Ontario, 1921–60 (per 1,000 live births)

Year	Canada	Ontario
1921	102.1	91.2
1925	92.7	78.9
1930	90.6	73.8
1932	74.6	61.8
1935	72.5	55.7
1940	57.6	43.2
1945	52.5	40.6
1950	41.5	34.5
1955	31.3	26.0
1960	27.3	23.5

Source: Statistics Canada. *Selected Infant Mortality and Related Statistics, Canada, 1921–1990*. Ottawa: Minister of Industry, Science and Technology (Ottawa: Statistics Canada, 1993). 8, 34–9 (table 2b), infant death rates by sex, Canada, and province, rate per 1,000 live births

childhood diseases including measles, scarlet fever, diphtheria, polio, and tuberculosis, slowly faded from the social and cultural experience of most non-Aboriginal families in Canada. It may never be possible to determine the precise contributions of improved nutrition, rising standards of living, changing housing conditions, vaccinations, and chemical interventions, but the combination of these changes fostered a new era of child health across the industrialized world that was without precedent. As tables 10.1 and 10.2 demonstrate, the infant and childhood mortality rates in Ontario, and for that matter in Canada more generally, fell by two-thirds over a generation. For the first time in human history, parents in the post-war period could have a reasonable expectation that none of their children would perish, or be severely disabled, due to infectious disease. Of course, tragic circumstances did happen, but they were becoming more exceptional. The children of the 1950s were indeed lucky enough to be "born at the right time."[36]

Table 10.2 Mortality rates (per 1,000) from all causes – Ontario (by age group)

Year	Under 1	1–4	5–9	10–14	15–19
1900	136.4	11.02	3.46	2.43	4.09
1942	40.1	2.34	0.92	0.77	1.46

Source: N.E. McKinnon, "Mortality Reductions in Ontario, 1900-1942," *Canadian Journal of Public Health / Revue Canadienne de Santé Publique* 35, no.12 (1944): 482.

The new antibiotic era would thus have multiple influences on the nature of paediatric hospitals. With an ever-increasing arsenal of chemical interventions, The Hospital for Sick Children witnessed a slow but steady shift in the emphasis of clinical tests and research, well recognized by Alan Brown on the eve of his retirement, from infectious diseases to congenital conditions. "It is extremely gratifying to observe," he affirmed,

> the phenomenal results following the use of chemotherapy and antibiotics. Throughout the American Continent, in all enlightened communities, it will not be long before all the common diseases will be eliminated as the result of modern treatment, and our chief difficulties will only have to do with congenital malformations, childhood accidents and diseases due to viruses – even the latter may, in the not too distant future, be brought under control.[37]

In effect, the self-evident success in saving young children from infectious diseases opened up a clinical space to begin to experiment with novel procedures to save a whole class of infants who had previously been written off. The treatments used for two groups of patients reflect this new emphasis well: surgery for children born with life-threatening congenital cardiac (heart) malformations and, second, the intervention to save premature babies. Within this new frontier of paediatric medicine, the surgical staff, long patronized under the leadership of Brown as second-class citizens within the hospital, would rise to the forefront of exciting, if experimental, clinical trials.

Frozen Hearts and Monkey Lungs

In the years leading up to the Second World Ward, the surgical staff at The Hospital for Sick Children remained quite modest in number. By the late 1940s, for example, there were only seven men on staff. Dr. LeMesurier, who served as chief for five years until the opening of the new building on University Avenue, purposely kept the surgical staff small, with each surgeon bearing a heavy workload and expected to be generalists. "Harelips to dislocated hips," one of the new hires in the 1940s recounted later in life, "[We] did everything."[38] When Alfred W. Farmer became surgeon-in-chief in 1956, the informal pre-war approach of a small number of surgeons performing a myriad of interventions became no longer tenable or even desirable. Farmer divided surgery into formalized divisions: neurological, genito-urinary, orthopaedic, general, and cardiac.[39] Each surgeon had to choose a specialty for his hospital work, though in their private practices many continued to perform a broader array of operations. Farmer recalls that, at the time, this policy "was most unusual in children's hospitals" and "was traumatic to them [his fellow surgeons] really. It upset some of them."[40] One of the younger surgeons to be introduced to the new system was William Mustard, who had trained as an orthopaedic surgeon, joined the surgical staff in 1947, and served as the attending physician at Thistletown in the early 1950s. He claimed that Farmer had told him "Well, make up your mind, are you going to be Chief of Orthopaedic Surgery or Chief of Cardiac Surgery? You can't be both."[41]

Mustard's choice of cardiac surgery was prescient, for these cases were emerging as an exciting new frontier of post-war surgery. An outpatient cardiac clinic had been created at The Hospital for Sick Children by 1920–1.[42] But there was, at the time, little to be done for the most serious cases. Put simply, there were two groupings of fatal or potentially fatal cardiac conditions. The first was congenital malformations of the heart, sometimes associated with genetic conditions. The other principal group involved patients with rheumatic heart disease, an autoimmune disease that causes the body's antibodies to attack vital organs instead of confronting invading bacteria. As Brown's medical reports of the time indicate, however, there was little in the way of effective treatment for either group despite the advances in the understanding of congenital cardiac disease pioneered by the Canadian Maude Abbott, among others.[43] Cardiac cases were given similar treatment to the chronic tubercular patients: home conditions were supervised, extra nourishment and rest prescribed, and some children sent to the Heather Club camp and even to Thistletown.[44] Rheumatic heart disease was a very serious condition that began in childhood and led to premature death; indeed, it constituted the second leading cause of death in Canadians aged ten to thirty-nine.[45] Children born with congenital cardiac malformations had an even worse prognosis: they were monitored and made comfortable until they died in infancy, childhood, or adolescence, depending upon the severity of the condition.

Heading the cardiac program at the hospital was the Scottish cardiologist John Keith. Keith embodied, in many respects, the characteristics associated with a certain generation of British-trained clinicians – overweening confidence, a military demeanour, and a certain intensity.[46] But Keith combined an old-school surgical superciliousness with a contemporary interest in the latest techniques of medical epidemiology. Along with George Smith, Alfred P. Hart, and Pearl Summerfeldt, he investigated rheumatic heart disease in a manner that would come to typify much of post-war research – the large scale epidemiological study. In 1948, in partnership with Toronto's Department of Public Health, some 75,000 Toronto children were examined. Over 1,000 children were referred for specialist examination, and Keith began to compile a massive registry including 423 patients with rheumatic disease and congenital malformations. It was, reputedly, the "largest data bank on inborn heart defects in the world."[47] A research associate remembers clearly Keith's "zebra" card system, where a patient seen by the cardiac clinic would have one patient file for the hospital and a separate checklist of medical characteristics on a striped sheet for research purposes.[48] Keith estimated that one-quarter of the cardiac clinic's patients had congenital heart disease, over one-third "rheumatic heart disease or a possible rheumatic infection," and one-third "murmurs or signs suggestive of heart disease [which were] ultimately proved to have entirely normal hearts."[49]

As the availability and use of sulfa drugs, and later penicillin, increased, the streptococcal infection underlying rheumatic heart disease could be easily treated provided cases were identified at an early stage.[50]

Buoyed by the sudden and effective solution to rheumatic cases, Keith and his team turned to the more problematic congenital cardiac malformations. There were attempts at surgical intervention over the previous decade, but surgery in infants was dangerous. There were many obstacles to overcome, including blood clotting during surgery, septic infection, and imprecise diagnosis.[51] Despite the overwhelming odds against success, surgeons began experimental operations on patients who were deemed to be "hopeless cases," those whose likelihood of survival was minimal or non-existent. In 1938, Robert Gross of Boston Children's Hospital completed the first corrective surgery for patent ductus arteriosus, an opening of the connection between the aorta and the pulmonary artery, the main vessel of the body and the main vessel of the lung, respectively. This opening was supposed to close at birth, but in some babies it remained open. The procedure was done for the first time in Canada, in Montreal, in 1940.[52] In 1944, Gross and Clarence Crafoord of Sweden developed procedures to ease coarctation of the aorta, "a congenital narrowing of a short segment of the aorta, which obstructs blood flow."[53] This latter condition inhibited proper blood flow, and thus circulation and oxygenation of the blood. Improperly or under-oxygenated blood would be recirculated throughout the body and cause cyanosis. The telltale signs of improperly oxygenated blood being pumped through the aorta to the rest of body were readily visible: children's lips, skin, and fingernails would appear blue. As a consequence, such cyanotic infants were widely referred to colloquially, at the time, as "blue babies."

The most common blue baby condition was tetralogy of Fallot,[54] a life-threatening anomaly involving heart abnormalities that impede proper blood circulation and oxygenation. Tetralogy of Fallot consists of four basic heart defects, including a ventricular septal defect (a defective wall between the ventricles), which permits unoxygenated blood to flow between the two heart chambers. The mix of oxygenated and unoxygenated blood then gets pumped to the body. At that time, fewer than a quarter of children born with tetralogy of Fallot ever reached adolescence. In Baltimore, surgeon Alfred Blalock and paediatric cardiologist Helen Taussig had inaugurated the era of paediatric closed-heart surgery by introducing a procedure to alleviate tetralogy of Fallot by use of a shunt to direct unoxygenated blood to the lungs.[55] Parents throughout North America immediately began to bring their affected children to Johns Hopkins for the potentially life-saving procedure.[56]

In Toronto, Gordon Murray was the first physician to begin performing closed-heart cardiac surgery on children and adults, for which he quickly achieved celebrity status. In the early 1930s Murray had been involved in the clinical development of heparin, a groundbreaking anticoagulant (a substance that prevents blood from clotting) which enabled the surgical reconnection of severed blood vessels. He began conducting vascular procedures on patients at the Toronto General Hospital in 1940. Like many leading surgeons of his era, he learned the Blalock-Taussig procedure in Baltimore, and operated on his first case at the Wellesley Hospital in 1946. His patient was a thirteen-year-old Toronto girl who survived the operation but died shortly thereafter.[57] Over the subsequent five years, Murray performed nearly 600 heart operations on patients of all ages. Families from around the country brought their terminally ill children to him, desperate for such a surgical fix. The Toronto General set aside six beds for his blue baby cases, an unusual situation, considering the inter-professional understanding that paediatric surgery would be centred at The Hospital for Sick Children.[58]

Later in life, William Mustard recalled that LeMesurier, the chief of surgery, approached him to say that John Keith had been "pestering him" about blue babies who were dying in oxygen tents at the hospital. Due to Mustard's battlefield experience operating on severed blood vessels, LeMesurier chose to send the young surgeon to Johns Hopkins to learn the new surgical technique.[59] After scarcely a month of training in Baltimore, Mustard returned to Toronto and began operating almost immediately. "When I got home," mused Mustard, "I sterilized the [instruction] book and took it into the operating room with me."[60] Meanwhile, Keith himself had visited Blalock with Arnold Johnson of the Montreal Children's Hospital following the war. Upon their return to Canada, both men established heart catheterization laboratories to enable more accurate diagnoses of heart malformations.[61] To further refine diagnosis, Keith, radiologist John Munn, and an electrical specialist developed a "diagnostic x-ray camera" to take serial X-ray plates of children. Blue babies were injected with iodine dye, and the camera captured its movements through the heart to facilitate more precise diagnosis.[62] As Gordon Murray began to focus more and more on adult cardiac surgery, Toronto's blue baby surgeries moved next door to the new Hospital for Sick Children on University Avenue with its state-of-the-art operating rooms.[63]

Paediatric cardiac surgery was extremely dangerous, with high rates of intraoperative and post-operative mortality. Several challenges confronted the surgeon, quite apart from the self-evident technical issues arising from the fragile state of underdeveloped newborns and the small size of the organ under manipulation. Blood, and the oxygen it transported to the body, needed to continue to circulate during the surgery, but surgeons could not

10.3 The advances in paediatric surgery required novel technical apparatuses. This photo shows an early example of an elaborate bypass machine that permitted blood to circulate and be oxygenated during cardiac surgery.

operate on a tiny heart pumping at full speed. To address this fundamental problem, surgical researchers began experimenting with ways to empty the heart of blood and to create a clearer operating field to perform surgical repair. One such technique, among many, explored in Toronto involved lowering the body's temperature, which would slow the heart and reduce the body's need for oxygen. Bring the body temperature low enough, and the surgical team could interrupt circulation and operate as quickly as possible on an open, but largely empty heart. The first successful "hypothermic" operation, as this procedure was called, was done in Minneapolis and the method was quickly taken on elsewhere.[64] In 1954, Toronto General surgeon Wilfred Bigelow, Mustard, and John Evans published their experiences operating on patients whose heart activity was suspended through induced hypothermia.[65] By that time, around two dozen patients had been operated upon for various conditions while in a hypothermic state, or as the *Toronto Star* popularized it (somewhat misleadingly), by "freezing" children's hearts.[66] The use of this early form of hypothermia was, however, short-lived, since few surgeons could accomplish the necessary operation in the under ten minutes necessary for these types of intracardiac operations.[67]

The successor to hypothermia was the employment of a bypass machine, so called because it would circulate blood and oxygen to the body while the heart was stopped during surgery and thus allow for intracardiac operations on an open heart emptied of blood. Blood would, in effect, bypass the heart in what contemporaries referred to, in the dryness of medical scientific terminology, as an "extra-corporeal" device. In 1949, Mustard, Chute, and engineer Campbell Cowan began work on an early version of the heart-lung bypass machine. Ultimately, Cowan designed the eponymous Cowan perfusion pump for artificial circulation. The pump "consisted of bulbs from blood pressure cuffs that were opened and closed by plates that squeezed them, mimicking the action of the heart muscle."[68] A prototype was even created by the federal government's Eldorado Company at Port

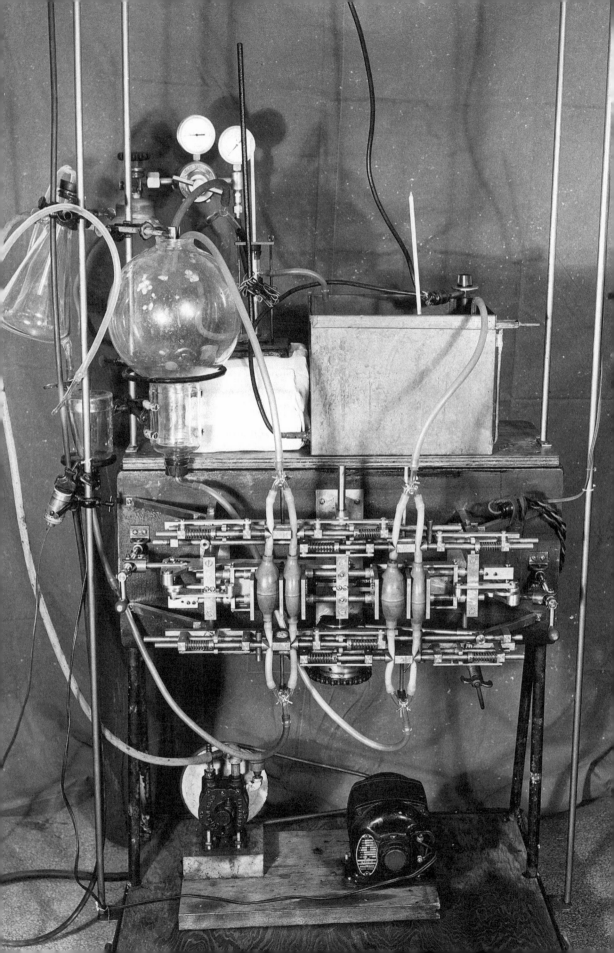

Hope with the aim of marketing it to hospitals throughout the continent.[69] Despite Cowan's early assertion that the pump worked "perfectly," however, the team's efforts ground to a halt when they could not resolve issues with the artificial blood oxygenator.[70]

Instead, the researchers turned to animal experimentation, using dogs' and monkeys' lungs as biological, rather than mechanical, oxygenators. Charles Best was drawn to the possibilities of their work and granted them space at the Banting Institute to conduct research.[71] In March 1949, Mustard successfully kept one dog alive using the Cowan perfusion pump and a lung (for example, oxygenation) from another dog.[72] Mustard's team carried out the same procedure on primates, using rhesus monkey lungs to oxygenate human blood. By 1951, Mustard and his team felt confident enough to make the leap to human surgical experimentation, and began to perform open-heart surgery on human patients. They successfully bypassed the heart and lungs of a human using the perfusion pump and monkey lungs.[73] Over the next few years, Mustard attempted experimental intracardiac procedures with the device. While his team demonstrated that the device functioned in a technical sense, mortality, however, remained very high. By 1954, Mustard had performed open-heart surgery using extracorporeal circulation on seven children aged nineteen days to two years. All seven infants had died, though some had lived for a few hours after the surgery.[74]

In this frontier of surgical experimentation, doctors identified "hopeless" patients whose condition rendered, in the medical world of the 1950s, the surgical trials professionally justified. For example, notwithstanding the fact that all seven infants had died during or shortly after surgery, Mustard and his colleagues concluded confidently, "We feel that this application of an extracorporeal circulation could be undertaken in less hopeless cases."[75] Sensitive to the potential criticism of what might be considered unnecessarily risky surgery, Mustard published an article in 1955 justifying the 25 per cent mortality rate for congenital cardiovascular surgery at The Hospital for Sick Children. He explained, somewhat defensively, that they did not refuse any patient "because of poor surgical risk," and accepted "moribund" patients as candidates:

> For example if one did not operate upon tetralogy of Fallot before three years of age the mortality figures would be much better for the surgeon but not for the patients, since a number would be dead before operation

was undertaken. We feel that in the infant any operative mortality which is less than 100% is certainly justifiable, since only those infants who would not live past their second or third year would be operated upon.[76]

Mortality, Mustard pointed out, was low for "uncomplicated cases" of patent ductus arteriosus; of a total of 176 operations, there was only one immediate death and one "later death." When all these cases were removed from the count, the mortality rate crept up to 37.5 per cent. In a few of these cases, he attempted an experimental technique to switch the main arteries of patients with "transposition of the great vessels," the second most common cyanotic heart malformation following tetralogy of Fallot. Transposition of the great vessels had been hitherto uniformly fatal: of twenty-nine cases recounted, there were twenty-five deaths, three late deaths, and one "trache-otomy ([still] alive?)."[77]

Still, amidst the gloomy outlook, parents of children with terminal conditions continued to give consent to these highly risky procedures, even though the surgeons enjoyed little success in 1955 and 1956. Indeed, in a 1957 published review of twenty-one cases of "open cardiotomy facilitated by extra-corporeal circulation," excluding transposition of the great arteries, only three were reported as "alive and well" at the time of publication. This rate of mortality, Mustard admitted, was such to augur against using the procedure with "good risk patients."[78] By this time, the death rate was taking a toll on Mustard himself. Later in life, he recalled how he loathed going to the Women's Auxiliary "quiet room" to deliver the inevitable bad news to parents:

We had a quiet room. God did I ever hate going into that quiet room. [One time] ... I had to go down and talk to his parents. I was crying so much. Call it a technical error, but it really wasn't a technical error. With the heart stopped still, you know, when you cut a piece of muscle out, and don't cut it out completely, and remove it, then sometimes you're in trouble like that ... God, when you operate on an infant that you thought was going to ... I'm talking about the first year of life – that you thought had every possible chance of survival, and the child for some unknown reason after the operation – it's happened to me twice – the heart has suddenly blown up ... but I had to see those parents. Oh Jesus, I hated it. And then you don't sleep at night. You go over and over the operations. I hated that, I ... hated it. Sleepless nights.[79]

By the closing years of the 1950s, however, mortality in complicated cases of congenital cardiac malformations began to decline.[80] By the late 1950s, researchers elsewhere in North America surmounted the problem of artificial oxygenation and began to report superior survival rates with new "bubble and membrane oxygenators."[81] These new mechanical heart-lung machines allowed surgeons to operate on an open heart for longer periods of time, permitting more complex procedures. With these new technical innovations, Mustard "abandoned his 'biological oxygenator,'" the monkey lung. According to his own account, he took home a bell jar that had held monkey lungs and turned it into a terrarium, which he kept at his summer cottage.[82]

The winter of 1956–7 appears to have been the turning point in cardiac surgery for Mustard. In 1956, he and his cardiac surgery team moved from their temporary set-up in the Banting Institute to "specially prepared facilities" in The Hospital for Sick Children. During their first year there, Mustard and his colleagues undertook work on the artificial heart-lung machine and possible approaches to correction of transposition of great vessels.[83] In 1957, Farmer introduced specialization, appointed Mustard as chief of cardiac surgery, and formalized the first paediatric cardiac surgery unit in Canada.[84] Mustard was joined by a second cardiac surgeon, George Trusler, the following year.[85] By this time, Mustard was performing cardiac operations on an almost daily basis.[86]

Surgical research necessitated more investment in space and personnel for animal care. In 1959, Research Institute Director R.R. Struthers called for the institute to invest more resources in surgical research.[87] The Animal House provided 3,050 square feet of space and accommodated an array of dark rooms, dressing rooms, operating theatres, refrigerated rooms, and a radioisotope laboratory.[88] The research also required a steady stream of animals upon whom to experiment. Prior to this, many animals were boarded "in the country."[89] In 1962, a "disastrous fire" at the boarding farm killed many of the animals, disrupting experimental research programs, including Mustard's.[90] The opening of the Gerrard Street wing of the hospital in 1964 afforded far more space for research, particularly neonatology, neurology, and cardiology, including Mustard's expanded operating theatres. Hospital researchers no longer had to trek to the Banting Institute to conduct certain components of their research; they could simply walk upstairs to the ninth floor of the new wing.[91]

As intracardiac operative mortality rates for tetralogy of Fallot began to decline in the final years of the 1950s, Mustard turned his attention to the even more dangerous congenital condition of children born with "transposition of the greater arteries." In this malformation, the aorta connects to the right ventricle and the pulmonary artery to the left, the reverse of their normal configuration. Oxygen-rich blood returns to the left atrium and the lungs, while oxygen-poor blood returns to the right atrium and the body. Like tetralogy of Fallot, untreated infants become cyanotic, and nearly all children born with this condition died before their first birthday. Sometimes accompanying defects allowed the blood on either side to mix, permitting some children to live for several years.[92] Ake Senning of Stockholm had introduced a procedure to correct the reversed arteries, but it was complex and had poor outcomes. Likewise, the surgeon Tom Baffes of Chicago devised a procedure to switch the veins, but it too was complex and had an "unacceptably high" mortality rate.[93]

After unsuccessfully attempting to correct the reversal of the arteries, and then to switch the veins rather than the arteries, Mustard thought laterally, by designing a technique to work with the existing deformity. He proposed inserting a "baffle" to transpose the two upper chambers to match the transposed chamber below, allowing the entire heart to, in effect, pump and circulate blood "backwards." Mustard described the procedure as an "Intra-atrial Transposition":

> because what you're doing is transposing the two atria to match the
> two ventricles which are already [congenitally] transposed ... And that's
> what you're doing is to match the transposition which is already there
> on the other side of the pumping chambers, you see. In other words,
> it's a silly expression but instead of the heart being half-ass backwards,
> you make it completely backwards.[94]

Mustard artificially created the condition and then tested the procedure on dogs, all of which died. He even built a five-foot plastic model of the atrial chambers with the baffle inside in an attempt to illustrate the conceptual approach to some skeptical colleagues. Regardless, the idea was difficult for others to comprehend, and Keith for one was very reluctant to approve it as an experimental procedure for humans.[95]

Keith finally permitted Mustard to try the experimental operation on Maria, who had been diagnosed as having transposition of the greater arteries and was a ward of the Children's Aid Society who had recently been taken in by foster parents in Whitby. A preliminary operation at two months of age established a hole between the left and right sides of her heart, allowing the vena side to mix. This preliminary procedure would buy her some time for her condition, which was terminal. Consensus at this time was to wait until the child was two years of age to engage in more extensive operations, but when the girl was nineteen months old her foster parents saw that she was deteriorating quickly, and Mustard convinced Keith to let him to try the theoretical procedure. Mustard completed the operation in a mere forty minutes. Speed was crucial as there was not much time on the pump. Looking at his finished work, Mustard temporarily forgot that he had reversed the organ; his first thought was "Oh my god, I've put it in upside down." The operation, however, was successful. Maria recovered with no post-operative issues and reportedly ran a mile a day as a young adult; fifty years later, she was still alive.[96]

Suddenly, the world of paediatric cardiac surgery had changed. After almost ten years of literally dozens of infants dying in experimental procedures on the operating table, Mustard had devised an operation which would subsequently, and quite literally, prolong thousands of lives over the next generation. The surgery was far from perfect, but thousands of children born with the fatal condition could live reasonably active lives well into adulthood, at which point a lifetime of pumping "backwards" often made them candidates for heart transplant surgery. The operation became known eponymously as the Mustard procedure, making Mustard one of the most celebrated paediatric cardiac surgeons of the twentieth century. When asked about the reasons behind the success of the operation, Mustard, known for his humour and pranksterism within the hospital, would simply retort, "you know, it is all rather ... [pause for effect] baffle-ing!"[97]

Premature Babies

The focus on terminal cardiac conditions in newborns led inevitably to a new interest in the status of premature babies. Paediatricians were well aware of the multiple physical and developmental problems associated with babies born before term, which at the time was defined as any baby born between twenty-six and thirty-two gestational weeks and with a birthweight of lower than 1500 grams. The medical approach to premature babies was a mix of sympathetic support for parents and a fatalistic resignation as the infants slowly succumbed to the "natural order of things." Prematures, not just at The Hospital for Sick Children, but elsewhere across the Western world, were often placed in a separate ward, or room, where they were left to die. Of course, those that showed signs of "thriving" would be supported and attended to, but the general approach was one of non-interventionism. Deaths of premature babies, however, was hardly trivial from an institutional standpoint: in absolute terms, 268 newborns perished in 1960 and 1961, constituting nearly half of all newborn admissions, and one-third of all annual deaths.[98]

The fatalistic attitude of doctors to premature babies began to shift in the middle of the twentieth century. A younger generation of practitioners began to question that wisdom of letting "nature take its course." The new paediatrician-in-chief, Laurie Chute, had a particular interest in newborns and the fact that so little research had been conducted into their causes of death. Chute brought over Paul Swyer, a young paediatrician doing a part-time research fellowship in child health at Great Ormond Street, to spearhead his research into oxygenation in premature infants. Swyer divided his time between the new ward – Ward 10A – for newborn babies, his research, and a part-time private practice. Swyer represented, along with Alice Goodfellow, a younger generation of fellows supported by the Research Institute of the hospital, which had been founded in 1954.

Swyer and the small group of neonatologists at the hospital confronted both a scientific and professional challenge. The professional obstacle lay in the fact that some of his more senior colleagues scoffed at the attention given to premature babies who would inevitably die. Many offered unsolicited critical comments on the ethical implications of helping a struggling premature baby, who would likely only face a long list of permanent disabilities if they survived. The scientific problem, by contrast, centred on the question of how to save the babies. The overwhelming majority of premature babies were succumbing to respiratory failure, a state that colleagues vaguely attributed to the status of being grossly below term weight. Swyer hypothesized that there were two central clinical challenges in the immediate hours after the birth of a premature baby: keeping the premature warm and providing immediate nutrition. He firmly believed that most premies were not succumbing to "natural causes" but rather, in fact, dying due to respiratory failure related to starvation. Yes, the immediate cause of death would be respiratory distress, but it was distress dramatically exacerbated by a lack of caloric intake. Deprived of nutrition, the premature baby's body was in fact feeding upon its own organs, hastening its demise. Swyer recalls vividly the protocol of premature babies born outside the children's hospital, either at home or at another medical institution, in the 1950s. The attending obstetrician or family physician would phone The Hospital for Sick Children, who would dispatch the hospital's "premature ambulance," if it was available. The premature baby would be placed in a wooden box and transported across town. By the time of arrival, some of the babies had already passed away; others were cold and malnourished.

Swyer and the hospital technician set about to build an incubator that could keep the premature infants warm while they were being transported to the hospital. At first, they could only build a small number of prototypes. They thus embarked on an ad hoc control trial: when the calls from the community came in, they randomly assigned premature babies to the existing wooden incubator or to the new, heated metal unit. When the children arrived at the hospital, "we looked at their blood gases, we looked at their survival rate, their condition on arrival."[99] They monitored survival rates over a six-month period and found that mortality rates halved for those in the new, heated units.[100] Armed with this data, the hospital approached the Ministry of Health, which agreed to fund a handful of the new incubators.

Manipulating the external and internal environments became key to re-establishing the homeostasis of the fragile underweight newborn. Oxygen tents and, of course, the iconic iron lungs for polio patients, had been an option within the hospital since the 1930s. Both cumbersome systems had been used to mediate the problems of respiration and insufficient oxygen flow. The polio epidemics of 1950 and 1952 provided recent examples of man-made respiratory assistance. The polio precedent would lead to experiments in mechanically assisted ventilation devices for prematures in 1962. In effect, the early neonatologists experimented with miniature iron lungs, using negative pressure to assist with ventilation for premature infants suffering from respiratory distress. Criticism would continue from colleagues, some of whom derisorily referred to the ward as "Swyer's vegetable patch." But by 1964, the senior staff had been convinced enough to dedicate its own Neonatal Unit (7G) as part of the new Gerrard Street Wing. Unsurprisingly, the neonatal unit worked closely with Mustard, Keith, and cardiology on the most fragile patients in the hospital, pushing the boundaries of what was considered to be the normal scope of paediatric practice and engaging with some of the most ethically and clinically challenging patients in the hospital.

Conclusions

The antibiotic revolution transformed medical care in general, and paediatrics in particular. Infant and childhood mortality had been on the decline from the 1920s, aided by public health initiatives that involved vaccination, improvements in personal hygiene, and infant nutrition programs. Such interventions, combined with a rising standard of living, helped reduce the prevalence of once dominant childhood diseases, such as rickets, diphtheria, and tuberculosis. Sulfa drugs, as well as vaccines for diphtheria, whooping cough, and scarlet fever, rendered many childhood killers diseases of the past. The Hospital for Sick Children became the epicenter of a virtuous circle of identification, prevention, and tertiary care, combining laboratory science, the public health department, and primary schools into a comprehensive approach to paediatric preventive care.[101] With such an arsenal of chemical interventions, childhood mortality continued its downward trajectory, and the average inpatient stay in the twenty-year period from 1939 to 1959 was cut in half, from fifteen days to eight days per patient.[102] Partly as a consequence of this and partly because of the baby boom, the annual number of admissions over the same period trebled, from 8,000 in the late 1930s to 25,000 by the end of the 1950s.[103]

The slow abatement of infectious diseases as the principal concern of paediatrics helped renew confidence in doctors' abilities to address more intractable congenital problems, such as the cardiac abnormalities of newborns and the respiratory and nutritional challenges of premature babies. Open-heart surgery, with its monkey lungs and frozen hearts, captivated the public's imagination and garnered international attention for Bill Mustard and The Hospital for Sick Children.[104] The life-saving technique was layered with dramatic moments and themes: the operation was performed on tiny infants and frail children whose hearts were stopped – and thus virtually dead – during the procedure, but within days of the operation children could be gallivanting about the hospital. As the journalist June Callwood summarized to an amazed public, the new era of experimental surgery

> requires a doctor to operate on persons who are neither living nor dead but in some spooky middle place plugged into a machine. There is one operation he does which is performed on dying 10-pound babies whose hearts are back to front, in which the infant is chilled, every drop of blood is drained, a heart little bigger than that of a chicken is connected properly, and then the blood is replaced and the baby warmed.[105]

Cultural tropes of inducing near-death through hypothermia and then bring-ing fragile infants back from the brink inevitably conjured up religious allusions and metaphors. Mustard, perhaps playing on the theological motifs redolent in much of the popular reportage around cardiac surgery, reputedly asked theologians "where the soul is during that hour" of operation.[106]

Surgical innovation also constituted a shifting ethical landscape of clin-ical intervention. Many infants and children perished on the operating table as a result of experimental therapies, their deaths justified since they were "hopeless" cases that would have otherwise died of their conditions. The high mortality rates of procedures to correct tetralogy of Fallot or transposition of the greater vessels would inevitably lessen, as surgeons learned "on the job" and developed experience over time. In this way, the deaths of the first generation of patients likely contributed to the survival of those who followed them into the operating room. Parents, informed that the high-risk surgeries were the only available option to save their dying child, were only too ready to consent. But this evaluation of risk was also informed by contemporary perceptions of social value and disability as understood at the time. As surgery became more effective in the 1960s, it was widely acknowledged that cardiac abnormalities commonly associated with congenital conditions – such as the high prevalence of tetralogy of Fallot in children born with Down Syndrome – were not selected for surgery. As one interviewee recalled, a senior surgeon, when faced with a Down Syndrome infant born with a potentially fatal cardiac condition, would often aver, "You know, you're a young couple, let nature take its course, and try again."[107]

By the early 1960s, The Hospital for Sick Children had become a leading international centre for the study and treatment of congenital health malformations.[108] As Edward Shorter has observed, three fundamental breakthroughs occurred in Toronto at mid-century which made it a renowned site for both paediatric and adult surgery: anticoagulation drugs, particu-larly heparin, pioneered by Gordon Murray; the successful canine cardiac bypass experiments of Mustard and Chute; and, finally, the use of hypo-thermia by Wilfred Bigelow.[109] Just as Toronto surgeons flocked to Johns Hopkins to learn the Blalock-Taussig procedure in the late 1940s, so too did a new generation of paediatric surgeons head to Toronto for the latest surgical techniques in the 1960s. Young clinicians from Germany and Swit-zerland, from Britain and Ireland, and from Australia and New Zealand streamed to Toronto in order to spend a year or two at the hospital. Over time, European and Commonwealth fellows would be joined by physicians from the Middle East, the Indian subcontinent, Africa, and the Far East. Their arrival would not only coincide with important scientific break-throughs but also reflect the influence of the hospital's Research Institute. They would arrive at a dynamic time in Canadian health care. Not only was paediatrics changing, but Canada itself was about to undergo a dramatic transformation in the way it organized and funded health services, as it stumbled towards universal Medicare.

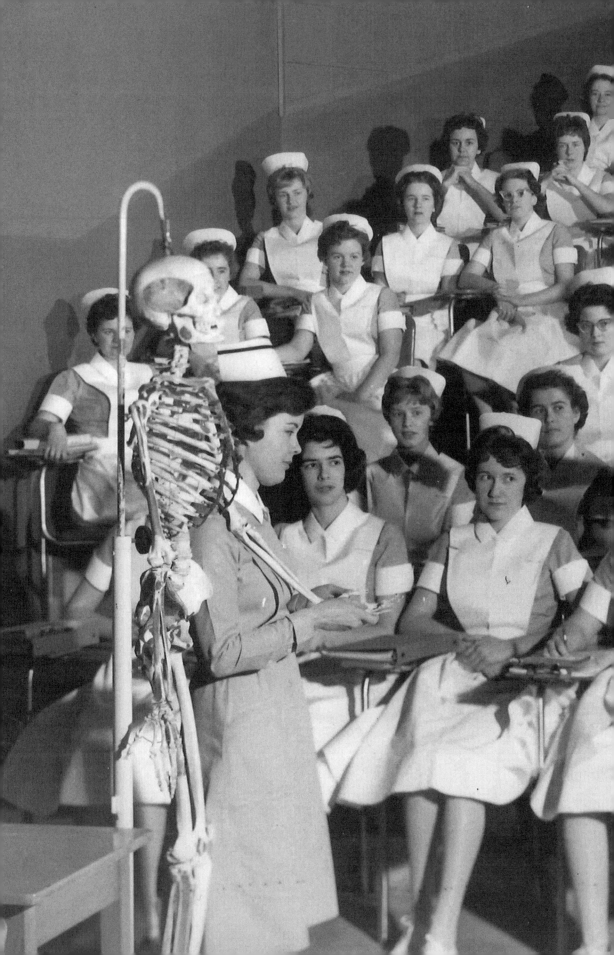

ELEVEN

A Sisterhood of Nursing

In 1958 we were frankly fearful we might lose our autonomy ... but
that fear never materialized. We're better off, in my opinion.[1]

Assistant Director Frank Hunnisett reflecting
on the advent of hospitalization insurance, 1967

When Tommy Douglas became premier of Saskatchewan in 1944, he positioned health care and free hospitalization as the centerpiece of post-war
reform in his adopted province. On the stump, he often invoked his own
childhood experience as a patient at the dawn of the First World War. Before
immigrating to Canada, he had suffered from osteomyelitis of the knee.
Although he had been operated on several times in his native Scotland, the
condition recurred shortly after the family arrived in Winnipeg, leading to
a new and longer hospital admission. At this time, Douglas was a "ward"
(that is public, non-fee-paying) patient. He recalled the perfunctory attention he received from staff physicians who informed his parents that his leg
would likely need to be amputated. As the story goes, a senior orthopaedic
surgeon took an interest in his case, believing the boy represented an excellent teaching possibility for the rounding surgical
students. Given the choice between amputation and
experimental surgery by a senior orthopod, the parents chose the latter. The surgeon operated three
times, for free, and was delighted when the surgery
ultimately proved successful.[2]

For Douglas, this life-changing hospital encounter
was a bittersweet insight into poverty and ill-health,

11.1 The 1960s and 1970s witnessed
the ascendance of college- and
university-based nursing programs,
which nursing leaders hoped would
be defined more by the education –
rather than the free labour – of
students. The nursing school class of
1963 is pictured here with instructor
Carol Ward.

for his working-class father had no insurance and it was only by chance that Tommy had kept his leg. As he grew into a young preacher and then politician, this personal story of paediatric care evolved into a moral parable: "I lay in a children's hospital in Winnipeg on and off for three years," he recalled in the legislature: "The only reason I can walk today, Mr. Speaker, is because a doctor doing charity work ... took an interest in my case."[3] To drive home the point, he concluded, "I felt that no boy should have to depend either for his leg or his life upon the ability of his parents to raise enough money to bring a first-class surgeon to his bedside ... I came to believe that health services ought not to have a price-tag on them, and that people should be able to get whatever health services they required irrespective of their individual capacity to pay."[4]

Under Douglas, Saskatchewan introduced hospital care insurance for all citizens, covering "standard ward level with no limitation on entitlement days as long as in-patient care was medically necessary."[5] The provincial plan included X-ray and laboratory services, as well as some common drugs, and even reimbursed residents a per diem amount towards the cost of "out-of-province" hospitalization. There were annual individual premiums of $5 ($30 per family).[6] All Saskatchewan residents had, in effect, "free" access to hospital care. Douglas, of course, was hardly working in a vacuum. During the war years, governments across Canada had been greatly influenced by what was going on in Britain, particularly the discussions leading up to the Beveridge Report (1942) which, among many other things, laid the plans for the post-war British National Health Service. With thousands of Canadian men and women serving in Britain during the war, and the civilian population at home being asked to sacrifice for the greater good of the country, it was inevitable that these ideas about state-run health insurance would recirculate in Canada. However, the then Liberal government in Ottawa trod gently on an issue that was considered the constitutional responsibility of provinces. Ultimately, in 1940, a Royal Commission on Dominion-Provincial Relations (the Rowell-Sirois Commission) recommended a federally sponsored health insurance system, but the wartime proposal died in infancy, a victim of provincial-federal wrangling. Douglas decided to go it alone.[7]

It is easy to forget the multiple interests that rallied against the early years of "socialized medicine" in Canada. Many will be familiar with the resistance of the medical profession, whose members feared becoming glorified civil servants working in an environment where fees, clinical interventions, and location of practice would be dictated by a faceless bureaucracy. A second anxiety, one more directly relevant to this book, concerned the independence of hospitals themselves, some of which had important denominational cultures and community support, such as the dozens of Catholic, and a smaller number of Jewish, institutions. Hospital Trustees across the country were only too aware that the creation of the National Health Service in Britain (which took effect in 1948) had been accompanied by the nationalization of all but a small handful of elite research institutions. Hospitals in Britain dating back two hundred years found themselves directly under the control of local health authorities. The voluntary system, described in the early chapters of this book, had come to an abrupt end.[8]

Within this passionate political debate, the free hospitalization of sick children in Canada occupied a complicated position. As described in previous chapters, children were already under surveillance by a range of medical and paramedical professionals paid by the state – school nurses, public health doctors, and educational psychologists. Indeed, vaccinations for measles, diphtheria, whooping cough, and mumps would become a memorable part of the school year for younger children, despite opposition from some religious groups. One could argue that public health interventions involving children became normative and widely accepted by the 1950s. In this way, municipal initiatives, from pasteurization to vaccination, had already validated the role of the state in the care of children. *Free* hospitalization, however, proved somewhat more controversial. It represented, to some skeptics, the thin end of the wedge, the first step towards a more sinister future in which the state controlled all of medical practice.

Nevertheless, the political wind was blowing in a particular direction. Provincial ministers of health were all too cognizant of the repeated majorities that Douglas and his Cooperative Commonwealth Federation (CCF) party had garnered in the late 1940s and 1950s, riding the wave of popularity that provincial health insurance enjoyed. Meanwhile, at the federal level, the post-war Liberal government had begun to assemble a range of entitlement programs that would form the backbone of the Canadian welfare state. For example, in 1944 the federal Family Allowance Act was introduced, which paid families a monthly amount per child under sixteen. The allowance was one very tangible example of how the government was intervening to help families care for young children.[9] The Progressive Conservative federal government of John Diefenbaker jumped on the populist bandwagon by implementing the Hospital Insurance and Diagnostic Services Act (HIDS) in 1958. This long-forgotten piece of legislation committed the federal government to reimburse provinces for 50 per cent of the cost of hospitalization and diagnostic services for designated common illnesses.[10] HIDS followed the pattern so common in post-war welfare state planning in Canada. In areas of provincial jurisdiction, the federal government dangled financial carrots by way of enabling legislation. In this way, provinces could receive substantial annual federal grants in return for following the general principles outlined in the act. The legislation did not *oblige* the participation of individual provinces, but rather promoted national policy objectives by making the provinces an offer few, if any, could refuse.

Hospital insurance was a case in point. Faced with a federal offer to pay 50 per cent of spiralling hospital costs, Ontario moved inexorably towards hospital insurance between 1956 and 1959. It began in 1956 with the establishment of an independent Ontario Hospital Services Commission to investigate and report on the issue of hospital insurance in the province. This was followed quickly by the 1957 Hospital Services Commission Act, which expanded the authority of the Hospital Services Commission to create a basic hospital insurance plan "without regard to age, financial circumstances or condition of health."[11] In 1959, the provincial legislature introduced a Hospital Insurance Plan, following the principles of HIDS, which permitted the flow of federal co-payments. By the close of 1960, over 94 per cent of the population was enrolled.[12] Thus, within a short period of time, the Ontario government had become the only provider of standard ward hospital insurance in the province. Henceforth, Blue Cross and other insurance companies offering health insurance were restricted to offering semi-private accommodation benefits and extended health benefits for employee groups. Malcolm Taylor, the doyen of the history of Medicare in the country, suggested that the fact that a reluctant Ontario adopted universal hospital insurance, "tipped the scales" for the federal hospital insurance program, allowing it to succeed from coast to coast.[13]

Needless to say, the advent of provincial insurance for hospitalization in the late 1950s had a profound impact on the daily operations and financing of hospitals across the country, including Toronto's Hospital for Sick Children. Many leaders in Toronto feared a complete takeover of the hospital by the provincial government, including the confiscation of Robertson's substantial legacy of and the royalties from inventions such as Pablum.[14] In his column in the hospital newsletter, *Paediatric Patter,* John Law,

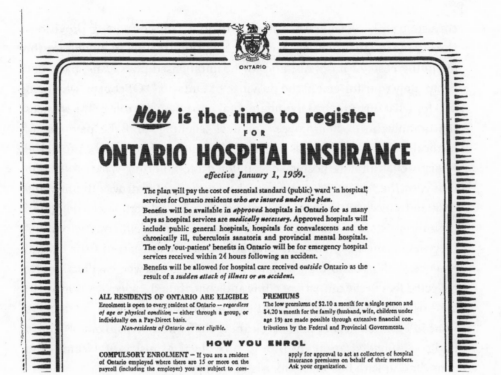

the director of The Hospital for Sick Children, sought to contain community anxieties that the hospital was being annexed by the government by characterizing the Ontario Hospital Services Commission (OHSC) in business terms, as the "largest customer" of the hospital. He may be accused of a rhetorical sleight of hand. By 1960, the OHSC was responsible for 94 per cent of the hospital's total annual inpatient revenue (approximately $5 million).[15] In a strict legal sense, the hospital remained independent of the government, but in what was increasingly a "single-payer" system, it would be drawn inexorably into the orbit of the state and its changing political priorities and fiscal fortunes.

11.2 In 1957, the federal government, sensing the growing popularity of public health insurance, agreed to co-fund hospital and diagnostic services. Here, the Government of Ontario encourages residents to register for the new system.

In 1966, the federal government of Lester B. Pearson passed the Medical Care Act, which followed the pattern of previous welfare legislation by offering cost-sharing for all medically necessary services, whether in hospitals or in the community. Provinces were required to abide by four principles: public administration of health insurance, portability between participating provinces, universality of coverage, and comprehensiveness of medical services. Three years later, Ontario introduced legislation consistent with the federal act in order to access the co-funding provisions. During the decade from 1959 to 1969, then, the structure of paying for the operating costs of hospitals, and for hospital-based physicians, had been completely transformed in the province of Ontario.[16] Of course, who paid, and for what services, had a fundamental impact on the role of the trustees, the organization of employees, clinical teaching, and the payment of medical staff. For example, as the money began to roll in from the provincial Ministry of Health, the hospital encountered a conundrum: What proportion, if any, of the fees owed to hospital-based medical staff was the hospital entitled to receive? The vast majority of the medical staff, including all of the surgical staff, continued to be, in effect, independent contractors, but they were using hospital space and infrastructure for part of their clinical practice. Within the hospital, a compromise was reached wherein practitioners collected fees in the outpatient clinic and contributed a specified portion to the hospital. Meanwhile, salaried staff – nurses, technicians, researchers, some full-time clinicians, porters, cleaning staff – were all paid out of "global budgets" decided annually by the provincial Ministry of Health after consultation with hospitals' boards of trustees.[17]

"It was our school for which we grieved"

As the building blocks of what Canadians now call Medicare were put into place, government planners and university administrators were faced with a growing crisis in health care personnel. In no realm was this felt more acutely than nursing. On a superficial level, the complement of nurses in Canada appeared to be healthy and growing steadily at mid-century. The number of registered nurses had expanded dramatically from 27,853 in 1941 to 78,340 in 1961, a faster rate of growth than the general population.[18] And yet many hospitals in the country appeared to be experiencing persistent personnel shortages, not only in rural settings but also in the principal urban centres. This paradox arose, in part, as a response to the emerging popularity of these new provincially run and publicly funded medical services and the growing emphasis on hospital-based care, which was more often than not based in urban centres. Put simply, HIDS had the impact of *encouraging* expensive hospital-based care, since it would ultimately be subsidized by the federal government.

In 1962, the Canadian Nurses Association (CNA) prepared a submission to the Royal Commission on Health Services (Hall Commission, 1961–4), which had been established by the federal government in Ottawa to investigate the possibility of federally supported, but provincially administered, universal health insurance. The CNA recommended not only a call for more trained personnel, but also better education for nursing students. This implied fundamental nursing education reform, whereby all nursing programs would be transferred to "designated educational facilities" – that is universities and community colleges. The stated concern was one of educational resources and access to new medical technologies, but lurking beneath the surface was a preoccupation among nursing leaders that hospitals were exploiting student labour at the expense of their clinical education.[19] At the time, the director of The Hospital for Sick Children responded internally to media criticism that hospital schools of nursing were inefficient, overly regimented, and housed students in "prison-like" dormitories.[20] In the wake of recommendations to move nursing training programs into university and college settings, deliberations ensued about what to do about The Hospital for Sick Children's own program. In 1968, a planned merger between the Toronto General Hospital's and The Hospital for Sick Children's nursing schools was floated, "caus[ing] much unrest within the [Nursing] School and Hospital proper." In response to the pushback, the hospital trustees initiated an investigation, led by University of Toronto's Abbyann Lynch. The final report, submitted to the trustees in December 1970, proposed closing the nursing school and transferring the program to an educational institution (Ryerson) in line with government recommendations of the time.[21]

The trustees, however, sensing the unpopularity of closing down the nursing school, ultimately voted to reorganize the program and continue to manage it in-house. The curriculum was changed from the "2+1" model to a two-year program for the students entering in 1968 and 1969, and the number of affiliated schools from outside Toronto was reduced to two. The new hospital curriculum had a stronger science foundation, modified entrance standards, and an approach that was less didactic and charged the student with personal responsibility for their learning – students were no longer acting as quasi-staff members, but rather as full-time students. The turquoise one-pieces that replaced the classic bib and apron were worn only for clinical experience, which was reduced and staggered over the course of the program.[22] Yet, the foot-dragging of the hospital would ultimately be overtaken by provincial fiat. In an effort to churn out more nurses through two-year programs, Ontario's Ministry of Health and Ministry of

Colleges and Universities decided to compel the transfer of nursing education to colleges of applied arts and technology as of September 1973. The hospital's internal staff publication, *What's New*, announced that the school of nursing "appear[ed] doomed."[23] In September 1973, The Hospital for Sick Children's, Wellesley's, and Women's College Hospital's nursing schools were transferred to Ryerson Polytechnic Institute, while the Nightingale's, Toronto Western Hospital's, St Joseph's, St Michael's, and Toronto General Hospital's schools of nursing were consolidated at George Brown College. The last nursing class of The Hospital for Sick Children to receive the pin and diploma was that of 1974. The class of 1975 began at the hospital and then relocated to Ryerson for their final year of training. As the alumnae association recalled, "Although HSC was only one of 56 hospital and regional Schools of Nursing to be closed, it was our school for which we grieved."[24]

"How to grow up in one hell of a hurry!"[25]

The closing of the nursing school at The Hospital for Sick Children in 1973 constituted the end of an important chapter in the history of the hospital, one replete with a vibrant subculture of nurse training that was deeply entwined with the University Avenue institution of the 1950s and 1960s. The epicentre of that culture was residence life, at a time when the overwhelming majority of student nurses were young, female, single, and lived onsite. Those that married were not permitted to complete the program. Indeed, given the young age at which women married in the 1950s, it is not surprising that Canadian nursing programs suffered an attrition rate of almost 20 per cent.[26] Whether due to changing social customs, or the emerging nursing shortages of the late 1950s, a liberalization of the policy occurred in the 1960s. Until January 1959, nurses were not allowed to marry until three months after completing the program. It was hoped that "consider[ing] each case individually on its merits and subject to certain rules" would help prevent the number of "secret marriages" that were proliferating. Of course, the hospital would insist that these marriages could only occur when the "approval of the parents ha[d] been obtained."[27]

Students from the 1950s remember common reasons for choosing the training school, namely, the love of children or a desire to carry on a family tradition of nursing. Many students came from outside of Toronto, including twenty-nine of thirty-seven graduates of the class of 1950, the last class to train entirely at 67 College Street.[28] This was perhaps in keeping with an overall trend of drawing students from the countryside, where women had fewer options for full-time employment. As one nurse, who graduated in 1960, recalled, "There were not many choices. You became either a teacher, a nurse or a secretary."[29]

Student nurses, graduate nurses, affiliating students, nurses' assistants, and ward aides resided in the overcrowded principal residence at 221 Elizabeth Street and seven additional temporary buildings, mainly converted houses. Students remember the "questionable characters" who lurked in the alley between the residences at 82 and 84 College Street in order to catch a glimpse of the young women. One nurse recalls that the women resorted to dropping water balloons from the upper floors in order to dissuade peeping Toms, though most soon learned to keep the blinds fully closed.[30] The first unit of the new Elizabeth McMaster Residence eventually opened in March 1952. Connected to the hospital by a tunnel, it featured accommodation for 175 student nurses, primarily in single rooms. The building also included an infirmary, a first-floor lounge, and sitting rooms and kitchenettes on each floor. Further renovations, completed in the fall of 1960, expanded the capacity to 300 rooms. Notwithstanding the improved residence, one nurse recalled, "[t]he worried look on my parents' faces when they dropped me off at our residence in September 1957, upon seeing the rundown houses, messy street and questionable characters roaming on Elizabeth Street."[31]

The intensity of living, eating, sleeping, and working together engendered lifelong ties and what has been described as the "sisterhood of nursing," an interesting turn of phrase given the ecclesiastical origins of many nursing orders. With no family nearby for support, fellow students and classmates helped each other through the "good days and the bad." Many of the memories from the post-war nurses' residence have been captured in oral histories, where retired nurses remember, among so many other things, the constant smell of toast, the struggle with uniforms, and even the formula for the best suntanning oil. The young women played bridge and euchre during free time, and recalled that the residence telephones were mainly used to speak with young men. In the school's final years, strict curfews and social regulation gave way to the honour system in which students were required only to sign in and out, and a handful of married students even "lived out." Graduate nurses were sources of support for students when the latter "felt their hearts would often burst with the suffering of their patients."[32] The fact that most senior nurses and instructors were graduates of the same nursing school strengthened the shared culture and community, one that was nurtured by a strong hospital alumnae association and even by family and kin connections. By the association's count, there were four sets of twins and thirty pairs of mothers and daughters among the thousands of graduates.[33]

Nurses' recollections of ward experiences often reflect a tension in the apprenticeship system of nurse training alluded to above – the hospital's need for labour and the school's commitment to education.[34] The tangible result was an immediate, and at times unsettling, introduction to life on the ward. "Our first visit to the patients was a disaster," one nurse remembered vividly, "[since] [m]any students were mentally unprepared."[35] Nurses recalled that they were given huge amounts of responsibility for patient care, often emphasizing their own youth and inexperience. "[W]orking with preemies in isolettes and worrying about whether they were alive," she retold, "and tapping on the tops of the isolettes to see if they were still breathing. I can't believe the responsibility we were given. I guess it was a good thing we were too naïve to realize it."[36] Some recalled years later the terror of being on the wards for the first time: "My first report as a new student on Infants 4D said I was unenthusiastic – heck I was just scared stiff!"[37] Others believe, in retrospect, formal support for nurses to handle traumatic experiences was in short supply. One graduate who returned as a "yellow daffodil" volunteer nurse while pregnant retold that "I was asked to special [sic] a new admittance still unconscious ... I will never forget my shock at seeing cigarette burns on the body and rope burns on wrists and ankles. I finished the shift, but not without throwing up in a waste basket. I now knew then why I could never go back – I just couldn't cope with ongoing pain and suffering among children. Even today, stories of child abuse still bring back the image of that little boy."[38]

At mid-century, formality and "respect for seniority" pervaded all relations; in keeping with the time, individuals were always addressed by their surname. The training school imposed military-like discipline and strictly observed the medical and nursing hierarchy. One graduate and veteran of the Second World War proclaimed, perhaps with some degree of embellishment, that the training "was never as strict in the Army as it was at The Hospital for Sick Children."[39] As the historian of nursing Kathryn

McPherson observes, this gendered, hierarchical "family" structure was common to most Canadian hospitals at mid-century.[40] Nursing students "soon learned that senior doctors expected a great deal of respect, even if we were doing charts we were sharply reprimanded" for not rising in their presence.[41] These ritual observances were encoded in the rules of the nursing school, as evidenced by a typed list of instructions on "professional etiquette" given to first-year nursing students, called "probationers," ca. 1938–41:

1. Always stand erect when spoken to.
2. If any member of the Office Staff, graduate, doctor or capped nurse enters the room where you are, remain standing until he or she leaves or tells you that you may sit down.
3. Never go through a door or enter elevator without looking to see who is behind you, and if one senior to you, allow her to enter or leave first ...
6. Realize that everyone entering the school before you is your senior, and show them her due courtesy.
7. Do not question authority, do what you are told by anyone in authority and never argue.
8. Sleeves must not be rolled up, only turned back, pull them down quickly if any of the Office Staff, graduate [or] Doctor speaks to you ...
13. If the head nurse is making rounds with the Superintendent or Doctor, do not interrupt her, go to the Senior Nurse for information.
14. If a staff Doctor or Staff Nurse is wanted at the telephone, speak to the head nurse or whoever is in charge ...
16. If any of the Office Staff, graduate or Doctor comes on the ward, find the nurse in charge at once.[42]

The document was accompanied by a handwritten note, presumably written by a student, which added, for good measure, "If any graduate or doctor is coming up or down stairs stop on stairs or landing until they have passed."[43]

Former nurses attest to the reciprocal respect on the wards, especially towards physicians. Yet, while nurses described the doctor-nurse relationship as "teamwork," it was a team divided by strict roles and observance of a professional, gendered hierarchy. That the nurses' role was parallel to that of a woman in the domestic sphere was stated explicitly by the revered head of nursing, Jean Masten, who reminded student nurses that "this is your house and you are the hostess. Treat each visitor as your guest."[44] As one former nurse explained, working relations varied from individual to individual. Doctors were "predominantly male," and

> It was the day when a staff man or a resident came on the floor, you hopped to your feet, you gave them your chair. It was "Yes doctor, no doctor, three bags full doctor," whatever the doctor said. And you learned the ones that you could ask questions and learn from, and the ones that you couldn't, and who didn't have the time, or the interest or the inclination. You learned more from the residents. As you worked there for a little while, you ended up teaching the interns because there was so much they didn't know ... And you never ever stayed sitting at a desk ... [If] you were sitting at a desk when a staff doctor came to the floor, you had better get to your feet, and you had better get the cardex and you better know what you're talking about when he wants to see his patients.[45]

While some doctors shared their knowledge, others were difficult to work with, and at times harassed or belittled nurses:

> There were the few doctors who had God complexes, if you want to put it that way ... [There were also] the ones who were very humbled by what they were able to do and were willing to talk to you about it. They would be willing to answer your questions and help you learn and the benefits of some of the things that they were doing. And that was amazing. There were the ones who, you know, made advances to a lot of the RNs [registered nurses] and thought that they were God's gift to the female population, if you want to put it that way. And you soon learned which doctors you didn't want to be in a room with alone. If you were doing rounds with particular doctors, you didn't go there by yourself.[46]

Certainly, in memoirs and recollections, nurses identified some individual surgeons as callous and prone to outbursts. One nurse recalled being "stunned in amazement," as she watched a doctor "hurl an instrument across the operating room, hitting the tile wall."[47] Another remembered being struck across the knuckles because she had dared to arrange instruments on his high stand.[48] Some recollections allude to bullying behaviour, upbraiding nurses who dared to cough or hiccup in the operating room.

Operating rooms were remembered as particularly trying sites for nurse trainees. One graduate recalled her terror upon scrubbing for the first time for an emergency appendectomy: "I thought, *Oh, dear God, protect me!* Anyways down in there, trembling in my boots, and set up for the appendectomy and thought, *How am I going to get through this?* And I practically had nervous diarrhea I think. It was terrible. But anyways he [former Surgeon-in-Chief Wansbrough] was absolutely wonderful and it was easy as pie."[49] Another remarked that while "My operating room rotation indicated to me that I was not 'cut out' for this kind of nursing ... Dr. Mustard joined me on the gantry. He drew pictures of his surgery to help me understand it."[50] Numerous former staff mentioned his supportiveness: "[Mustard] asked me, 'Do you want to feel a Patent Ductus before I close it?' He explained, 'It will feel like water cascading over rocks in a brook' ... [and] it did."[51] Staff have spoken of a culture shift from the Alan Brown era – the time of "the man in the Great White Coat" – to that of A.L. Chute. One long-time Women's Auxiliary member described Brown as "someone you were scared to death of mostly. I mean everyone was scared of him ... Dr. Brown was not approachable at all ... when [he] came on the floor you just felt like Lord High Commissioner had appeared you know, [the head nurses] had to have his coat hung up and everything ... Oh he never did anything for himself, he just ... people kowtowed to him."[52] One colleague "reported that when [Alan Brown and Surgical Chief Dr. D.E. Robertson (d.1944)] entered a ward it was 'like the arrival of God and Jesus Christ.'"[53]

Although one nurse recalled that, with all of the regulations, she was "convinced [she] had entered a nunnery,"[54] the 1950s and 1960s were actually decades of change for nurses and nurse trainees. Much of the liberalization was brought about by long-standing Director of Nursing Jean Masten, who held the position for over two decades before retiring in June 1961. Masten, who is regarded with universal praise in documentary sources, had guided the design and organization of the new hospital and residence building. Under her leadership, the school did away with the three-year contract which students had previously been required to sign, as well as eventually eliminating the morning assembly and prayers after breakfast. Following the example of several other schools, she eventually ended the cap-less six-month "probationary period" to reduce the stigma, and in 1953, students began wearing caps upon beginning at school.[55] Masten brought in the first coloured staff uniform, a "blue multi-buttoned and stiff collared military type uniform for administrative and education staff members," the wearing of which was later also extended to student and graduate nurses.[56] A series of social rituals, including quarterly parties, mother's graduation teas, and father's day banquets, marked a student's advancement through the program, a progression that was symbolized by the adornment of uniforms. At the end of the first year, the school crest was added to the sleeve. At the end of the second year, students exchanged black stockings and shoes for white, acquired the school pin and a blue band on their cap, and, as one student recalled, engaged in the ritual of "stringing black stockings and shoes in a long line and parading through the internes' quarters. We tied them to their bedroom doorknobs while they slept."[57] At long last, students obtained a black band on their cap and attended graduation ceremonies that were traditionally held at University of Toronto's Convocation Hall. Student nurse uniforms later changed from all-white with apron and bib to a one-piece turquoise uniform, and staff nurses adopted one-pieces in other pastel shades.[58]

The uniformity of the dress code and regulations was subtly reinforced by the common ages and cultural backgrounds of many of the recruits. Graduation photos show a sea of white women with Anglo-Saxon names. This was a reflection in part, of course, of the demographic from whence the hospital drew its population. However, historical research has also demonstrated that black nurses, like Jewish nurses a generation before them, were effectively excluded from the major hospitals in Toronto before the mid-1950s, despite the sizeable African-Canadian population in Ontario that existed since the time of Underground Railroad. In response to the nursing shortage emerging in Canada, nursing experience was added to the "exceptional merit" clause of the federal Immigration Act of 1952, which permitted "non-traditional" immigrants to enter Canada to work in occupational areas facing significant labour shortages. This change allowed African-Caribbean nurses to begin to migrate to Canada in the 1950s, often after receiving training in Britain. Many Canadian young women of African descent who had been born and raised in Ontario were forced to travel to the United States for nurse training.[59] Graduating class photographs of The Hospital for Sick Children, while incomplete, indicate that the school graduated about one "visible minority" student nearly every year during the 1960s out of a class that, by that time, exceeded 150. The first African-Canadian graduate of the nursing school at The Hospital for Sick Children appears to have been Elizabeth Harrison, in 1965. A picture of her trying

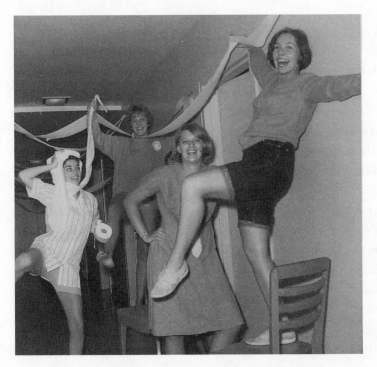

11.3 This personal photo of senior nurses preparing to welcome nurse trainees captures, in a small way, the rich culture of nursing life that was an indelible part of the hospital until the Nursing School was closed in 1973. From left to right: Martha (Douglas) Kowal, Judy (Cole) Nesbitt, Dee (Schuster) Cavanagh, Margaret (Farquhar) Garber.

on a cap, with a Women's Auxiliary member, while she was a trainee was shown in the *Globe and Mail*.[60]

Miriam Gibson directed the nursing school for thirty-five years before retiring in 1962, by which time her teaching staff had grown to twenty-two.[61] The post-war curriculum conformed to the requirements of the provincial Council of Nurse Education, formalized in 1953. Applicants to the school "were required to be in good physical and mental health, and hold a secondary school graduation diploma with the required science option."[62] The first six months were a pre-clinical introduction to basic nursing practices. Students rotated through the hospital on a "Block System," which included the operating room for six to eight weeks, the diet kitchen for two weeks, and the outpatient department for four to six weeks. During a month-long "Senior Duty," students learned ward administration from the head nurse and department instructor. The curriculum consisted of 1,200 to 1,400 hours of lectures over a three-year period, including classes on microbiology, pharmacology, nutrition, and biochemistry. Student nurses from nineteen other Ontario hospitals gained paediatric nursing experience through twelve-week rotations. Hospital for Sick Children nurses also affiliated with other hospitals to obtain experience with adult, psychiatric, obstetric, and tuberculous patients. For example, students went to Toronto General for adult care (eight weeks), either the Toronto General or Women's College for obstetrics (sixteen weeks), and either the Toronto Psychiatric Hospital or St. Thomas Ontario Hospital for psychiatric care (twelve weeks). Public health experience was obtained through the city health department or the Victorian Order of Nurses. As of January 1960, students could avail themselves of an optional rotation at Red Cross outpost hospitals.[63] At the old College Street hospital, the training school was located within the residence itself. In the new building,

> [t]he nursing education department was located in the Hospital proper. The philosophy supporting this change in location had to do with the belief that the integration of classroom and clinical experiences could be more readily achieved if the school were part of the Hospital. Several class-rooms and a large well-equipped demonstration room constituted the Department.[64]

The opening of the Gerrard Street Wing in 1964 added a floor for nursing education, making space for a library, classrooms, and teachers' offices. These expanded facilities reflected the size of the nurse training school, which increased dramatically in the 1950s and 1960s. The student body as a whole grew from around 100 in the pre-555 years to around 150 in the 1950s and 180 in the 1960s. The province-wide expansion of nursing schools is readily visible in the increase in affiliating students, from just over 600 to 800 or 900 by the end of the 1950s, peaking at 950 in the 1963–4 academic year.[65] Yet, despite the dramatic increase in size of the nursing school, the hospital, like many medical institutions of the time, struggled constantly with personnel shortages and retention throughout this period.

Administrative Leadership

During this period of rapid growth and transition to hospital insurance, John T. Law became the hospital's first professional administrator, taking the helm from J.T.H. Bower, who had retired in 1957 after thirty years at the hospital. Originally from Rochester, New York, Law was a former public health lecturer and administrator at Yale-New Haven Medical Centre. Law was recruited to act as director, a position formerly known as superintendent, by J. Grant Glassco, the chairman of the board, and brought with him two decades of experience in American hospitals. Law served as the first executive director from 1967 to 1970, leaving to pursue a master's in health administration at the University of Toronto and returning as vice chair of the board of trustees in July 1971 with responsibility for long-range planning. He left this position in order to establish The Hospital for Sick Children Foundation, of which he became president in 1972. Law understood modern hospitals as comparable to "big business," and the chief administrator to the president of a corporation, though he admitted that medical staff "are not employees of the hospital in the same sense that people working for most corporations are."[66] As described by Claus Wirsig, Law's fellow administrator, Law's vision for the institution "developed and acquired an outward-looking thrust that few [could] match anywhere."[67] Law was a new class of manager for a new era of state health insurance, the head of what was often being described as the largest children's hospital in the world.[68]

Law preoccupied himself with modernizing the relationship between the hospital and its staff, who were notoriously poorly paid. In the early years of the new hospital on University Avenue, the hospital set up a personnel office and thereafter introduced pensions and group insurance, Blue Cross insurance, the Quarter Century Club for long-time employees, salary and wage scales, a hobby fair, and an employee health unit. By March 1962, he boasted that 738 staff members were in the pension plan and 582 had joined the group life insurance plan. Law continued to seek improvements, such as instituting a forty-hour work week. "The status and remuneration of the hospital worker have improved greatly in recent years," he affirmed in *Paediatric Patter*, "with comparable pay for types of work, compared to other industries."[69] Reflecting provincial trends, of the nearly 2,000 individuals on payroll in the early 1960s, around one-third were nursing staff members (619 in 1962), and one-quarter service staff (481 in the same year).[70] About 85 per cent of all staff were women.[71] Although unionization of municipal employees was at its height during the 1960s, The Hospital for Sick Children avoided either a nurses or a staff union during this decade and the next. Indeed, by the beginning of the 1980s, it appears to have been "[t]he only large non-union hospital in Ontario."[72]

Law's second challenge was to re-orient and redefine the role of the board of trustees, to whom he was ultimately responsible. Now that the government determined annual operating budgets, as well as a portion of capital expenditures, the role of the trustees was called into question. Trustees still retained legal responsibility for the quality of patient care in the hospital and saw themselves as serving a parallel function to boards of large corporations – concerned "with plans and policies," not day to day operations.[73] A report by Duncan L. Gordon, chairman of the trustees, however, reflects the insecurity about the shifting role of the trustees under provincial health insurance and into a more corporate medical surrounding:

> The atmosphere changed when we moved to our new premises [on University Avenue] and it is not possible to recreate it in the larger institution. Any institution which is growing will at some point in time have to face the fact that it can no longer be run on an informal basis and a formal organization will have to be developed to permit its government.[74]

Following his corporate model of the hospital, Law suggested that the board should focus on long-term planning, improving the relationships between their institution and the university, and finding ways to evaluate progress in medical research and treatment.[75]

Of course, one of the principal roles of the trustees was also to provide a network of the most wealthy and influential members of the Toronto community. Their fundraising was central during these anxious years of transitioning to Medicare. Before health insurance, charitable donations were mainly used to support patient care; however, gifts and bequests were now channeled to numerous other areas of the institution, namely research and the establishment of new sub-specialty services, such as paediatric pharmacology, immunology, and genetics. Meanwhile, fundraising for construction and renovation projects became more complicated. Hospitals relied on federal, provincial, and municipal grants as well as local initiatives to finance new construction which was not directly covered by the Ontario Hospitals Commission. Law felt that the new system made capital campaigns even more challenging. He attributed this in part to an increased number of funding drives, higher taxes and costs of living, the increased amounts of money required for construction, and the initial public perception that the government had taken responsibility for all operating *and* capital costs. The hospital's record of successful campaigns was purported to have worked against it. As the *Globe and Mail* reported, "Canvassers have repeatedly been turned away or have received reduced contributions because people generally believed the institution would easily top its objective."[76]

One of the principal policy issues with which the board and medical staff had to grapple was the near monopoly over paediatric care and education that the hospital exercised in the city. Internal and external studies demonstrated that the hospital operated with a daily capacity that was far higher than the ideal rate. The main hospital had reached 100 per cent occupancy – 609 beds and patients – by February 1960.[77] To put these figures in perspective, contemporary hospital experts advised that occupancy should range between 80 and 85 per cent for "maximum efficiency."[78] Overcrowding in the medical wards at 555 University was especially bad for infants, where beds were occasionally placed in dressers' rooms, an ominous allusion to the overcrowding in the final years of the old College Street hospital.[79] Increased demand for hospitalization was especially pronounced among infants and preschoolers, for whom more beds were "urgently" required.[80] Of course, an overtaxed Hospital for Sick Children raised the inevitable question about whether one children's hospital could do everything. As the trustee minutes acknowledged, the overcrowding begged "the question as to whether we will admit all cases presented for admission if hospitalization is requested or if admission should be of a more selective nature, allowing many of the more ordinary cases to be admitted and treated in hospitals elsewhere in the City and the Province."[81] In Toronto, it was apparent to many that the city – particularly its booming suburban population – was becoming sufficiently large to support two medical schools and, by implication, two children's hospitals.

During the 1960s, provincial civil servants initiated discussions about situating another university medical school in the Greater Toronto Area, the most practical option being one associated with the new York University on the northwest edge of the city. Indeed, oral interviews with retired practitioners insist that leading figures in the Ministry of Health at the time were already "sounding out" individuals as potential heads of departments of a new medical school for Toronto.[82] A second medical school, with its own children's hospital, however, threatened deeply vested interests at the University of Toronto and The Hospital for Sick Children. The Hospital for Sick Children had always retained a monopoly over public children's wards under Brown. To be sure, there were a handful of paediatric beds scattered throughout the city, but it was understood that these were ancillary to the principal hospital. As long-time paediatrician Harry Ebbs remembered, during the Brown era, there had always been a "tug-of-war" over paediatric beds. Toronto Western Hospital had "for years" wanted to establish expanded accommodation for children, but "this was resisted fiercely" by Brown.[83] The uncompromising attitude eased somewhat under Laurie Chute. Chute supported establishing paediatric units in other hospitals and vastly increased the number of paediatricians with admitting privileges and cross-appointments from other hospitals. When 555 University first opened there was a surplus of beds, and Chute responded by "add[ing] to the medical staff practically all persons who obtained their certification in paediatrics."[84]

However, the advent of health insurance changed the dynamic, as demand for hospitalization surged in Toronto and elsewhere. In the wake of HIDS, the board of trustees held a special meeting to consider a possible further expansion of the hospital. They decided to increase their own hospital's bed capacity one final time and to modify the admissions policy. Lest non-urgent cases overwhelm the wards, a selective admissions policy would be implemented, and thus paediatric beds would have to be opened elsewhere. The medical policy committee deemed 700 to 800 to be an optimal number of beds for the hospital, and resolved that, once the hospital had built the second unit of the nurses' residence, added 100 beds, and expanded "ancillary services," the hospital "will have discharged its responsibilities to the community" and could reasonably do no more.[85] This bed limit was embraced for logistical reasons – a hospital with over 800 to 1000 beds was thought to become "unwieldy and less efficient"[86] and also out of recognition that further growth would interfere with "the character of the institution ... as a skilled specialty and research institution."[87] The previous surgeon-in-chief, W.E. Gallie, had felt especially strongly that if the hospital expanded beyond 750 beds, "the Hospital would inevitably lose its character as a great medical centre and tend to become a mere treatment centre."[88] A three-part building project was undertaken in part to increase bed space. The first part of the project was the construction of the aforementioned Gerrard Street wing, officially opened in May 1964, which provided additional research and patient care space and raised the total number of beds to 810.[89]

Chute and the senior medical staff proposed a more restrictive admissions policy, similar to that at Boston Children's Hospital and Great Ormond Street, where "patients [we]re carefully selected and only the type of patients who can benefit from special facilities of the hospital, [we]re admitted." Chute even proposed changing the slogan to "Where No child *who Needs Our Special Services* Knocks in Vain."[90] This awkward alternative was not implemented, but the senior medical staff did resolve to "gradually ... convert our procedure to the basis of a reservation system," while "continu[ing] for the present at least to admit all children who reach our doors who are in

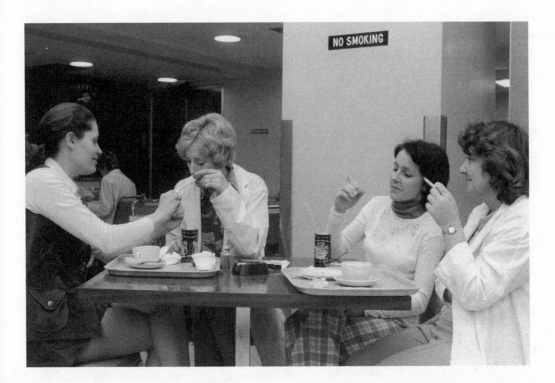

NO SMOKING

need of hospitalization."[91] However, as there were only 176 designated paediatric beds in Metropolitan Toronto outside of The Hospital for Sick Children at the time, the complete adoption of such a policy would have to be delayed until more accommodation was added elsewhere. The public reception of this subtle, but fundamentally important, policy shift had to be handled gently. Allan Ross, while supportive of the report, "reminded the Trustees that in some ways the Hospital would be losing its "franchise" which it has held for so many years in caring for the sick and crippled children of the province and beyond."[92] Reflecting the sensitivity of the issue, the board determined that "the change in the Hospital's admitting policy will take place gradually and without public announcement."[93] When faced with a "critical state of overcrowding" by 1961, Law stated publicly that the hospital's "main purposes" were henceforth "the treatment of unusual and difficult cases" and "act[ing] as a research centre for children's diseases and disabilities"; he suggested that existing facilities should be used for general paediatric cases.[94]

11.4 Although still dominated by a discernable hierarchy of male doctors, the hospital was in fact overwhelmingly a female institution, with thousands of women in paid and volunteer positions, from nurses to lab technicians to cleaners. Here, in the early 1970s, several women relax in the cafeteria.

Meanwhile, at the municipal and provincial level, debate continued over the siting of new paediatric beds. The Committee for Survey of Hospital

Needs in Metropolitan Toronto published a seventy-five-page report on paediatric hospital requirements in 1962. This was the first of a twenty-part series on hospital needs in the Metropolitan Toronto region. The report opened with a map of sixteen hospitals providing hospital beds for children in Metro Toronto. In total, there were 928 children's hospital beds. The Hospital for Sick Children provided two-thirds of these (610 beds). It was projected that, by the middle of the 1960s, there would be 1,248 beds in total, of which the hospital would continue to supply approximately two-thirds (801 beds) (see table 11.1). The committee asserted that the occupancy rate of The Hospital for Sick Children (86.5 per cent in 1961) was "entirely too high" to accommodate the fluctuating demand for paediatric beds and prevent cross-infection. The committee concluded, "It is readily apparent that the additional beds now under construction are urgently needed."[95] Other hospitals with "more than a token children's service [were] being used beyond the desirable rate of occupancy and, in some cases, [were] extremely overutilized to the point of being dangerous." In contrast, hospitals with "only a token children's unit" had low occupancy and were used mainly for tonsillectomies and emergencies.[96] They recommended that the province support the expansion of paediatric hospital facilities, with a goal of 1,700 beds by 1970 and 2,000 by 1980. The survey committee weighed the option of a second children's hospital, but ultimately recommended the establishment of additional wards "in certain strategically located general hospitals." The committee was emphatic that "the services at the general hospitals for children are to offer relief, and support, to the Hospital for Sick Children, not to compete with it as specialized referral centres." The Hospital for Sick Children would retain its primary research role and responsibility for "highly specialised

Table 11.1 Hospital beds for children in Metro Toronto, 1962

Hospital	Children's beds
Hospital for Sick Children	610 (65.7%)
TEGH & Ortho Hospital	46
St Joseph's Hospital	77
New Mount Sinai Hospital	22
Northwestern General Hospital	43
Scarborough General Hospital	35
North York Branson Hospital	16
Doctors Hospital	32
Humber Memorial Hospital	12
Toronto Western Hospital	14
Queensway General Hospital	6
Toronto General Hospital	3
The Wellesley Hospital	3
Women's College Hospital	4
St Michael's Hospital	5
York Downs Hospital (Bethesda)	–
Total	928

Source: Committee for Survey of Hospital Needs in Metropolitan Toronto, *Hospital Accommodation and Facilities for Children in Metropolitan Toronto*, Part Six of a study by the committee (Toronto: The Committee, 1962), 68.

services such as cardiac surgery."[97] In anticipation of a medical school at York University in the near future, they recommended establishing a large unit of 200–300 beds that would, in effect, *eventually* substantiate a second children's hospital.

In June of 1964, Director Law used his column in *Paediatric Patter* to cautiously encourage the development of other paediatric facilities in Toronto. He drew parallels to the United States, where paediatrics were concentrated in general hospitals and plagued by low occupancy and duplication of services:

> Toronto is about to decentralize paediatrics. This is desirable and necessary. A number of hospitals have decided on or are considering the addition of paediatric units. It is hoped that they will be of sufficient size. It is hoped also that the people responsible for the development of these facilities will proceed cautiously and benefit by the experience elsewhere with decentralization. Toronto has the opportunity to avoid problems; other committees are in the position of attempting to solve problems in this regard.[98]

In 1966, he wrote to the Ontario Hospitals Service Commission advising that Toronto needed additional paediatric facilities, reiterating that The Hospital for Sick Children had added 200 beds and was stopping there. The board's budget and finance committee, by contrast, regarded the opening of new children's facilities with some degree of anxiety, observing that Medicare, relations with the ever-expanding University of Toronto medical school, and the development of other paediatric centres all posed complex challenges to the institution. The committee asserted that "[t]he establishment of childrens' [sic] wards in the new hospitals in the suburban areas will provide competition and problems for this hospital ... It is too early to predict the outcome of these developments but it is safe to say that they will result in great change in this Hospital."[99] Ultimately the city witnessed the creation of a new children's centre, rather than a full-fledged children's hospital, which was opened at the North York General Hospital in 1968 with 121 beds.[100] In some respects, this made much more sense than locating a new children's centre, or hospital, within the city centre, since the city's population was relatively stable, and it was the outer suburbs that were exploding by the end of the 1960s. Logic, however, coincided with self-interest: The Hospital for Sick Children would continue to be the only paediatric institution in what had recently become the most populous and powerful city in Canada.

Conclusions

Medicare was accompanied by fears that the autonomy of the hospital, the scope of practice of its medical staff, and the support of the community would all be compromised. But, after a bumpy transition period, many hospital administrators, including The Hospital for Sick Children's John Law, strongly preferred this new system of universal health insurance to the former regime. Speaking to a conference of Canadian and American hospital administrators, the American-born Law affirmed that hospitals in Canada now enjoyed

> improved facilities and equipment, greater financial security, more adequate staff and improved salaries for staff. Administrators are "better off" because they benefit from all of the things mentioned, but most important to me, based upon my long experience in the United States, we are not obligated in our system to pauperize people as a result of large hospital bills.[101]

Such was the paradox of the voluntary hospital in the era of state medicine. Rather than succumbing to the vices of an inflexible state and the dictates of bureaucrats, key stakeholders noticed that the interest of volunteers expanded, rather than diminished, in the era of universal health insurance. Moreover, the new funding model enabled the improvement of care and facilities as well as "the equalization of wages and salaries of hospital employees with those for similar occupations in the population generally."[102] However, government financing exacerbated the existing trend of spiraling costs for equipment and personnel. By only insuring hospital-based services, the 1957 Hospital Insurance and Diagnostic Services Act encouraged the concentration of health services within medical institutions, the most expensive location for care. Budgets swelled during the 1960s, as service usage increased and diagnostic and therapeutic technologies proliferated. In Law's opinion, patients became even less aware of the real cost of hospital care, and medical staff expected "an endless supply of money."[103]

The historical trajectory of The Hospital for Sick Kids was often informed by what did *not* happen, even though most believed it would.

There was no more poignant example than the failed attempt to create a second medical school in the GTA and the parallel, inter-related initiative to found a second fully operational children's hospital in the centre of the city. Stakeholders at the University of Toronto lobbied effectively against the proposal to create a new medical school at York University.[104] Ultimately, the extra medical school was established around the lake in Hamilton, at McMaster University, and plans for a medical school at York University were shelved indefinitely. Of course, the failed attempt to create a second medical school in the city of Toronto did not mean that a second children's hospital was impossible. But the continued preference of The Hospital for Sick Children for a managed decentralization to secondary children's wards or centres in established hospitals, rather than a purpose-built or converted children's hospital within the city, would prevail.

The general improvement of wages and work conditions at The Hospital for Sick Children, and its status as a mecca of paediatric training and innovation, was partly dependent on the generous financial support of a province, and public, which enjoyed almost uninterrupted boom times in the 1950s and 1960s. Senior medical staff recall arriving at the hospital and being called to the board and told, in the words of one retired senior doctor, "Anything you want, you can have. Okay? Anything, you need a recording device, fine, you need a secretary, just let me know, we'll work it out ... walk into my office anytime you like and ask things."[105] Being dependent upon the state was wonderful when the government was flush with cash. Toronto was overflowing with money, and resources seemed almost endless. But the wheels of the post-war economy eventually came off. Just as the hospital closed down its nursing school in 1973, a financial shock rippled through western economies bringing the two-decade-old post-war boom to an end. The remainder of the 1970s would be an era in which the older model of a single children's hospital welcoming all patients would become untenable. As budgets dried up the hospital would turn to new forms of fundraising — including the ubiquitous telethons — to fund new research in genetics and other fields. After such a revolutionary period in the 1960s, the hospital seemed to drift in the 1970s, unable to respond effectively to changing technologies and demographics. Ultimately, it would end the decade embroiled in the biggest scandal in Canadian medical history.

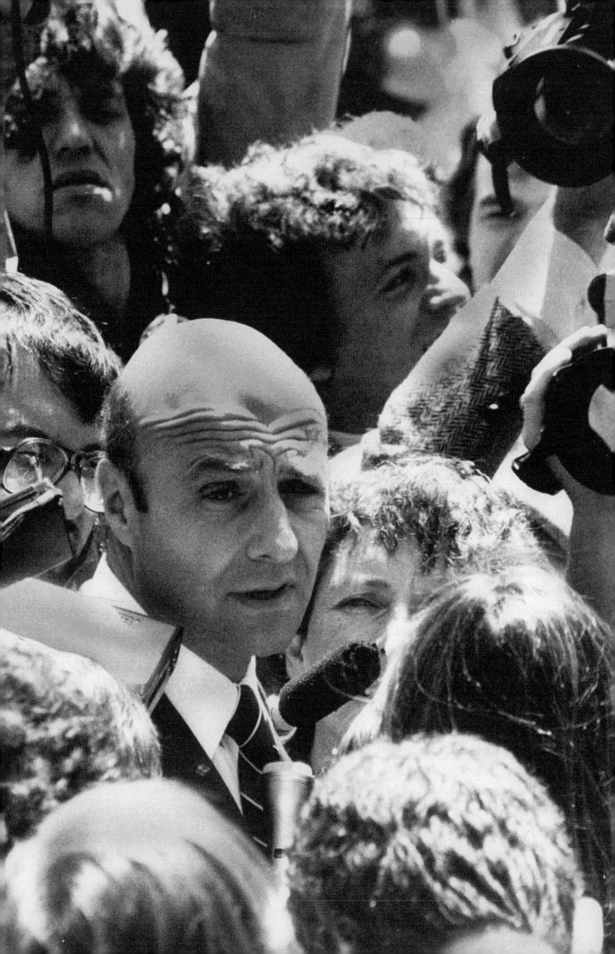

TWELVE

Tragedy and Transformation

... during the tragic saga triggered by the Nelles investigation, some
highly qualified people communicated to me their deep concern about
a growing arrogance and apathy within the hospital, stemming perhaps from the fact that this excellent reputation had never been
seriously questioned.[1]

Former Ontario Attorney General Roy McMurtry,
Memoirs and Reflections, 2013

In late January 1980, an eight-year-old boy, Steven Yuz, was readmitted
to The Hospital for Sick Children for abdominal pain and vomiting. The
senior fellow in radiology misread the results of a barium enema as normal,
and "contrary to established practice" a staff radiologist did not verify the
resident's conclusions.[2] No other physical symptoms were detected and,
in light of the "history of emotional difficulties" attributed to the boy,
Yuz was diagnosed with "psychogenic vomiting." His rare condition –
non-fixation of the bowel – went undetected. After a junior resident
ordered a discontinuation of intravenous fluids, Yuz
became dehydrated and suffered a heart attack. He
was moved to intensive care, where he received ten
times the recommended dosage of an anti-infective
drug for a yeast infection. He died on 20 February
1980. The circumstances surrounding his death were

12.1 A scrum around Toronto lawyer
Austin Cooper, one of the lawyers
representing Susan Nelles. The
potential of a nurse-killer at Canada's
most famous hospital led to a media
frenzy and, much later, suspicions that
the police had acted far too hastily.

detailed by a coroner's inquest and an external investigation, which identified a sequence of errors and a breakdown in patient care responsibilities and supervision.[3]

What made headlines in the Yuz case, however, was not merely the train of medical errors that led to his untimely demise. Rather, it was also the public perception that the details of his death had been covered up. The five-day inquest that followed revealed that substantial portions of his medical records had inexplicably disappeared. Sixty-eight pages of a blood specimen book had been ripped out and two other entire books were found to be missing, as well as several doctors' order sheets. The public became increasingly disquieted that no one was able, or willing, to pinpoint which individual physician was responsible for his care. Yuz's parents took out a malpractice suit against the hospital and medical staff members. They accepted $40,000, but continued to fight for a disciplinary hearing and revocation of the licences of the doctors implicated in the incident.[4] After a decade of back-and-forth to determine if the hearings would be private or public, they were held publicly. Ultimately, two doctors were found guilty of professional misconduct and given reprimands.[5]

In some respects, the Yuz case was the proverbial canary in the coalmine, an individual tragedy that spoke to significant systemic problems that had crept into the hospital over a decade. The incident revealed, to a presiding judge, "a lack of clear definition in the Hospital ... as to who was in fact the responsible physician, particularly where the patient is receiving assistance from various quarters."[6] The McGregor Committee, an external review committee, asserted that the hospital needed to clarify the roles and responsibilities of disparate physicians, concluding that "patient care in the department of paediatrics is being jeopardized by an overworked staff and confused lines of responsibility in both day-to-day administration of the ward, and in the ultimate responsibility for individual patients."[7] A senior administrator, J.D. Snedden, acknowledged in the spring of 1980 that "[t]he death of Stephen Yuz has left a cloud over HSC. Everyone within the Hospital has been aware of an erosion of public confidence and a lowering of staff morale resulting from the inquest."[8] As his words went into print, however, the clouds of a much larger medical scandal had already begun to gather. For 1980 also marked the beginning of the deaths of multiple infants under suspicious circumstances, an event indelibly imprinted on contemporary Canadian history.

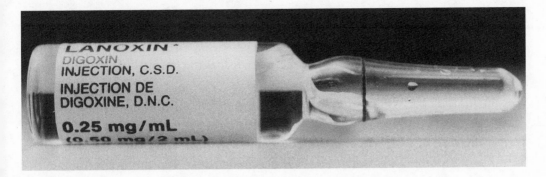

Digoxin

The infant deaths at The Hospital for Sick Children have entered the collective memory of Canadians and must certainly be seen as a cardinal event in Canadian medical and legal history. The paper trail that the series of events unleashed was without precedent. The deaths precipitated one preliminary court hearing, two inquiries (the closed Dubin Review and the public Grange Commission), two hospital-invited scientific analyses (the Bain report and the Atlanta report), a formal review of one of the external scientific reports (the Haynes report), several lawsuits, a small handful of books, live televised coverage, and endless newsprint.[9] The preliminary inquiry into Susan Nelles was reputedly "the longest pre-trial hearing ever heard in the Canadian courts," involving forty-one days of evidence and over one hundred witnesses,[10] and the Grange Commission may have been the first continuously televised commission proceedings in Canadian history.

12.2 Digoxin, whose criminal employment was allegedly the cause of death of as many as three dozen children at The Hospital for Sick Children in the early 1980s.

Between June 1980 and March 1981, sixty-four infants died on two cardiac wards (4A/4B) at The Hospital for Sick Children, a mortality rate significantly higher than usual, even for a ward specializing in high-risk infants. A certain proportion of these infants, depending upon whose account one places the greatest weight, appeared to perish under unusual circumstances. When a handful of nurses brought what they perceived to be an unusual spike in deaths to the attention of hospital medical staff, senior officials reassured them that the deaths were due to "natural causes." Some staff members, not unreasonably, attributed the increase in deaths to the frail condition and younger-than-normal age of 4A/4B admissions. The theory of "clustering" was also posited. This was a statistical phenomenon that suggested it was entirely understandable that deaths might well happen not in a spaced-out and sequential manner, but rather in groupings that might appear, at the time of their occurrence, to be unusual. Other staff members, however, suspected that there might be other contributing factors, such as the continuing shortage of nursing staff or even the recent arrival at the hospital of seriously ill cardiac patients transferred from Winnipeg.[11]

Over the winter of 1980 and 1981, suspicion and disquiet around the deaths continued to augment. Autopsy findings revealed high levels of digoxin, a cardiac drug, in the blood of two of the infants. After this finding was reported to Coroner Dr. Paul Tepperman, the Toronto Metropolitan Police Department's Homicide Squad initiated an investigation in March 1981 on the assumption that that they were investigating possible murders. The police obtained information about nursing practices, staffing, and patient care on the wards from "physicians and representatives from nursing and the Hospital Administration," as well as medical records personnel.[12] Through an investigation of the timing of the deaths and the staffing of wards 4A/4B, the police concluded that one nurse – Susan Nelles – was the common link between the most suspicious cases. On 25 March 1981, only three days after the investigation began, she was arrested, charged with the deaths of four babies, and held for five days before being released on $50,000 bail. The arrest triggered a media frenzy, capturing the attention of an anxious and bewildered public, many of whom assumed "the police wouldn't have charged a nurse with such unspeakable acts unless they were absolutely sure she was guilty[.]"[13]

Faced with the prospect of a serial baby killer – a young female nurse no less – the baby deaths became a national sensation. As the non-public preliminary inquiry dragged on, however, the ground of certainty and evidence began to shift. In January 1982, during the preliminary inquiry itself, a number of patients on 7F, neonatology, mysteriously became ill. Two cohorts of patients were transferred to intensive care, and one, Jonathan Murphy, died. These patients were initially diagnosed with neonatal sepsis, but later epidemiological and laboratory investigation "showed that these illnesses were the result of a recurring medication error involving the substitution of epinephrine for vitamin E."[14] Epinephrine was not even supposed to have been on the ward. More worryingly, other medication errors were detected; blood tests revealed low, below-threshold levels of digoxin in several patients on the ward who had not been prescribed digoxin. One patient had an above-threshold (that is, a level that could be reliably read) level of digoxin "as a result of a medication error on the part of a nurse."[15] Yet another inquest was called, but the death was not treated as a homicide. As a judge concluded, an "extraordinary number of mistakes" underlay this parallel event:

> the epinephrine was not supposed to be on the floor at all, one nurse picked it up by mistake, yet returned it to the shelf, somehow it got placed next to the Vitamin E, several nurses used it in separate administrations, etc. ... it turns out that some of the infants to whom the epinephrine was administered were found to have in their body measurable quantities of digoxin as well which they had never been prescribed.[16]

Just a few months earlier, in October 1981, three-year-old Rafiki Cruise, a tracheotomy patient, died of asphyxiation on ward 7B while hospitalized for "a routine bronchoscopy."[17] Following an inquest in January 1982, the coroner's jury made recommendations pertaining to the recording of nursing procedures, patient conditions, and monitoring equipment. There were apparently two other similar incidents on the same ward before Cruise's death that shared a commonality: "[I]t appeared that during the critical time there was inadequate supervision and leadership at the nursing level."[18] When Cruise's mother approached the administration to find out in what way The Hospital for Sick Children was acting on the coroner's jury recommendations, the treatment she received was, according to the Dubin Committee, "insensitive and casual." She persisted, and further changes were implemented "which would prevent a re-occurrence of what had happened to her child."[19]

Amidst these overlapping controversies and inquests, the preliminary inquiry into Susan Nelles began in January 1982. At the hearings, all of the nurses who had had contact with the four babies were brought before the hearing, and all verified that Susan Nelles "was a normal, stable person, both emotionally and mentally."[20] Nearly four dozen nursing staff members, including thirty-two RNs, nine RNAs, and two Ward Clerks, testified, as did two dozen medical staff members, laboratory technicians, pharmacy assistants, switchboard operators, members of the Toronto Metropolitan Police Homicide Unit, parents, and other personnel. Nevertheless the prosecution continued to press the point that Nelles was a lone killer, citing her immediate request for a lawyer, instead of tearfully pleading her innocence upon questioning, and for not breaking down with emotion following every patient death, as some evidence of criminality. Much was made of a passing observation by cardiologist Rodney Singleton Fowler, who remembered "a very strange expression" on Nelles as she wrote up a death certificate for one of the infants in question, Kevin Cook:

I knew that she [Nelles] had given the digoxin before so I was anxious to see what she looked like at this time and she had a very strange expression on her face and she had no signs at all of grief and she had been looking after this child and I thought this was very, very strange that this would be her appearance at a time such a terrible thing had happened.[21]

Fowler admitted that he had not spoken to Nelles that day and had not seen Nelles following any other patient deaths. He admitted that he had no way of knowing what she was feeling, and had not spoken with her at all following the death, but simply thought that "she had no signs of grief."[22]

As the trial proceeded, however, the prosecution's theory began to unravel, particularly after it was determined that Nelles was not on shift at the time of the death of Janice Estrella, the fourth charge affixed to her. Apparently, nurses were initially assigned shifts and then often traded those shifts between themselves, a practice not fully appreciated by the police who were accused of relying too much on incomplete documentation and the recollections of medical staff. Indeed, Susan Nelles had not been on duty for several days preceding and on the day of one key death that had been attributed to digoxin, that of Stephanie Lombardo. As a key chart demonstrated, only one nurse – Phyllis Trayner – was on shift for all of the deaths. If someone other than Nelles had killed Lombardo, there had to be either more than one killer or a conspiracy between at least two nurses, something that began to stretch credulity, and at any rate ran counter to the initial line of prosecution.[23] As the Crown's case began to fall apart, Judge David Vanek discharged Nelles on 21 May 1982. He concluded, in a damning eighty-three-page judgment,

1. The evidence is entirely circumstantial;
2. There is no evidence of any motive;
3. In the case of Janice Estrella, there is no evidence to go before a jury that the accused was the person who murdered this child;
4. While the accused had access to each of Pacsai, Miller and Cook and therefore had opportunity to administer the dosage of digoxin that caused death, in none of these cases did she have exclusive access and opportunity; in each case other persons also had access to each of these infants at relevant times and the opportunity to administer the digoxin to them that caused death.

5. There is no evidence of any acts or conduct on the part of the accused in relation to any of the four babies that is out of the usual course of her duties as a registered nurse at the hospital, or which isolates and identifies her as the person who caused death by the administration of overdose of digoxin to any of them.

6. The accused is an excellent nurse and enjoys an excellent reputation among her peers.

7. Each item or piece of evidence in support of the Crown's case, if consistent with guilt, is equally consistent with a rational conclusion, grounded in the evidence, that the accused is not the guilty person.

8. In addition, there is powerful evidence in disproof of the allegation that the accused is the person who caused the death of the four babies. This evidence is composed of proof that the accused could not be the person who caused the death of Janice Estrella or who administered an overdose of digoxin to baby Lombardo that likely caused his death, together with the strong likelihood that one person caused the death of all five children: Lombardo, Estrella, Pacsai, Miller and Cook.

9. There is evidence that points in a different direction.[24]

Having dismissed Nelles, Judge Vanek, far from concluding that the deaths were an unexplainable epidemiological event, identified deliberate overdoses of digoxin as causes of death in the four cases under consideration. As *The Fifth Estate*, one of the many television shows to devote considerable investigative time to the deaths, highlighted, "It was this finding that gave credibility to the theory that babies had been murdered, a theory that was never again seriously questioned by most of the media, the public, or government officials."[25] Vanek himself recalls that his decision landed "like a bombshell," particularly since the preliminary trial had been under a publication ban:

> [I]t was the first substantial account of the events to reach the public. The newspapers published long extracts from my written reasons. A colleague of mine commented that my judgement drove coverage of a war off the front pages of the newspapers.[26]

In retrospect, the judge regretted making the further link to digoxin, acknowledging, in his own reflection on the trial later in life, that "there was no need for me to make any such finding" for the purposes of the preliminary inquiry.[27] Nonetheless, the lingering sense that a murderer was "on the loose," and that the lone children's hospital in Toronto could not be fully trusted, haunted the institution for many years to come and would set the tone for the acrimonious Grange Commission that would follow. Augmenting the furor was the expansion of the scope of the tragedy. After months of devising new tests to identify digoxin in post-mortem infant tissues, sixteen other cases were found to be potential "digoxin deaths." When the police investigation recommenced following the hearing, it was expanded to include forty-three "suspicious" or "unexpected deaths" on the wards, although the hospital identified only thirty-six that deserved further clarification.

Shortly after the collapse of the Nelles case, former chief of paediatrics, Harry Bain, completed a review of the medical charts of thirty-six children under investigation. He concluded that thirty-four of the thirty-six deaths were the result of natural causes, and attributed Jordan Hines' death to SIDS and Kevin Pacsai's to "transient adrenal insufficiency." He allowed that Cook "might have received a dose of digoxin but he was not sure the medication caused the death, and moreover he believed the digoxin level test results to be unreliable."[28] At this point, however, public trust in the hospital had been compromised and allegations of a cover up had been alluded to in the press. Pressure remained intense for an external review. The Ontario government responded to the growing pressure by appointing a formal external review of the practices of the hospital, chaired by Justice Charles Dubin.[29]

Meanwhile, stung by the criticism of the hospital, senior medical staff "requested" that the Ontario Ministry of Health and the Atlanta-based Centers for Disease Control (CDC) undertake an epidemiological study "to describe mortality patterns at the hospital, particularly among patients with heart disease, and to identify possible risk factors associated with the deaths."[30] The mandate was not to establish the causes of the thirty-six suspect deaths during the epidemic period, although the police and, and later, the Grange inquiry, had already named digoxin as the culprit. The CDC investigators, however, further contributed to the belief that malfeasance had occurred by concluding that there was a marked increase during the "epidemic period." In total, three-quarters of the suspicious deaths took place between midnight and 6 a.m., many were "unexpected," tests indicated that seven were likely due to digoxin overdose, and for four of the seven who had not been prescribed digoxin for four hours before death, "a single overdose of digoxin was administered intravenously within approximately two hours before death."[31] As if to drive the point home, the study found that "the person associated with the largest number of deaths, Nurse A, was not the nurse who was originally arrested (Nurse B) [Susan Nelles]."[32] The report was submitted to the Ontario Ministry of Health and the attorney general in mid-February 1983. It was also shared with The Hospital for Sick Children, but withheld from full publication so as not to interfere with the police investigation, which was nearing completion. Some members of the public felt that this withholding of the report only placed further suspicion onto the hospital.[33]

By this time, even these most basic "facts" had come under question as senior epidemiologists began to question the CDC report itself. The hospital asked R.B. Haynes and D.W. Taylor of the McMaster University's Department of Clinical Epidemiology and Biostatistics to review the Atlanta (CDC) report. The McMaster team concurred that there had been an increase in mortality but were "critical … [of] the methodology used by the authors of Atlanta."[34] The Haynes report found that the Atlanta authors had mistakenly included all of the dead babies in a supposedly random sample of the ward population, thus obtaining a false result. These specialists in epidemiology concluded "that the question was not whether there was an unusual increase in mortality [as there clearly was an unusual increase], but what was the cause of that increase."[35] As the long police investigation dragged on and the preliminary inquiry and scientific studies failed to produce answers, members of the public, parents, and opposition Members of Provincial Parliament (MPPs), including opposition leaders David Peterson and Bob Rae, pushed for the creation of a full public commission of inquiry into the deaths, the hospital's response, and the police investigation, in order to remove, to borrow Peterson's words, "that black cloud [hanging over Sick-Kids] as well as find the perpetrators of these crimes."[36]

Needless to say, such an inquiry was not universally welcomed or even considered productive. Supporters of the hospital felt that such a commission would further damage the reputation of the hospital and provide little more information than the Dubin inquiry had revealed. Others, by contrast, believed that only an inquiry could clear the hospital's name. The attorney general for the Province of Ontario, Roy McMurtry, initially resisted the growing chorus calling for a second publicly funded inquiry, reiterating that such an investigation should not take place alongside an active police inquiry. Moreover, as he rightly predicted, "a public inquiry into deaths which are believed to have been deliberately caused is simply without precedent in this province" and would conflate the purpose of an inquiry with the goal of a criminal investigation.[37] Nevertheless, political calculations trumped such legal considerations, and he relented. The initial announcement did not augur well for the future: news of the royal commission and the name of the judge – but not the commission's terms of reference – were leaked to the press, much to the annoyance of provincial legislators and parents. The director of The Hospital for Sick Children greeted the announcement of the Grange inquiry bleakly, fearing "the prospect of another disruptive period of interrogation and intensive media coverage." He held out hope, however, that it was to be the last inquiry during the "period of interminable investigations."[38]

The Grange Commission

Entitled the Royal Commission of Inquiry into Certain Deaths at The Hospital for Sick Children, the nearly $3-million inquiry involved 176 days of hearings and 500 exhibits. Data management became so extensive that the court took the unusual step of using a computer to retrieve evidence and notes during and after the hearings. As with many public inquiries, its terms were initially contested, and there was considerable legal wrangling over the nature of evidence and the conclusions that could be drawn. Ostensibly, the principal mandate was "to inquire into and report on and make any recommendations with respect to how and by what means children who died in Cardiac Wards 4A and 4B at the Hospital for Sick Children between July 1st, 1980 and March 31st, 1981, came to their deaths." Further, now that there was a growing concern that the police had rushed prematurely to arrest a now seemingly innocent health care practitioner, the commission was also "to inquire into, determine and report on the circumstances surrounding the investigation, institution, and prosecution of charges" against Susan Nelles.[39]

Pursuant to the twin objectives, Justice Grange opted to organize the inquiry's hearings into two distinct phases – one concerning the deaths and another the police investigation. During the course of phase one, however, concern mounted over the legality of the terms of reference. Grange was originally permitted to assert if a death was accidental or deliberate, and, initially, to name individuals responsible for causing those deaths, despite his mandate to report on the deaths "without expressing any conclusion of law regarding civil or criminal responsibility."[40] The counsel for Nelles, Trayner, the Registered Nurses' Association of Ontario, and other Hospital for Sick Children registered nurses successfully challenged the judge's prerogative to "name names." After consideration of the interventions, the provincial court of appeal removed the judge's ability to "identify a perpetrator" – that is, to name any individual who had accidentally, or deliberately, given any fatal overdose, which would, of course, have been tantamount to expressing criminal or civil responsibility. Even trickier, Grange was also prohibited from admitting evidence intended to identify a perpetrator, unless it was primarily given in order to shed light on the cause of a patient's death. Just as Nelles was taking the stand, the order-in-council was formally amended so that the proceedings would not "express any conclusion of law regarding civil or criminal responsibility."[41] As Justice Grange articulated in March of 1984 in the hopes of clarification, "Not only is no one accused of anything but I am not allowed to make an accusation against anyone. All I am allowed to do is make the findings of fact as to how, and by what means, these children met their deaths."[42]

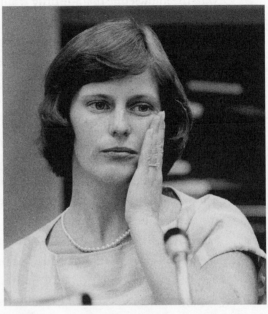

12.3 In what was considered to be one of the longest and most controversial court cases in modern Canadian history, nurse Susan Nelles was charged, and then acquitted, in four baby deaths at The Hospital for Sick Children.

During phase one, fifty-one witnesses testified before the commission. Of these, thirty-four were Hospital for Sick Children staff members, including fourteen nurses. It opened with "expert testimony" on digoxin from toxicologists, pharmacologists, and biochemists. The hospital's own chief of cardiology, Richard Desmond Rowe, took the stand for seventeen days, followed by senior cardiologist Robert Freedom. The commission heard from an array of doctors and external experts, including the authors of the Atlanta report and several parents of deceased patients. In total, during phase one the commission heard from twenty members of the medical and scientific staff of the hospital and over a dozen external medical and scientific experts.[43] What became clear from this non-televised session of the commission was that the scientific community was deeply divided over the tests to determine digoxin levels in infants.

Digoxin (digitalis) was a cardiac drug used to regulate heart rhythm. It was commonly prescribed to children with a variety of life-threatening cardiac conditions, but needed to be administered in precise dosages. Overdoses would result in the slowing of the infant heart and, ultimately, cardiac arrest. The theory of intentional overdose of digoxin thus was based on a theory of one or more individuals injecting digoxin, most likely in the intravenous line, with the knowledge that the drug would slowly, but surely, kill the vulnerable infant a few hours later. The "expert" witnesses, however, provided conflicting evidence and arguments both for and against the "digoxin theory," or the notion that a number of the deaths were the result of intentional digoxin overdose. When faced with conflicting testimony, Grange favoured that of cardiologist Dr. Hastreiter and pharmacologist Dr. Kauffman, who were satisfied that the toxicological data supported the digoxin murder theory.[44]

The first nurse, clinical nurse specialist Carol Browne, testified over four days in December 1983. From January through May 1984, a further fourteen nurses testified, the treatment of whom became a subject of much contemporary, and retrospective, controversy. Nurses' groups complained about the "aggressive" interrogation of the nurses. "For more than nine months, [Elaine Buckley] Day argues, Canadian cable TV viewers watched nursing authority and expertise devalued or brought under suspicion."[45] The Registered Nurses Association of Ontario (RNAO) counsel fought to convince Grange of the relevance of expert nursing perspectives to contextualize the actions and conduct of nurses. The RNAO endeavoured to procure a nursing expert to testify about normal nursing practices which, during the hearings, were presented by non-nurses "as being suspicious or improper." The association also sought expert testimony to explain medication errors, which they alleged were "a systemic problem" and not completely the fault of individual nurses, as well as quality assurance programs, which were not thoroughly dealt with in the Dubin report.[46] Amidst the climate of fear and paranoia, the RNAO struggled to find "a nurse willing to try to qualify as an expert witness." Paul Lamek, counsel to the commission, argued against the inclusion of an expert representative of the nursing profession and practices, and *Toronto Star* reporter Sarah Jane Growe proposed that "the legal objection was really a rejection of the whole idea of an expert nurse."[47]

Dr. Marion McGee of the University of Ottawa finally obtained an opportunity to testify during the final days of witness testimony for phase one, 14 and 15 May 1984. Despite being an associate dean of health sciences and director of the School of Nursing, McGee was not included in the appended list of "scientific and medical" experts in the Grange report, but is named in the category of "other experts" within the text of the report.[48] Nurses felt that they were being unfairly targeted and painted with suspicion throughout the investigation and inquiry. As McGee herself later levelled, "nurses were the focus of illegitimate scrutiny and ... all systems were not scrutinized equally. Whether it was conscious or subconscious, there was an obvious aspect of male chauvinism and sexism involved."[49]Alice Baumgart, the dean of nursing at Queen's University, famously slammed the inquiry as "the highest-paid, tax-supported sexual harassment exercise that that we've ever witnessed."[50] The gendered dynamic of this quest for objective truth was not lost on the nursing community: "Did the men who asked nurses if they had murdered their patients really have any understanding of nursing?" one nurse asked in an open letter to a nursing journal at the time. She went on to inquire, "And if they did have a concept of nursing, whose concept was it? I know for sure it wasn't mine."[51]

Sarah Jane Growe, who wrote a book on the Grange Commission, characterizes it as a forcible "loss of innocence" for the nursing profession. The overarching theme within her chapter on the hearings was the belittling of nurses by lawyers and the media, and their abandonment by the hospital administration. Growe insists that the nurse witnesses were "scarred ... for life" by "the way the inquiry was carried out," that is, the ways in which nurses were identified as the primary suspects by both the homicide squad and commissioner.[52] To make matters worse, the Grange Commission became not only a media sensation, but a televised media sensation. Starting on 9 April 1984, the fifth day of Susan Nelles' six days of testimony, Justice Grange permitted "continuous live television coverage" until the end of the commission. All of the previous hearings had been recorded, but not broadcasted.[53]

Commenters, nursing and non-nursing alike, invoked metaphors of victimization and sacrifice to characterize the treatment of the nurses of The Hospital for Sick Children and the profession itself. Their contentions were joined by numerous voices of discontent with the inquiry in the news media. Some nurses referred to the inquiry as an "Inquisition" and to themselves as "Joan[s] of Arc."[54] Alice Baumgart, MPPs, journalists, and members of the public slammed the inquiry as little more than a "witch hunt." One nurse, calling for professional unity and mutual protection, stated flatly that "[t]he information coming from the media leaves me with the impression that society is burning the nursing profession as a witch."[55] Elaine Buckley Day used this language shortly thereafter in an article entitled "A

20th Century Witch Hunt."[56] Frances Kitely referred to the commission as "a non-murder murder inquiry," and her comments immediately made local headlines.[57] Weeks later, the coordinator of the RNAO, Allie Lehmann, voiced similar criticisms during a CBC interview, referring to nurses as "sacrificial lambs in this entire process" and stating,

> I think it is quite evident form the kind of examination that went on today that lawyers for the Attorney General and the police are trying to blame nurses for their own inept investigation. And rather than look at a lot of other Hospital personnel that may have been associated with the infant deaths, it's only nurses that are taking the rap and they are being grilled very comprehensively.

She objected to attempts to paint nurses such as Bertha Bell as uncooperative witnesses, arguing that "[t]hey were treated quite shabbily and they did not have any legal counsel during the preliminary or during the police investigation."[58] Other commenters challenged the essential premise of a royal inquiry into a criminal matter, citing violations of civil liberties. The Canadian Civil Liberties Association unsuccessfully sought to argue to the Ontario court of appeals that nurses' rights had been violated.[59]

When the 224-page report was released on 3 January 1985, Judge Grange concluded that eight of the thirty-six deaths under review were due to deliberate overdoses of the heart drug digoxin, identifying five deaths as "highly suspicious," and ten as "deaths suspicious of digoxin toxicity." Grange acknowledged the scientific dispute over the digoxin theory, but concluded that "[t]he suggestion that the drug overdoses were the result of error was preposterous ... Accidents will happen, of course ... but the theory of multiple, repeated, concentrated, fatal error must be rejected as untenable."[60] In the end, critics asserted that, "the Commission's results satisfied almost nobody, not the parents, not the public, not the police, not the attorney general's office, and least of all the nurses."[61]

A Medical and Economic Malaise

The roots of the administrative and clinical drift in the hospital must be understood, in part at least, in the context of the harsh economic climes of the decade. By the early 1970s, the post-war boom had run its course. Nearly three decades of uninterrupted economic prosperity, low interest rates, and high employment cascaded into a decade of stagnant economic growth and high inflation. The reversal of fortunes resulted in a new era of fiscal restraint that came as a shock to hospital administrators and medical staff across the country. The Ontario Hospital Services Commission had already begun to reduce permitted increases in hospital budgets from 8.5 per cent in 1970 to 7.6 percent in 1971 and to 7 per cent in 1972.[62] Although these might seem generous by today's standards, they must be understood in the context of increases in health care expenditure that regularly reached the double digits in the early 1970s. As the global fiscal crisis erupted in 1973, the Ministry of Health imposed budget reductions totalling $1,025,000. Ultimately, sixty-one active beds were closed on the tenth floor (wards 10A and 10B) of the hospital.[63] Over the next few years, the fiscal and personnel situation went from bad to worse. By the hospital's own numbers it was 140 nurses short in the summer of 1973.[64] To add insult to injury, in 1975, the much-anticipated centenary year of the hospital's founding, the Ministry of Health imposed a 2 per cent constraint and froze staffing levels. This was felt in a $600,000 reduction in the operating budget of the hospital. Secretary-treasurer J. Douglas Snedden's columns in the in-house publication *What's New* and in annual reports routinely praised the staff's devotion during what he referred to, diplomatically, as "challenging" times. As Snedden foretold, this would affect facilities maintenance, hiring, and, most significantly, nursing attendance. "All Staff Must Cut Costs to Save Jobs," was the heading for one of his more disquieting internal memos.[65] It would be a common refrain for the rest of the 1970s.

As the decade dragged on, hospitals, nursing unions, and the provincial government engaged in a war of finger-pointing over the shortcomings in provincial hospitals, tensions that were heightened by the rapid unionization of nurses across the province and the country. During the 1970s, there were over two dozen nurses' strikes in Canada, though Ontario nurses had lost their right to strike, and Hospital for Sick Children nurses remained non-unionized.[66] Hospital administrators found themselves in the paradoxical situation of spending more and more on personnel while simultaneously being faced with ever-worsening personnel issues. The Ministry of Health found itself with a ballooning budget and constant complaints of deteriorating services. Teaching hospitals were squeezed on both ends, as the Ministry of Health directed them to reduce staff levels for direct patient care, while community hospitals operating on what they called "bare bones" budgets transferred acutely ill patients to tertiary care institutions. The Hospital for

Sick Children responded by closing two wards (5B and 5C), ceasing to hire per diem nurses, and supplementing nursing care with funds from its global budget, even at the risk of incurring a serious deficit. In an even more controversial move, the hospital applied to The Hospital for Sick Children Foundation for funds to maintain staffing levels in the neonatal ward. By 1976, budget constraints threatened the closure of ten hospitals in the province, further bed reductions across the board, and budget and staff reductions.[67]

While the government insisted that the primary challenge was one of "mismanagement" of existing personnel rather than underfunding, hospital administrators, in turn, complained that the graduates of the two-year community college nursing program were unprepared for work on the ward.[68] In March 1976, at a forum on health care at the Toronto Hotel, The Hospital for Sick Children's chairman, Duncan Gordon, stated rather sharply that the new programs were graduating nurses who were "completely useless" and needed an additional two years of clinical experience, during which time they were "overpaid" at a salary of $13,000 annually. The executive director of the Ontario Hospital Association, R. Alan Hay, unwisely supported this very public assertion, which was then reported in the *Toronto Star* the following day.[69] A bitter fight then erupted over the working conditions at the hospital, with nursing leaders defending the new nursing program and criticizing the senior male board members and administrators for impugning nurses' skills and scapegoating them for rising health care costs.[70] Letters from disgruntled nurses also reminded the interlocutors that it had been the Government of Ontario that had "forced nurses into a two-year program in a Community College," against the wishes of many nurses, who recognized the need for more clinical experience during training. They also called attention to the fact that "a large number of nurses" in Toronto had been taking "days off without pay to help their hospital out of financial difficulty."[71] One registered nurse expressed her impatience in a letter to the *Toronto Star*, stating that she hoped "to get Gordon as a patient on my ward. I have reserved for his derriere my biggest shiniest, sharpest horse needle"![72]

What was happening in hospitals was a microcosm of a more general trend in the broader Canadian labour force. The 1970s represented the height of unionization in post-war Canada, of which nurses and other public sector employees were important constituencies. By the early 1980s, 40 per cent of Canadian workers were unionized and 60 per cent were "covered by union contracts."[73] Unions bargained hard to maintain real (that is, inflation-adjusted) wages by asking for double-digit increases in collective bargaining.

Meanwhile the collective agreements of double-digit pay raises further fuelled inflation, leading unsympathetic onlookers to blame unions for contributing to the ongoing "stagflation." As the consumer price index peaked at 15 per cent in 1975, the Liberal government of Pierre Elliott Trudeau, after having hammered the Progressive Conservatives in the 1974 election for proposing wage and price controls, passed the Anti-Inflation Act which capped pay increases in public sector collective bargaining. The measures contributed, in part, to restraining inflation in the short term, which dipped to 6 per cent before returning to double digits in 1980. Seen in this broader context, the unionization of nursing was reflective of these general trends, as provincial nursing unions were created separately from existing professional associations.[74] Fiscal restraint led to cutbacks within hospitals, but little in the way of creative responses from hospitals to adapt to the new hospital management environment and changing technologies. The result was poor supervision, a lack of comprehensible lines of reporting and medical authority, and, quite possibly, undertrained and overstretched nursing staff. McMurtry's allusion to the "arrogance" of the hospital's senior staff in this chapter's epigraph might have been rather harsh, but there was a palpable sense of a hospital structure invented during the heady days of the post-war boom, which had failed to adapt to changing social, cultural, and medical norms of accountability and transparency. A great transformation in the entire management of the hospital was seemingly long overdue.

Conclusions

The memory of the mysterious deaths on wards 4A/4B at The Hospital for Sick Children continues to linger a generation later, seared in the minds not only of the parents of the children who died, but also of hospital staff, many of whom remember vividly the traumatic atmosphere of the time. From a more distant historical perspective, it is fascinating how, over time, the basic facts have become less, not more, clear. Research into the spontaneous production of digoxin has led some scholars to believe that the theory of intravenous administration of digoxin – the centerpiece of the prosecution and, for that matter, the Grange Commission – may never have occurred at all. They argue that both the tests used to determine digoxin levels at the time, as well as the expected posthumous levels, were both inaccurate and, in retrospect, scientifically suspect. For these critics, which included most notably Peter Macklem, then dean of medicine at McGill University, digoxin was, and is, a naturally occurring chemical that ought to be found in elevated levels in deceased infants. In Macklem's opinion, contemporary tests for digoxin were designed for living subjects and had not been used for exhumed tissue. The radioimmunoassay (RIA) test results of the time were not reliable because no controls existed – that is, there were no controls of living infant tissue to compare against the samples of exhumed infant tissue. Another overlapping line of retrospective research has turned to the chemicals used in certain medical products of the time – particularly syringes – which had led to unexplained spikes in deaths in children's hospitals in Britain and the United States. Of course, these theories themselves are open to criticisms and qualifications, but they lead to the remarkable, and somewhat destabilizing, possibility that the baby murders may not have been murders after all.[75]

Focusing narrowly on digoxin theories, however, may well deflect attention from the many other problems that riddled the hospital in the early 1980s. The deaths on 4A/4B overlapped with several other unexpected patient deaths that resulted in coroner's inquests and revealed deep-seated problems with the institution's patient care system, and particularly its delivery of pharmaceuticals. These faults were compounded, in the minds of the affected parents, by a sense of aloofness on the part of the hospital, a reflection of an older paternalistic medical culture of elitism and non-disclosure. As a consequence of these multiple factors, public trust in the hospital had eroded by the middle of the 1980s. It would take years of hard work before the hospital could move from under the "black cloud" and build bridges back to the community, as well to heal the internal divisions within the hospital itself.

Meanwhile, Susan Nelles, whose life had been turned upside down, took out a case against the Crown, the attorney general, the chief of the Toronto Metropolitan Police, and several members of the Homicide Squad for negligence in the investigation and in the laying of charges, and in the prosecution, for false imprisonment, malicious prosecution, and infringement of her Charter rights. The case would eventually find its way to the Supreme Court.[76] The Nelles family complained bitterly about their treatment by the police and prosecution. Nelles's father succumbed to a heart attack following the preliminary hearing, which friends and family linked to the stress of the ordeal.[77] Once the case against her was dismissed, she approached several hospitals in Toronto, none of which would offer her a position. After meeting with The Hospital for Sick Children several times, she was offered a position on the burn unit, and later on the dialysis unit, where she worked for a further five years before moving to Belleville.[78] During this time, and to make matters more unusual, her brother, David Nelles, was a young paediatrician at The Hospital for Sick Children in the years after the Grange Commission. So sensitive was the hospital to the Nelles name, that they took the unprecedented step of using his first name when he was paged over the intercom. To compound the family tragedy, he died of a stroke only a few years later at the age of thirty-six.[79]

Quite apart from the tragic personal impact, the Nelles case was also noteworthy as an early challenge under the newly minted Canadian Charter of Rights and Freedoms. Much was made of the decision by Nelles to remain silent, which was used by the prosecutors as evidence of guilt. Subsequent cases upheld the principle that all defendants had the right to remain silent, and this decision could not be interpreted as some sort of implicit admission of wrongdoing. The case against McMurtry for malicious prosecution, which wound its way to the Supreme Court, proved ultimately unsuccessful. But the Supreme Court decision was significant insofar as, for the first time in English Canada, Crown immunity from prosecution was challenged; the individual attorney general, Crown attorneys, and police officers were no longer "absolutely immune from civil suits in that they were liable for malicious prosecution." As a legal scholar has summarized: "Since Nelles [1989], an accused can therefore hold the attorney general and/or the prosecutors personally legally accountable by a civil suit if there is proof on a balance of probabilities of a malicious prosecution."[80]

Many of these legal battles continued until the end of the 1980s, marking almost a decade of intense public scrutiny. As one staff lamented, "Over the last three years we've been poked and prodded, investigated and criticized, taken apart and written about more than any other hospital in recent history. But now that we have been taken apart and examined, who is going to put us together again?"[81] In the wake of the Dubin report and the Grange Commission, which both criticized the hospital's "exceedingly complex system of administration" and what were critically referred to as "fiefdoms,"[82] the hospital hired David Martin, a fifty-three-year-old accountant, as president and CEO. Martin, who had made a name in Toronto for the "turnaround" of the Toronto East General Hospital, was recruited in 1986 to perform a more substantial reorganization at The Hospital for Sick Children. It would prove to be almost as painful as many of the events that had preceded it.[83]

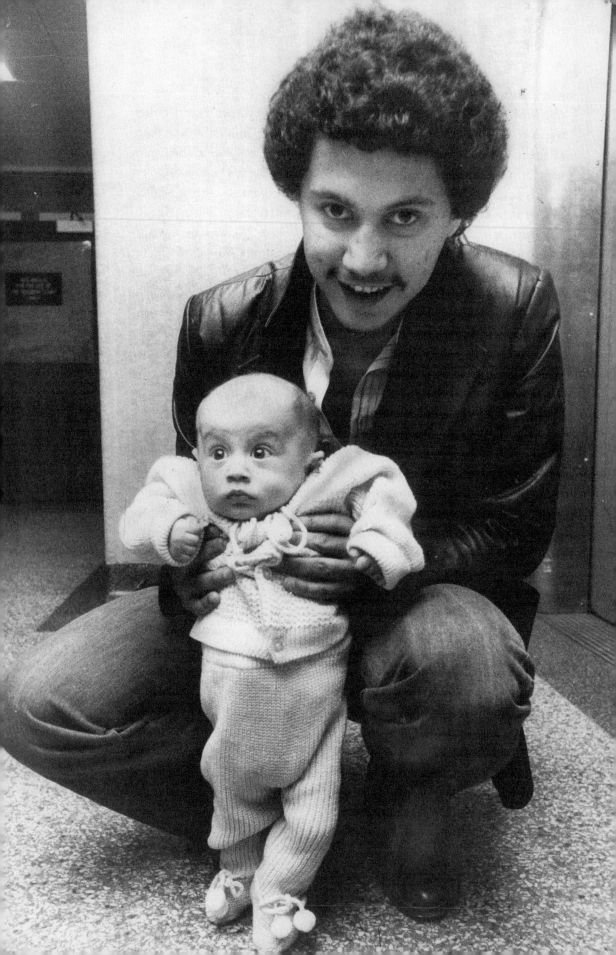

THIRTEEN
The Atrium

I'll never forget hanging around in the corridors at night, wanting to
be with my child, yet knowing there was no place for me on the ward.[1]

Eb Zeidler, *Globe and Mail*

A Baby Named Herbie

Baby Herbie Quinones spent most of his early life in the Brooklyn Hospital
in New York, where he suffered from tracheomalacia, a condition of the
"excessive collapsibility" of the trachea and its connective tissue.[2] Resulting
from this, Herbie had experienced thirty "dying spells," including twenty
in the first two months of 1979, when he was still an infant.[3] His neonatol-
ogist, Jose Luis Rementeria, read an article by Robert Filler, a surgeon at
Toronto's Hospital for Sick Children, who had developed a novel technique
to correct the condition. Filler's operation, in which the aortic arch of the
heart was relocated by sewing it to the breast bone (to relieve the pressure
on the trachea), had been performed six times, all but once successfully.[4]
Peter Kottmeir, the director of paediatric surgery at Downstate Medical
Center in Brooklyn, examined Herbie and suggested that this operation
could be done by a surgeon in New York. According to Rementeria, however,
"[t]he parents thought about it all night, but they
elected to send Herbie to Toronto because Dr. Filler
ha[d] had more experience with the operation and
ha[d] had good results."[5]

Rementeria and the Brooklyn Hospital contacted
Filler, who offered to perform the operation for free

13.1 Herbert Quinones of New York
City poses for a photograph with his
infant son. The narrative of a poor
child in the United States having his
life saved by Toronto surgeons
became a parable of sorts about
universal health insurance.

instead of the usual $1,000 charge for out-of-country patients. As news of the boy's needs spread, Air Canada offered free flights, and the Four Seasons Sheraton free accommodation. However, the Quinones still had to contend with the potential daily hospital rate of $475 for non-Canadian residents (which, over the course of two to three weeks, would quickly amount to thousands of dollars). As recipients of New York Medicaid (the American public health system for low-income people not able to access private health insurance), their son's life was held in the balance while state bureaucrats struggled to decide "what type of treatment to give him, where he should get it and who should pay for it."[6] Medicaid was then paying $200 per day for his ongoing hospitalization in the NICU in Brooklyn.[7]

As the Medicaid review drew out inconclusively over six long weeks, the *Toronto Star* picked up the story, informing Torontonians that "[t]he delay – blamed by Medicaid officials on a failure to follow assistance application procedures correctly – has almost cost Herbie his life."[8] Newspapers recounted that Herbie's young parents, Letitia (who spoke only Spanish) and Herbert Senior, lived in what was referred to, rather indelicately, as the "Puerto Rican ghetto" of New York,[9] scratching out a living on the $100 per week Herbert Senior earned working at a Brooklyn fish market. Gina Godfrey recalled seeing the story in the newspaper and urging her husband, Paul, then Metro chairman, to take action. The Godfreys proceeded to organize friends and coordinate fundraising. Paul Godfrey opened a special account at the city hall branch of Canadian Imperial Bank of Commerce, and, with the publicity in the Toronto area, funds continued to pour in. The initial goal of the Toronto Help Herbie Fund was $5,000, the expected cost of hospitalization for two weeks. A *Toronto Star* story on February 17 urged immediate action: "Dozens of Toronto residents called *The Star* yesterday and Saturday, asking whether they could help. Several, who had asked to remain anonymous, have offered large cash donations."[10] Within a week, the coffers were overflowing with $13,000, which rose to over $17,000 by the end of Herbie's stay.[11]

By the time of his arrival, the plight of young Herbie had gone viral. As one *Globe and Mail* reporter recalled, rather tellingly, "Medicine had become a media event" as Herbie was rushed from the airport to the hospital on 24 February 1979.[12] The hospital's own internal staff publication, *What's New*, covered the story with its usual whimsy: "Although he was greeted by a jostling mob of strangers wielding bright lights, cameras and microphones, Herbie surveyed the scene with a detached nonchalance remarkable for his seven months, probably inwardly labelling Canadians as a hysterical race."[13] Herbie underwent a successful operation, and three weeks later, on 20 March 1979, flew home with his parents. Up to that point, he had reportedly spent only four days of his entire life in their home. The successful operation, and the circumstances whereby a dying American youngster needed to be saved by Canadian health-care know-how, was reported coast to coast by American papers, including the *Boston Globe*, *New York Times*, *Chicago Tribune*, and *Los Angeles Times*. Following this national coverage, Medicaid eventually picked up the $5,000 tab, publicly stating that it was doing so out of recognition that Filler was the most skilled expert for the case.[14]

Having reached the mainstream American press, the story prompted a comparison of health-care systems north and south of the forty-ninth parallel. A spokesman of then-Senator Ted Kennedy, a champion of universal health care and no stranger to political grandstanding, pointed out, "There are thousands of 'Herbie stories' in the United States," with tragic endings due to the iniquities of the American health care system.[15] This observation was trumpeted in the Canadian House of Commons, when Members of Parliament took the opportunity to indulge in heavy doses of sanctimony:

> MR. DAVID ORLIKOW (WINNIPEG NORTH): Mr. Speaker, I would like to move a motion under the provisions of Standing Order 43, regarding an urgent matter. In view of the successful operation in Toronto yesterday on the little boy, Herbie Quinones, who was unable to obtain medical services in his own country due to his parents [sic] lack of financial resources, I move, seconded by the hon. member for Winnipeg North Centre (Mr. Knowles): That this House recognize and applaud the citizens of Toronto for their generosity and, furthermore, that this House urge the United States to adopt our medicare system so that there will be no more little Herbie cases in the United States.
>
> MR. SPEAKER: Order, please. This motion seems to be a little beyond our administrative jurisdiction.[16]

The outpouring of financial support for Herbie Quinones led to inevitable questions about what to do with the surplus in the bank account. Since New York Medicaid had decided, rather reluctantly, to cover the surgery, the $17,000 still resting in the "Help Herbie Fund" was used to create an ongoing fund for similar children. The timing was apposite: 1979 just happened to be the International Year of the Child, and Paul Godfrey was a powerful and well-connected man within Toronto. He established the fund on behalf of the Municipality of Metro Toronto, presenting the first annual donation of $50,000 from Metro Toronto to the Herbie Fund in June. The provincial ministry of health matched this with a one-time donation of $50,000. Over the first twelve months, the fund had received ten foreign applications (from the United States, Jamaica, Trinidad, Israel, Sri Lanka, and St. Vincent). In 1982, the ministry of health repeated its grant of $50,000. An internal publication tellingly commented on this second donation as a demonstration of the government's "continued confidence" in the hospital, amidst the ongoing "digoxin affair."[17]

However, the establishment of the Herbie Fund was like opening up Pandora's box. How would the hospital define a scheme for children from around the world to receive medical interventions that were not available in their home countries or provinces? Initially, children were eligible up to their eighteenth birthday (later reduced in accordance with hospital admission policies). An eligibility committee evaluated candidates according to medical necessity, the availability of the procedure or treatment in their home country or province, the appropriateness of it being done at The Hospital for Sick Children, the family's financial situation, and possible funding alternatives. The child's doctor had to apply for assistance and send the child's medical records to the hospital. As Filler himself acknowledged, "We select children with problems we can fix quickly with a minimum of follow up."[18] Perhaps unsurprisingly, the hospital committee tended to choose patients with acute surgical conditions that, while life-threatening, could be corrected with time-limited intervention. During the first decade the most common cases were heart operations, craniofacial surgery, and orthopaedic procedures. The first patient supported by the Herbie Fund was thirteen-year-old Jennifer Branch, who, accompanied by her father and sister, was rushed to Toronto from St. Vincent after her aunt contacted York mayor Gayle Christie. The girl underwent a seven-hour operation to treat her serious rheumatic heart disease, but died.[19]

Herbie Fund patients inspired other community fundraising initiatives to bring international patients to Toronto. In July 1979, Toronto's Arab and Muslim communities raised the funds to cover hospital costs for fifteen-year-old Rashida Didouh of Morocco, whose father had sold everything to buy a one-way ticket to Toronto for an operation at St. Michael's Hospital to correct her hereditary heart defect. Two years later, Tudor Negrea, a recent Romanian immigrant living in Scarborough, opened a trust fund to bring eight-year-old

Tudor Rusescu to Toronto to have a leaky heart valve corrected. Negrea had heard of the boy while visiting home, and an East York postal worker stepped in to foot the airfare for Tudor and his mother.[20] Numerous high-profile Herbie cases attracted considerable media attention, such as the separation of conjoined twins Lin and Win Htut (Burma), Heera and Shiva Ramkhalawan (Trinidad),[21] and Tinashe and Tinotenda Mufuka (Zimbabwe).[22]

Operation Herbie, which started off as a volunteer group in the community rather than a hospital-led fundraising initiative, focused on galas – such as the 1986 Herbie Hoedown, a $250-per-person "wild western extravaganza" – as a source of fundraising.[23] The first annual Mistletoe Ball, "a successful annual black-tie event that targets mostly a corporate crowd," was held in 1983.[24] Coordinated by well-known society women, the ball never raised less than $100,000, and became a "staple of the Toronto social scene around Christmas,"[25] attracting the "cream of the crop" and "the Toronto WASP crowd." As Rosemary Sexton remarked, "There were no NDP types spotted."[26] Cartier Canada sponsored the ball for six years throughout the boom time of the late 1980s. Despite these fundraising successes and efforts to retain only children with quick fixes, the fund was continually depleted. In 1988, when it spent all of its $700,000 on twenty children, the fund was in "critical condition" and seeking provincial support.[27] One patient, a girl from Mexico, incurred an unexpected $170,000 in medical costs, at a time when the average cost of a Herbie patient was $15,000. During this period, Metro Council was supporting the fund with over $100,000 annually, and the gala brought in an additional $100,000. The annual Metro grant was discontinued in 1995, and since then the fund has depended entirely on voluntary donations.[28]

The intensity of the spotlight on these children became itself a subject of growing scrutiny and disquiet; some commentators expressed concern over the media exposure of the children affected, asserting that "hospitals have the most to gain" from sensational or intensive news coverage.[29] An article in the *Canadian Medical Association Journal* in 1988 drew strong responses from readers,[30] one of whom alleged, "Only someone from a distant planet could have failed to notice that the hospital exploited the story [of the Htut twins' separation] to the hilt, apparently to try to rebuild public confidence, battered by the 'baby deaths' and the Grange Commission."[31] This was adamantly denied by the hospital, whose spokesperson asserted, "It was our hope that surgical separation could take place without public attention."[32]

Table 13.1 Out-of-province and out-of-country patients at The Hospital for Sick Children

Year	Total	Ontario	Other provinces	U.S.	Other countries
1966	26,224	25,975	166	65	18
1969	27,621	27,306	190	94	31
1977	30,697	30,123	345	147	82
1978–9	23,378	22,925	273	104	76
1980–1	23,212	22,618	368	119	107
1984–5	21,911	21,272	379	106	154
1986–7	20,849	20,303	236	118	142
1987–8	20,433	19,906	284	84	159
1988–9	19,865	19,347	289	60	169
1989–90	18,603	18,107	279	61	156
1990–1	18,362	17,921	302	42	97
1993–4	16,705	16,355	222	32	96
1995–6	16,816	16,361	290	40	125

Sources: AR 1966, 7; AR 1969, 26; AR 1977–8, 6; AR 1978–9, 25; AR 1980–1, 12–13; AR 1984–5, 13; AR 1986–7, n.p.; AR Poster 1987-8; AR 1988–9, n.p.; AR 1989–90, n.p.; AR 1990–1, n.p.; AR 1993–4, 26; AR 1995–6, n.p.

Yet despite the criticisms and a perception, among some, that The Hospital for Sick Children was becoming the destination for more and more international patients, the reality was quite the opposite. Despite many high-profile cases, a consistent proportion (95 to 96 per cent) of admissions came from Ontario, with usually no more than 1 per cent of patients arriving from outside the country (table 13.1). As one publication quipped, "Patients come from Ajax and Addis Ababa."[33] This may have been true, but most came from Ajax. Indeed, although the hospital continued to become known as a destination for paediatric patients with very complex conditions, its ability to offer surgical intervention to all patients was undermined by persistent – and increasingly acute – shortages of critical care/ICU nurses in the late 1980s. By 1990, the hospital was so short of critical care nurses that it was on the verge of cancelling elective surgery indefinitely. The same year (1990), less than half of the 22 paediatric ICU beds were open at any given time, a situation that took nearly a year to turn around, in part by offering a pay hike for nurses with more than two years' service and a special retention bonus for those who worked in the ICU.[34]

Children's Miracle Network

Operation Herbie arose from an ad hoc, unforeseen chain of events that made Herbie a national sensation when, as Ted Kennedy alluded, there were thousands of other potential cases of familial tragedy and financial constraints. What was more commonplace in the 1980s, however, was the rise of a more premeditated and intensive epoch in voluntary hospital financing. And no method became so emblematic of the 1980s expansion of fundraising than the annual telethon. Of course, telethons have a long lineage, including the much-celebrated (and, later, much-lampooned) Jerry Lewis Labor Day Telethon for muscular dystrophy. This star-studded television event — replete with musicians, football stars, patients in wheelchairs and, of course, an increasingly fatigued Lewis (who claimed not to sleep during the twenty hours of the "marathon") — set the stage for later imitators. In 1983, the Salt Lake City–based Osmond Foundation began a telethon to raise funds specifically for children's hospitals. Early successes prompted them to found the Children's Miracle Network to coordinate telethons annually across English-speaking North America. The first telethon raised $4.7 million in 1983 and quickly grew in size. In the first six years, the Children's Miracle Network raised a staggering $170 million; twelve years later, the total had eclipsed $1.8 billion.[35]

The structure of the Children's Miracle Network proved seductive for individual hospitals struggling to meet the ever-rising costs of medical technology, drugs, and personnel. The network gave each participating medical institution twenty minutes of local television time interspersed with forty minutes of "national" programming. Pooling resources minimized the operating costs of a telethon for individual hospitals, and participation helped hospitals leverage corporate sponsors. Moreover, the Osmond-sponsored organization was praised for its practice of devolution, for keeping funds local (all participating hospitals retained and allocated their own funds), relying on donated studio time and space, and, perhaps in a not-so-veiled critique of Jerry Lewis, ensuring a degree of "dignity and class." The producers professed to focus on "success stories, kids who [had] been helped by hospitals to live normal lives" rather than exploiting "suffering kids."[36]

Canadians, one could argue, were already primed for charitable giving on a new media-saturated level. Media appeals already existed in the form of radiothons, and the national conscience had been moved by Terry Fox's 1980 Marathon of Hope, which raised over $10,000,000. Observers in the 1980s commented on the increasingly competitive nature of charitable fundraising, with organizations that supported research and public awareness of particular conditions competing with individual institutions. The telethon occupied a prominent place for many organizations. For example, the Ontario division of the Canadian Cerebral Palsy Association derived 90 per cent of their funding (over $1 million annually) from telethons. Increased telethon competitions meant that established telethons, such as those for the Muscular Dystrophy Association of Canada, began to "feel the pinch" as other organizations invented their own telethons, working within the tight restrictions governing charitable fundraising in Ontario. The Variety Club of Ontario, for example, had begun a telethon for "crippled children" by 1984, as had the Easter Seals.[37]

Toronto's Hospital for Sick Children joined the Children's Miracle Network in June 1985. They were not the first paediatric institution in Canada to participate; by this time, four other children's hospitals were already involved, including the Children's Hospital of Eastern Ontario in Ottawa, the Children's Hospital of Winnipeg, the Izaak Walton Killam Hospital for Children in Halifax, and the Janeway Child Health Centre in St. John's. Hosted by news anchors Lloyd Robertson and Liz Grogan (as well as Pamela Wallin and Pat Marsden) in partnership with CFTO TV, the Toronto event took place at CFTO's studio but involved taped and live segments in the hospital. In-house publications featured call-outs for talent in what was becoming a signal social event of the hospital's calendar. The telethon was a unique form of variety show, rotating between musical and dance performances, patient stories, celebrity appearances, and interviews with staff and board members. The first telethon began with $300,000 up front from corporations and sponsors, and brought in $800,000 in individual donations. The second iteration, in 1986, involved 700 volunteers from the hospital and Women's Auxiliary, 400 "friends," and 300 celebrities and luminaries. Volunteers also ran satellite pledge centres in other Ontario cities.[38]

The appeal of the telethon model lay in the way it invited viewers into the heart of institution and interwove patient stories, humanizing the sometimes hidden activities of a hospital. As one contemporary observer remarked, the telethon provided "a unique opportunity to showcase their hospitals' work to a mass audience."[39] At the centre of the appeal were vignettes, which showcased particular patients and which CFTO crews obtained in the hospital in the spring months leading up to the event. Short "mini-docs" featuring families' stories, interspersed among the performances,

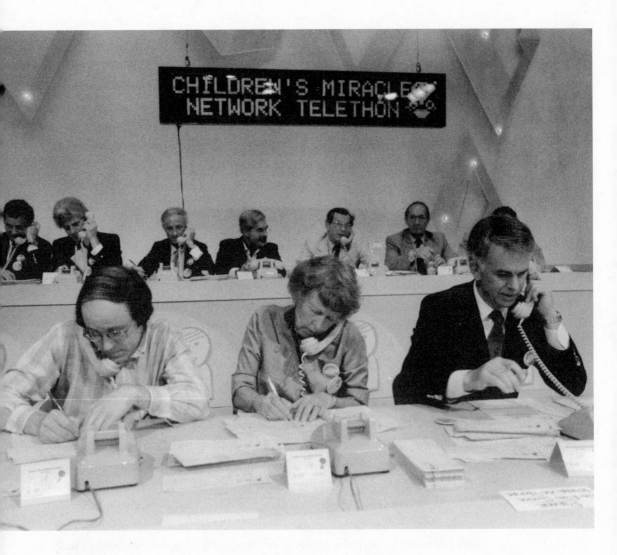

invited the viewer to witness a patient's journey. For example, the first telethon featured the case of Maria, a toddler with Crouzon syndrome,[40] following her, her parents, and the craniofacial team through the process of corrective surgery in April 1985. The second

13.2 Drs. Denis Daneman, Adelaide Fleming, and Bill Crysdale work the phones and take pledges during the annual Children's Miracle Network Telethon.

mini-doc ("A Gift to Last") had a more sombre tone, emphasizing the uncertainty and distress borne by parents of Sandy Harrison, a leukemia patient who had received a bone marrow transplant from her sister Jennifer. Teen sisters Sarah and Susan of Aurora had each undergone surgery for congenital heart defects, and regarded The Hospital for Sick Children as their "second home." Mini-docs were structured around vignettes of recovery and fortitude, but the telethon could not dictate the recovery of its highlighted patients. The story of four-year-old Jennifer, who had undergone chemo-therapy at home for nasal tumours, emphasized the close relationship between mother, grandmother, and daughter. Jennifer had finished her final treatments in February, but just a few weeks before the telethon new lumps had been identified; she was expected to undergo another round of chemo and, this time, radiation. She sat on the couch in a little dress while her mother, looking strained, spoke with Lloyd Robertson, who expressed his pleasure at seeing the girl, because "right up until last night we weren't sure if she was going to be here."[41]

The telethon also took the viewer out of the hospital and into the com-munity, interviewing people about their connection to the institution and its meaning to the many communities it served. Reflecting Toronto's self-proclaimed title as the most "ethnically diverse city in the world" and, indeed, Canada's newfound embrace of multiculturalism, the telethon included segments featuring traditional dances of different "national" groups as well as four hours of non-English, non-French programming to reach out to "Canadians of many origins," to borrow the euphemism of the time.[42] Local hero Johnny Lombardi, the founder of CHIN multicultural radio and television in Toronto, was an enthusiastic participant. CHIN coordinated this multicultural "telethon within a telethon," featuring performances and "radio personalities from Chinese, Greek, Italian and Portuguese commu-nities." For several years, it also put on its own radiothon in thirty-two languages.[43]

In the early years, Toronto's Hospital for Sick Children Foundation manifested some ambivalence towards the larger Children's Miracle Network, deciding to go it alone for its second annual telethon, held 14 and 15 June 1986. This time, 90 per cent of proceeds would be directed towards the capital campaign for the new patient care centre (see below). This telethon was not run with the CMN telethon in Utah, but was hosted by CFTO TV, with the phone banks located at CFTO studios. CFTO TV organized the adver-tising and donated several hundred thousand dollars' worth of space, time, and equipment. The telethon was designed to put the "fun" back in fund-raising, and included a student dance marathon, a "jungle jog and baby crawl" at the Toronto Zoo, a celebrity auction, and a teddy bears' picnic on Centre Island. In financial terms, this approach met with another resound-ing success: $1,521,900, of which over $980,000 came from the telethon itself, and the balance from corporate events and existing pledges.[44] How-ever, the timing for this second telethon could have been better — it took place on the first weekend of the physicians' strike in Ontario over the elimination of extra billing. The hospital was thus placed in a situation in which it was simultaneously calling for spontaneous donations while only emergency surgeries were being conducted in the operating rooms. Whether or not the coincidence was seen as an omen of sorts, the foundation reverted back to the Children's Miracle Network for subsequent telethons throughout the decade.

The Atrium

The money raised in these telethons kick-started the newest chapter in the physical evolution of the hospital. The University Avenue hospital had been state-of-the-art in the early 1950s, showcasing the latest in medical technology. But it had also embodied the philosophy of the time – hospitals were intended for medical staff, medical research, and medical procedures. The families of patients were, in many respects, an afterthought. As mentioned earlier in this book, the restrictions on patient visitation began to ease in the post-war period, and the 1960s saw a greater involvement of families in medical encounters. The simple trope of handing over children to the "care of strangers" was receding, but the physical environment had not appreciably changed. As David Martin, the president and CEO of SickKids in the 1980s recalled, "On any given night at The Hospital for Sick Children, more than 150 parents c[ould] be found sleeping in lounges, or on cots squeezed in between cribs."[45] Indeed, the 1985–6 annual report featured a full-page image of a father sleeping awkwardly on a couch underneath a doll display case. After uncomfortable nights, parents had "to line up for the limited washroom facilities provided for [them]."[46] The new atrium's architect, Eb Zeidler, was not only a designer for the new patient tower but had also been a parent who had, in the 1960s, found himself "pacing the halls ... and wondering about the condition of [his] five-year-old son."[47]

The new Patient Care Centre, as it was first called, was thus intended to express the hospital's new philosophy of "family-centred care." In this new, post-Grange era, parents were formally invited to shape the planning stages of the latest extension of the hospital, offering their input on the various preliminary designs, and serving on bodies such as the bioethics committee and the family advisory committee. These new hospital-family relationships were described tellingly, in the business parlance of the early 1980s, as "partners in a consumer-oriented world."[48] As Paediatrician-in-Chief Robert

Haslam explained, "We have designed this hospital for children and their parents, rather than the staff."[49] This was in stark contrast to the restrictions in place when Haslam had begun his career elsewhere three decades prior, when he and his colleagues "actually used to stage covert operations to sneak parents in at night for a visit."[50]

The soon-to-be-iconic tower in which these new rooms were situated was part of a substantial refit of the footprint of the hospital. A construction plan adopted in 1983 and developed in 1984–5 with Zeidler Roberts Partnership and Karlsberger Hospital Consultants was the signature structure of a three-phase renovation. First, it proposed a new Elizabeth McMaster Building on Elizabeth Street, containing offices, research labs, and a family hostel (finished in October 1985). Second, the above-ground parking garage and nursing residence of the post-war period would be razed to make way for a new patient tower and four-level underground parking garage (all completed by 1992). Third, the relocation of beds and services to the new tower would facilitate conversion of some of the University Avenue hospital wings to research and out-patient clinics. The new tower – sometimes confusingly referred to as the "new hospital" even though it was attached to the 1951 hospital structure – would include new facilities for admitting, an emergency department, ambulatory radiology, fourteen operating rooms, paediatric and neonatal intensive care units, and a fast-food-style cafeteria.[51]

Financing the extension of the hospital, of course, proved to be another huge challenge. The 1982 annual report stated that the Hospital for Sick Children Foundation had provided the only funding for capital projects during the past decade; the ministry of health had contributed no tangible support for new construction. In the previous five years alone, the Foundation had given $15,000,000 for renovations, laboratory facilities, and major equipment. Recent construction projects had included the Alan Brown Building (119 apartment units for residents, fellows, and staff). Newly appointed trustee Reva Gerstein chaired the campaign committee for the new Capital Campaign, which initially aimed to raise $50,000,000. Gerstein wasn't just a University of Toronto psychologist (as she was sometimes described); she was also the first woman to sit on the boards of several large corporations in the 1980s, including Avon, Maritime Life Assurance, and McGraw-Hill Ryerson. The campaign rolled out in three stages: first, "within the Hospital family" (including staff, alumni, the auxiliary, and retirees); second, a corporate campaign; and finally, a public campaign and groundbreaking in May 1986.[52] With $1.85 million initially committed by the trustees, the board hoped to bring in $35 million from individual and corporate donors. A new mascot was debuted during the campaign, "with subway ads, T-shirts and television commercials showing teddy bears – with Bandaids on their bottoms – trying to squeeze into a sardine can, above the slogan 'We're feeling the Squeeze – Help Us Build It For The Children.'"[53]

The premier of Ontario, David Peterson, and television anchor Lloyd Robertson launched the public campaign amidst an array of festive events on the hospital front lawns on 8 May 1986. The public campaign, billed as "the biggest such campaign by any institution in the world," kicked off with an unusual "Great Media Race," in which media representatives from across the country "raced" (in costumes ranging from an RCMP Mountie to Princess Diana) across the Atlantic from Great Ormond Street to Toronto's Hospital for Sick Children. Upon arrival, the chairman of Great Ormond Street laid the first stone, taken from the original London hospital, emphasizing the symbolic and historical connection between the two institutions.[54] Following the event, the minister of health for Ontario, on cue, announced publicly that the province would provide $60,000,000 for the project. Although the Ontario (and Canadian economy) was booming again by 1986, the campaign was launched alongside nearly a dozen Metro-area hospital campaigns, "triggered by the aging of a number of hospitals, all outgrowing their original design at the same time."[55] These hospitals were issuing competing pleas in a climate of reduced corporate generosity. As *Report on Business Magazine* noted, "corporate stinginess" ruled the day, as average Canadian corporate donations had dropped from 1.5 per cent of pre-tax profits in 1958 to 0.5 per cent in the mid-1980s. The report, however, highlighted the tactics of successful campaigns that appealed to corporate "self-interest":

> If the right name opens doors, nothing opens wallets like a little judicious ego-stroking ... Sick Kids will, for the right price, put individual plaques bearing the donor's name on locations such as medication rooms ($10,000), patient rooms with adult accommodations ($25,000), and nursing stations ($75,000). Elevators sold out at $150,000 a shot. This "donor recognition program" has givers so enthused that they are flocking to the architect's model of the new Sick Kids, on display at the campaign headquarters, to see where their plaque will hang.[56]

Such an approach yielded dividends. As of October 1986, $27 million had been gathered through such functions as an art auction, a West Indian breakfast with the Caribbean community, and the Kids for Kids Campaign; by March 1987, the Capital Campaign had raised $33,437,421. Fundraising continued after the beginning of the initial demolition, with the Brazilian Ball of 1990 helping push the Capital Campaign over its goal of $50,000,000.

13.3 Hospitals reflect the social and cultural preoccupations of their eras. With its dancing pigs, exposed elevators, and private rooms, the SickKids Atrium, constructed in the 1980s, reflected a new vision of what a children's hospital could look like.

Although most were unrestricted donations, some were earmarked for specific units: the Shriners pledged $1 million for the burn unit, and a run of *Les Misérables* staged in the SkyDome raised funds for oncology. Nearly all (90 per cent) of the proceeds of the second annual telethon, mentioned above, which raised over $1.5 million, went to the Capital Campaign. That year, the ministry of health committed an additional $32.5 million to capital costs, bringing its total contribution to over $100 million, or nearly half of the anticipated cost of the project.[57]

The actual construction and demolition, by contrast, proceeded less smoothly. To make way for the new tower, the hospital razed the above-ground parking garage that then existed, and the McMaster Nursing Residence, a task complicated by the presence of asbestos, an insulator widely promoted by the federal government in the 1960s but later found to be potentially carcinogenic when airborne. During the demolition of the nursing residence in November 1987, a hospital research technician, Marilyn Cannon, was killed on the sidewalk by a falling four-ton concrete slab. A coroner's inquest followed, finding the demolition company "somewhat deficient" in ensuring public safety.[58] The provincial ministry of labour laid charges against the company, which were later dismissed in court. The demolition and construction projects were further marred by tragedy when worker Michael White fell to his death through a roof opening while installing skylights in the Atrium. Delayed somewhat by strikes, the new patient care centre was 60 per cent complete as of March 1991 and 85 per cent by the following year.[59] During the construction years, the hospital had to contend, once again, with shortages of critical care nurses so severe that complex elective operations (mainly cardiac), had to be repeatedly cancelled and delayed, creating a waiting list of dozens of patients. The *Ottawa Citizen* reported that SickKids was performing operations only in "life or death" situations, with over 200 children on the waiting list for elective procedures. This issue reached the floor of the provincial legislature. Newspapers

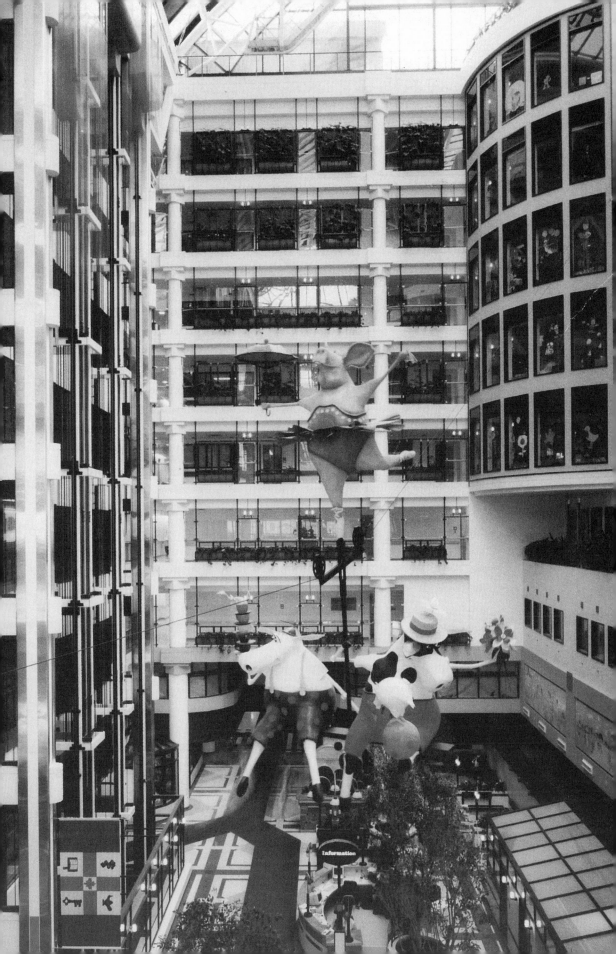

described the "strains of daily tragedy" and inadequate salaries that contributed to the shortages.[60]

In January 1993, the $232,000,000 patient care unit, increasingly referred to as "the Atrium," opened debt-free amidst a climate of fiscal restraint following the recession of the early 1990s. In the end, the province provided over half of the funding ($105 million), direct public donations $56 million, and donations and bequests to the Foundation a further $71 million.[61] In an echo of the unveiling of the 1951 hospital, 600 volunteers shepherded 15,000 visitors on scheduled tours during an eighteen-day open house. All in-patients were moved to the tower during the second week of March. In-patient units featured single bedrooms with private bathrooms and accommodation for one parent, with playrooms in each nursing unit.[62]

> Every child's room has a day bed for a parent to remain comfortably overnight, a full private washroom, storage space for both the child's and parent's clothing, a private TV and a private phone. Every room looks outside or into the Atrium. Single rooms were chosen to provide privacy for the child and family; to allow families to remain as a unit; to maintain as normal a family routine as possible; to enable parents to be involved with their child's care; and help with infection control. Children who are repeatedly admitted or hospitalized for long periods of time have an opportunity to select pictures for their wall from a binder.[63]

The tower boasted a twelve-bed bone marrow transplant unit; previously many children (over a dozen a year) needed to be sent to the United States for specialist treatment. In addition, the hospital acquired its first MRI unit, expanded its PICU to twice its former bed capacity, and established an ER observation unit as well as a trauma/orthopaedic/neurosurgical unit.

Quite apart from these multiple aspects of family-centred care, for the public the amazement lay in the stunning architecture of the Atrium itself. Entering from Elizabeth Street, visitors were ushered into the eight-floor tower boasting four exposed elevators, an indoor waterfall, a balcony for Atrium performances, as well as an extensive fast-food court. Above all, the colour and endless whimsical distractions spoke to an emerging embrace of the healing powers of physical space in the hospital environment and provided a sharp contrast to more sterile hallways of the 1951 structure.[64] The reception, at the time, by family, visitors, and the media was adulatory. Most people had seen nothing like it in any other hospital: "We should bathe in the glory of the new Atrium," effused Paediatrician-in-Chief Robert Haslam.[65] Haslam, pursuing the popular religious metaphors being invoked, described the move to the 817,000-square-foot patient care centre as the end of a "long pilgrimage." Coverage in the newspapers struggled to find appropriate superlatives: "Pediatric care finds its Jerusalem" was the crusading choice of the *Globe and Mail*.[66] Of course, opening up a hospital that was so ornate compared to any other in the country was bound to cause some underlying tensions and resentment, particularly as 1993 would represent the beginning of six years of severe health

Table 13.2 Number of beds in service, 1990–5, at The Hospital for Sick Children

Year	Beds in service	Avg. daily census	Avg. stay (days)
April 1990–March 1991	520	387	7.5
1991–2	511	363	7.1
1992–3	489	309	6.8
1993–4	457	308	6.8
1994–5	430	286	6.2

Source: Annual Reports of The Hospital for Sick Children.

and social welfare restraint in the country. But boosters preferred to accentuate the positive: "[I]n this bleak economy, we need something to lift our spirits. Come to the new SickKids."[67]

Behind the self-evident pride and delight of parents, patients, medical staff, and of course the architects themselves, were fundamental changes to clinical care that would profoundly affect the operation of the new hospital from the outset. As then-President David Martin reported, it was hoped that the new building would shave costs "by reducing lengths of stay and allowing us to expand facilities for day surgery and pre-admission testing."[68] Increasingly, the hospital was emerging as a tertiary care centre, particularly for oncology and haematology, neurosurgery, immunology, burn care, and neonatology. During the planning process, the inpatient capacity was reduced. The hospital had retained a U.S. consultant firm to establish the number of necessary beds, but as one senior administrator recalled, "[T]hey were way over the number of beds. You could see that the whole way of treating patients and children, it was swinging towards day surgery."[69] The hospital could accommodate a maximum of 574 beds, but initially only opened 450. Keeping in mind the discussion in the late 1950s and early 1960s about the optimal size of The Hospital for Sick Children (figures which ranged from 600 to 800 beds), it is worth noting the downward trend of inpatient capacity, where the "census average" dropped below 300 by 1995 (see table 13.2).[70]

The advent of the newly configured hospital was paralleled by a less structural, but no less important, transformation in the administration and management culture of the children's hospital. In the wake of the Dubin report and the Grange Commission, which both criticized the hospital's "exceedingly complex system of administration" and what were critically referred to as clinical "fiefdoms,"[71] David Martin was recruited in 1986. Martin introduced a corporate management philosophy and model of governance. His approach to the hospital reorganization was bold for its time and, for many long-standing members of the hospital, controversial. It sought to implement widespread "program management," by which he and his team meant a new clinical-administrative environment wherein senior physicians and nurses were incorporated into the management structure and empowered with decision-making over the allocation of resources.[72] To confront a significant annual debt (then estimated at $8 million), Martin streamlined the administration, reducing the number of senior administrators from twenty-two to five vice-presidents, reviewing all senior staff, and sacking many who were deemed insufficiently "adaptable."[73] "We shall be in the throes of change for many months to come," Martin informed staff in an open letter in December 1986.[74] This was no idle warning. Over 200 jobs were cut from 1991 to 1993, and in addition, there were both wage freezes and cuts to long-cherished programs.[75]

In one of his more controversial moves, Martin recruited Mike Strofolino, a former professional football player, as VP Finance in 1987 (then COO, in 1990). Strofolino proved to be a polarizing figure: for some, he was a tough and determined manager who could carry through what would ultimately be a long-needed root-and-branch administrative overhaul of the institution; for others, he was an outsider ill-suited to manage change in a delicate paediatric hospital setting. As one retired administrator put it bluntly, "The doctors hated him."[76] Martin and Strofolino sought to revise the hospital's future by discarding older institutional values (loyalty, long service) and practices (rare firings, a lack of accountability). In particular, the new team aimed to combat a culture that they felt was too asymmetrical — health-care practitioners, to them, complained endlessly about the lack of resources and were concerned only with patient care. For Martin and his team, the hospital was both a medical *and* a not-for-profit corporation that needed to work efficiently to meet its own goals of patient care and research. Martin believed that the physicians couldn't just endlessly criticize administrators; they had to take responsibility themselves for the very decisions regarding the allocation of resources. As the cuts deepened in the 1990s, however, physicians and nurses grew disenchanted at the pace of change. "I was there for forty years," recalled one senior physician. "The last ten years were terrible. When the accountants came in in '86, the whole environment of SickKids changed ... People were summarily fired. People who worked there for years, given their heart and soul, were taken one day and thrown out."[77]

From a management standpoint, however, the success was palpable. Within a few years, the budget had been rebalanced and senior medical staff, whether they liked it or not (and most did not), placed in decision-making roles. A victory had been declared, as highlighted by a glowing chapter in a book, sponsored by the *Financial Post*, which trumpeted the changes at The Hospital for Sick Children between the mid-1980s and mid-1990s as a case study of how to successfully turn around a public institution in crisis.[78] Despite the split in opinion – both at the time and in retrospect – few can argue that the nature of medical management had changed fundamentally. Budgeting and accounting – on various levels and involving health practitioners – became integral to decision-making. A new era of health-care management in the hospital had truly arrived.

Conclusions

The 1980s was marked by a new and intensive era of hospital fundraising, in which Herbie Quinones was but one of many examples of the fleeting fame that sometimes awkwardly accompanied media exposure for life-threatening illnesses. As a result of his operation, Herbie survived into adulthood, living in New York. He returned to Toronto on several occasions for follow-up appointments, and was always greeted as a returning celebrity and adopted son. In 1981, for example, he performed the kick-off at the College Bowl Festival to celebrate the national university football championship game. The newspapers made much of how he had become a Blue Jays fan, supporting the team even against his hometown Mets. Yet, as time went on, Herbie became distanced from the "ritz and glamour" of fundraising. At the 2002 Mistletoe Ball, one reporter observed: "one person seemed slightly out of place, even awkward and embarrassed." It was twenty-four-year-old Herbie himself.[79] In a retrospective, thirty years after Herbie's life-saving surgery, *Toronto Star* reporter Dale Brazao followed up on the story that he had helped bring to Toronto. He found Herbie still living in Brooklyn, having recently lost his job as a mail clerk. Unemployed, Herbie could not afford to visit Toronto for the thirtieth anniversary celebrations of the fund named after him.[80]

The physical legacy of fundraising efforts of the 1980s – the Atrium itself – remains an impressive hospital space today, a fascinating manifestation of post-war architectural and social trends. The principal new entrance, on Elizabeth Street, ushered patients, families, and visitors to the new visual representations of philanthropic giving. Inescapable in the Atrium were the ubiquitous family, Foundation, and corporate plaques and logos that seemed to adorn every bridge, door, meeting room, and hallway, paying testament to the support of the community. At its opening, the Foundation commissioned artist Robert Caico to design pieces to recognize donors on the ground floor of the Atrium, including a five-ton Ventulus Harmonium, "inscribed with the names of 350 organizations that took part in the Kids for Kids campaign," as well as a 40' × 14' Wall of Honour and "scrolling Book of Honour," inscribed with the names of donors.[81] Although aesthetically incongruent, these tributes to philanthropy paid testament to the remarkable depth of support for the hospital, even in the wake of the Grange Commission and the unresolved matter of the digoxin affair.

Physical space, of course, not only reflects changing architectural tastes; it helps shape social relations – between patients and practitioners, between families and the hospital, between corporate giving and the public institution, as well as between employee groups within the institution itself. There were now play areas for patients as well as for their siblings during family visits. Parents could henceforth sleep in the rooms of their children, as well as participate on more and more hospital committees. In some ways, even the addition to the commercial aspects of the food court, "Main Street" and the controversial placement of fast-food chains, facilitated a less visible, but no less real, democratization of employee relations, where all ate together, regardless of rank or function. The entire new hospital design, as architecture historian Annmarie Adams has observed, mimicked the suburban shopping malls of the 1980s,[82] with, perhaps, a nod to Disney World. Over time, uniforms had become more informal (too informal for some senior medical staff), and medical staff began to refer to each other by their first names. Gone too were the demarcated dining areas where physicians dined separately from nurses and non-medical staff. All lined up for the same coffee, doughnuts, sandwiches, and burgers. One new aspect of segregation, however, was introduced: after years of internal debate, smoking was finally prohibited throughout the entire hospital.[83]

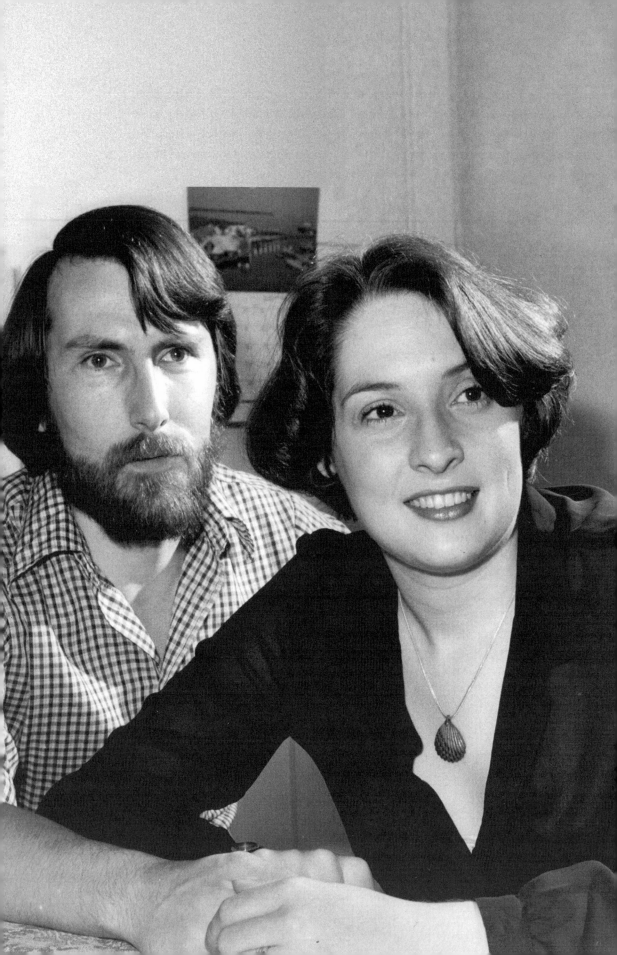

FOURTEEN

A Genetic Wilderness

Chromosome seven represented "a vast genetic wilderness somewhere between one and two million base pairs wide."[1]

Helen Pearson, "One Gene, Twenty Years," *Nature*, 2009

Susan McKellar was not supposed to live beyond childhood. Born in 1955,
she had spent most of her school years suffering from diarrhoea and coughing
up mucus in class. Susan was born with cystic fibrosis (CF), a genetic condition that condemned most children to death before they finished adolescence.
Despite her multiple and chronic symptoms, she did not receive a formal
diagnosis until the age of twelve. Already on the upper end of the life expectancy, Susan immediately began to attend the CF clinic at The Hospital for
Sick Children, which had garnered a reputation of having some of the longest
life expectancies for patients born with the condition. She continued to pursue as normal a teenage existence as possible, under the cloud of expectation
that she was unlikely to live much longer. However, she continued to defy
the epidemiological odds. In her own words, "When I turned 17 I suddenly
realized that I wasn't going to die right away and that I had better make some
plans for my life."[2] She studied nursing, began working as a psychiatric nurse
at the Clarke Institute in Toronto, and got married. An
article in the *Montreal Gazette* described her as a "viva-
cious, chestnut-haired psychiatric nurse" who believed
her faith kept her grounded amidst the deaths of her
friends. The drug plan available through her job covered the estimated $3,000 annual cost of the fifteen to
twenty pills she took at every meal.[3]

14.1 Former patient, and cystic
fibrosis advocate, Susan McKellar,
who defied the odds and lived well
into adulthood. She would challenge
long-held stereotypes about the
disease and overcome social
prejudices about parenthood for
those with terminal conditions.

Susan McKellar came to the attention of the Canadian public in 1980 when, at age twenty-five, she appeared on David Suzuki's *On the Nature of Things*. Her advocacy work made her the face of cystic fibrosis, which was in the process of being transformed from a childhood killer to a disease of young adults. By the early 1980s, about one-quarter of Canadian CF patients were no longer minors. A few years later, reportedly half of the hospital's clinic patients were over sixteen. This posed a new problem for clinical care. In her husband's words, "She objected that it was always treated as a childhood disease and patients treated as children, even in their adult years."[4] Susan and another student represented Canada at the First International Meeting of Young Adults with CF in Brussels in 1982. She formed support groups for adult patients and became the first patient to sit on the National Cystic Fibrosis Foundation board.[5]

After being advised that she should not have her own children, she apparently, in the words of her father, "fired [her doctor] immediately" and sought a second opinion.[6] The question was as much about the current state of medical ethics as the physical implications of childbirth among adult CF patients. Lurking in the background, of course, were emerging debates over the appropriateness of patients with terminal illnesses to bear children and, indeed, the emotive considerations regarding those women and men who were carriers of potentially life-threatening genetic disorders. Nevertheless, in 1985, at age thirty, Susan McKellar became the first Canadian woman with CF to bear a child; Christopher was introduced to the wider public on the second telethon at The Hospital for Sick Children in 1986. He was followed four years later by a second son, Cory. When Christopher was three months old, the family was featured in a hospital telethon mini-documentary ("The Wish"), where Susan shared her experience "living in the moment" as a new mother with a chronic, terminal illness. She did not reach her final goal – to live to see her sons as teenagers – dying shortly after a lung transplant at age 42.[7]

The New Genetics

The life of Susan McKellar humanizes an important moment in the history of paediatric care and indeed a chapter in the fast-evolving scientific research into genetic disorders. Human genetics itself emerged in the 1950s. Most notable, of course, was the famous discovery of the "Double Helix" by

Watson, Crick, and Franklin in 1953. Three years later, two Swedish-based researchers, Joe Hin Tjio and Albert Levan, revolutionized cell preparation techniques. Long restrained by technical shortcomings in the analysis of the human chromosome, the Swedish-based researchers were able to demonstrate visually that all humans possessed forty-six chromosomes in twenty-three pairs.[8] Other scientific breakthroughs came fast in the late 1950s. The same year as the Swedish innovation (1956), researchers found that they could determine the sex of the foetus by the presence (or absence) of the Barr body in cells drawn from amniotic fluid. From the late 1950s, departments of genetics began to identify – through blood-type sampling and, later, karyotyping – chromosomal anomalies, such as the most common trisomies (21, Down syndrome; 18, Edwards syndrome) as well as haemophilia A. Moreover, amniocentesis provided the capability to identify chromosomal anomalies *in utero*, a technique that was pioneered in the late 1960s and became generalized in North America in the early to mid-1970s.[9] This new diagnostic protocol, combined with the liberalization of abortion laws in Western countries (Canada's own abortion laws were decriminalized in 1969), provided the scientific and social space for the rise of genetic testing and the selective termination of foetuses with what people considered to be either life-threatening, or disabling, conditions. The Toronto General Hospital and The Hospital for Sick Children, for example, initiated a joint genetic counselling service in 1971. The Hospital for Sick Children introduced carrier-screening clinics for Tay-Sachs disease in 1972–3. By 1974, there was an amniocentesis laboratory, chromosome clinic for testing, and tissue culture service lab for suspected genetic disorders.[10]

In Montreal, cytogenetic research began to be practised in 1959 at the Sainte-Justine hospital and in 1960 at the Montreal Children's Hospital. From the early 1960s, Toronto's Hospital for Sick Children followed suit, engaging in the dominant genetics pattern of research, based on "family studies" of specific disorders. This often involved tracking down family members of individuals with particular chromosomal anomalies – Down syndrome, for example – and testing family members for potential "markers." In these early years of genetic testing, identifying infants with trisomy syndromes became relatively straightforward. Blood samples eventually replaced bone-marrow extractions, and advances in visualizing chromosomal anomalies on a karyotype became routinized in major North American hospitals. However, other diseases – like cystic fibrosis – which had become accepted as being genetic, still required the identification of the "rogue" gene or genes. Without a complete map of the human genome, the scientific quest became the laboratory equivalent of finding a needle in a haystack.[11]

Around 1970, The Hospital for Sick Children appears to have made a strategic, long-term investment in genetics research. Its vision was under-pinned by the remarkable success of the Research Institute under the leadership of Aser Rothstein. With funding kick-started by the royalties from Pablum (among other patented discoveries), The Hospital for Sick Children was receiving the most amount for hospital research of any hospital in Can-ada, and, by the end of the 1970s, ranked second (to the Boston Children's Hospital) in all of North America for paediatric research. The Hospital for Sick Children created a department of genetics and a division of genetic research attached to the hospital's Research Institute. Louis Siminovitch was appointed geneticist-in-chief in 1968 and began staffing his unit with a new team of scientific investigators. Siminovitch was dedicated to the then relatively novel investigations into somatic cell genetics. Of course, with an estimated 3 billion chemical base pairs, the global study of the human genome was, in the 1970s, still the stuff of scientific theorizing and futurism. Still, new technologies drove what was sometimes dubbed the "new genetics" and laid the groundwork for later discoveries. By the mid-1970s, novel tech-niques, such as artificially recombinant DNA, were being used to determine the sequence of progressively larger fragments of the genome.[12]

This new molecular era involved a procedure whereby a gene was found by searching for markers in the genome that were consistently inherited in affected families. Scientists would then use these markers as "signposts" to a mutant gene itself. They were thus working from the phenotype (the physiological expression of a disease), through family trees and genetic reconstructions, back to the genes themselves. As a consequence, this sci-entific process was sometimes dubbed working "in reverse," or simply "reverse genetics." Other researchers preferred the term "positional cloning" to describe this complicated process whereby a "candidate region" of a particular chromosome is searched intensively for the relevant gene. The goal was to march systematically along parts of a particular chromosome, comparing DNA fragments until one matched a gene. The trek, sometimes referred to as "chromosome walking," was painfully slow at times, particu-larly in regions that were challenging to clone. Ultimately, the goal was to identify what genes were producing proteins that were causing, or contrib-uting to, the expression of a disease. These scientific approaches overlapped with the revolution in computing technology in the late 1970s and early 1980s, which was mobilized to manage data and calculations. The automation and computerization of many of these techniques accelerated DNA sequencing and improved accuracy.[13] Suddenly, a scientific race was on, with teams around the world scrambling to identify the genetic basis of some of the most famous and intractable childhood diseases.

In retrospect, it is easy to become immersed in the dizzying array of novel scientific and computer techniques that accelerated the search for rogue genes and to overlook the social and clinical context of research experimentation. Understanding the genetic breakthroughs that would occur in the hospital requires that one reflect on the comparative advantage of The Hospital for Sick Children at the time – an advantage that did not lie simply in the fact that it had smarter scientists than comparable research centres in North America and Europe. Rather, a combination of universal health insurance (where the patient population was not restricted by who had, or did not have, health insurance), a huge patient catchment area (which was approaching 4 million persons in the late 1980s), an institutional practice of not throwing away old medical records, as well as a sophisticated and supportive patient advocacy network (in the form of the Cystic Fibrosis Foundation of Canada), created a virtuous circle. Patients were drawn to The Hospital for Sick Children as the largest and leading paediatric institution in the country; physicians worked cooperatively with basic scientists by alerting patients' families to the ongoing trials. The Cystic Fibrosis Foundation of Canada updated members on research results and calls for new research subjects, as well as raised funds for research. In this way, the research endeavour became less and less about the caricatured isolated wet lab and white-coated scientists and more about complex social networks that intersected with the hospital, patient communities, and Medicare. As some of the key scientists would later emphasize, their large, interdisciplinary research teams (geneticists, biochemists, technicians, etc.) benefited from what some estimated to be "the largest cystic fibrosis clinic in the world."[14]

The Centre of the Genetics World

The 1980s marked the decade in which paediatric genetics research took flight. In 1982, DNA markers on the X chromosome had been linked to Duchenne muscular dystrophy. The following year, the causal gene was narrowed to a specific part of the X chromosome. As the pace of, and excitement

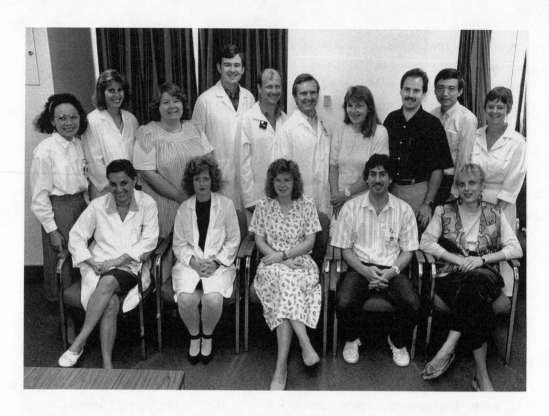

14.2 The "Centre of the Genetics World," as one researcher referred to the team at The Hospital for Sick Children, pinpointed the cystic fibrosis gene, among other discoveries. The discovery was a remarkable scientific feat but also a lesson in how research triumphs may not always lead directly to therapeutic advances.

around, genetics research began to augment, Ron Worton took the helm of genetics at The Hospital for Sick Children in 1985, refocusing on staff trained in the latest technologies of molecular genetics. He apparently accepted the chair of genetics on the condition that Lap-Chee Tsui be retained as part of his team. It was an exciting time in the Research Institute. Stephen Scherer (a graduate student during the late 1980s) emphasized the culture of overachievement at The Hospital for Sick Children, recalling that "it was a time when there was a sense of electricity and arrogance in the air. Genetics was the hottest field in science and SickKids was arguably the centre of the genetics-world."[15]

By 1985, multiple research teams, including the group at Toronto's Hospital for Sick Children, had narrowed the field regarding the CFTR (the cystic fibrosis gene), mapping it to chromosome seven. Despite this advance, chromosome seven represented "a vast genetic wilderness somewhere between one and two million base pairs wide."[16] A mistaken announcement that Robert Williamson's team (based at St Mary's Hospital in London, England) had identified the gene prompted some international teams to abandon their work. According to his own recollection, Tsui stated that Williamson's team wouldn't share their data; however, his own team could tell that it was incorrect from newspaper photographs of Williamson "holding a gel containing a chemical footprint of the suspected gene."[17] Francis Collins in Ann Arbor, Michigan, and Lap-Chee Tsui at SickKids persisted, partnering their laboratory efforts in 1987. Through the advanced technique of "chromosome jumping" (whereby scientists could effectively jump ahead and analyse periodic segments of the chromosome for hints of whether there was a possible match, at which point the team would revert to systematic "walking"), the team raced ahead and cloned the CF gene in 1989.[18]

A media frenzy ensued across the North American scientific and medical communities. News of the discovery leaked, appearing in the North American press on 22 August 1989, several weeks before scheduled scientific publication, an event that the editor of *Science* described as "no surprise," given that the endeavour involved "some two dozen researchers at two institutions and perhaps a half-dozen funding agencies involved in two countries."[19] The flagship journal abandoned its embargo policy (whereby scientists were forbidden to release news of scholarly articles prior to publication), patent applications were rushed in, and press conferences hastily scheduled in Toronto and Washington, D.C., for August 24. "It was an enormous splash," Manuel Buchwald recalled later, "and the psychological impact was that Canadian scientists can do truly competitive international science. That was the importance of that discovery, more even so than the scientific thing: it was the response of the larger world to this discovery. And it had never happened before in Canada."[20] Although the sense of Canadian pride was palpable, there was no little irony in the fact that the research program was turned down by the Medical Research Council of Canada for funding as being "too ambitious" for a Canadian-based research project; rather, it was funded principally by the (American) National Institutes of Health and the United States Cystic Fibrosis Foundation.[21]

Tainted Blood

The importance of genetic research for paediatric institutions reached new heights in the last quarter of the twentieth century. Whereas previously hospitals like SickKids had been savaged by epidemics such as measles and polio, the advent of effective vaccination campaigns in the middle of the twentieth century had reoriented the hospital more and more to the treatment of congenital conditions. However, any sanguine expectations as to the end of infectious disease outbreaks were put to rest by the AIDS epidemic of the 1980s. HIV/AIDS was transmitted by unprotected sex and by intravenous drug use; but it could also be conveyed through the blood supply. As the AIDS epidemic evolved into a serious medical crisis in North America, public health officials began to question the oversight of the blood distribution network that had then been the responsibility of the Canadian Red Cross. At The Hospital for Sick Children, two units were particularly reliant on public supplies of donated blood – cardiac surgery, of course, but also the haemophilia unit. However, as the AIDS epidemic burst onto the public health scene, the monitoring and testing of the blood supply in Canada proved to be slow to respond and riddled with bureaucracy. As the *Globe and Mail* journalist André Picard documented in his powerful book *The Gift of Death*, blood services oversight became a national public health nightmare.[22]

The tainted blood scandal that shook the country affected The Hospital for Sick Children in specific ways. Although haemophiliac patients had been tested from 1985, the fear lingered that some 17,000 other recipients of blood products at The Hospital for Sick Children in the years 1978 to 1985 may have been exposed to HIV-infected blood. In the emotive environment of the first decade of the AIDS epidemic, the hospital faced a conundrum: how to go about encouraging families of children who had undergone blood transfusions during the early 1980s to consent to testing? As a hospital's spokeswoman acknowledged, "it was a tough call" to "creat[e] tremendous anxiety" among the public when the risk of infection was "very low."[23] In 1993, Susan King and her colleagues (Dr. Brian McCrindle of cardiology and Marion Stevens of quality assurance) launched the HIV Information Project. The project team began with a preliminary notification study of a high-risk group: 1,783 cardiac surgery patients (who received large quantities of blood) who had been operated on between January 1980 and November 1985. No other hospital in the country had completed such an initiative, and they sought to unroll it as gently and effectively as possible by contacting patients through community physicians, rather than direct correspondence. However, the press picked up the story, triggering an avalanche of anxiety and, ultimately, a press conference. The front page of the *Toronto Sun* screamed "AIDS ALERT: Sick Kids Hospital Warns of '79–'86 Blood Risk."[24] Suddenly, a question of best public health practices became an exercise in managing the media. King went on air, "advising parents that if their children had been in hospital as infants and were sick with unexplained illness they should be tested for AIDS."[25] The Hospital for Sick Children opened a hotline, and "hundreds of parents flooded a bank of four telephone counsellors with a nonstop barrage of phone calls."[26] The hospital received over 500 calls *per hour* during the hotline's first twelve hours, and 1,000 voicemails overnight.[27]

The media attention altered King's initial study design, as patients and families learned of the risk incidentally, rather than through their physicians. Although it might seem unusual in retrospect, many were not fully aware of their transfusion status. Few felt that they personally were at risk of AIDS, only seeking testing once informed of their risk through the study. The ultimate finding that seventeen of the 1,783 children were infected was groundbreaking, "ma[king] headlines around the world."[28] These discoveries prompted the team to notify the remaining 15,000 "lower-risk" transfusion patients. The following April, the hospital's team sent letters to those who had received blood products from January 1980 to November 1985, "informing them of the risk of HIV infection from blood products at that time."[29] The media coverage also prompted various provinces and health-care organizations to recommend that transfusion recipients get tested. A House of Commons subcommittee advised, to little effect, that all hospitals follow The Hospital for Sick Children's example and contact individuals who had received blood transfusions before comprehensive testing of the blood supply began in November 1985.[30] Despite the ethical impetus, hospitals around the country were extremely wary of the legal liabilities involved in doing so.

Needless to say, the relative novelty of AIDS patients in a paediatric setting challenged clinical procedures and reflected evolving perceptions of the disease. A protocol for AIDS patients' care at the hospital was first developed as early as 1983. The first Hospital for Sick Children patients affected were young haemophiliacs, and later babies infected perinatally by their mothers. The haemophilia clinic sought parental permission to test patients in 1985, and initiated sexual counselling for adolescent patients. Not all parents were willing to cooperate. Some refused to give consent; others asked not to be told the results.[31] The issue was far from hypothetical: by 1987, over one-third of the haemophilia clinic's 120 to 150 patients were HIV-positive, and at least one had developed AIDS.[32] Infectious disease specialist Dr. Stanley Read spoke publicly "in an attempt to allay some of the public's fears about AIDS and its infectivity."[33] In response to public fears of haemophiliac children, the hospital offered to send doctors to speak at schools to reassure teachers, children and parents.[34]

The Ontario Ministry of Health responded to the rising public concern by funding a comprehensive care program for HIV-positive patients at the hospital. Stanley Read and Susan King began an outpatient clinic in late November 1988, which involved staff from the haemophilia program, adolescent medicine, psychiatry, clinical nutrition, neurology, gynaecology, nursing, psychology, social work, nutrition and food services, pharmacy and chaplaincy. In 1989, it was reported that fifty patients with AIDS attended regularly. Of those patients, thirty-five were haemophiliacs infected by blood products, and five were patients infected by transfusions prior to screening. Another five were infants of infected mothers, and five more were teenagers who had become infected through drug use or unprotected sex. At that time, three babies were reportedly doing well on AZT (the first anti-retroviral drug approved by the FDA).[35]

The Krever Commission, charged with examining the tainted blood scandal in Canada, learned that at The Hospital for Sick Children, the presence of infants and children with AIDS precipitated considerable disquiet on the wards. One mother recalled that "nurses initially approached [one patient] dressed in gowns and goggles, which frightened him, staff left his food on a tray outside his room."[36] A clinic coordinator, who joined the unit that year, recalled the children

> being very sick, very uncomfortable and very unhappy. Often they were alone or with a family member other than their parents because the parents were too sick to be at the hospital with them. They had chronic diarrhea, bloated abdomens, skinny little arms and legs, as well as poor appetites. Many required feeding-tubes for sustenance. The stigma was so bad, even among health-care providers. People were scared to get "it"; double gloving, gowning, some even declined to care for children with HIV.[37]

Through outreach from the haemophilia and HIV/AIDS clinics, CHAS (a children's HIV/AIDS support group) was begun by parents and clinic staff to promote education and reduce isolation experienced by families. In May 1989, the hospital held a one-day conference on ethical issues in paediatric AIDS, where it was announced that parents of patients who were old enough to give informed consent would not be informed of testing results.[38] The response of the hospital raised profound issues in terms of the ethical duty of hospitals to patients and their families. André Picard would praise the hospital for the stance it took to inform families, despite the danger of significant legal ramifications. Such praise, however, would be in short supply in terms of the hospital's response to another ethical dispute that would rock the institution and the University of Toronto.

University-Industry Partnerships

By 1993, the federal and provincial governments were mired in debt, with Canada posting one of the highest per capita debts of any G7 country.[39] At the nadir, over one-quarter of the entire federal government's revenue was devoted to merely servicing the accumulated debt.[40] Large structural changes were overdue and could not be solely addressed by the imposition of the much-hated goods and services tax (GST), which, after all, had been intended to be revenue neutral. As a consequence, the new Liberal government in Ottawa slashed federal spending, including federal transfers for co-funding health care. The federal share of funding insurable services had declined from the landmark 50 per cent (in the 1957 Hospital Insurance and Diagnostic Services Act and the Medical Care Act of 1966) to close to 33 per cent.[41] As health care remained a provincial responsibility, the fiscal challenges were effectively downloaded to the provinces, which then cut hospital budgets and social assistance programs. In Ontario, with the arrival of a Progressive Conservative government under Mike Harris (in 1995), the provincial government at Queen's Park sought to implement its "Common Sense Revolution," which reduced government spending to address its own accumulated provincial debt. The fiscal overhaul in Ontario targeted hospitals in particular, with a view to reducing the perceived overcapacity of beds in the central city core, one that had persisted to the disadvantage, many argued, of the growing population in the suburban regions of Metropolitan Toronto. The Health Services Restructuring Commission (HSRC) was created in 1996 with a four-year mandate to recommend "changes necessary to make the provisions of health services in Ontario more efficient and effective."[42] As a book on hospital restructuring observed, it was distinguished by "having the unprecedented and seemingly unconstrained authority to restructure public hospitals."[43] The HSCR's report recommended the closure of forty-five hospital sites, dozens of amalgamations, and a reduction of $1.1 billion in hospital budgets between 1995 and 2003.[44] Many hospitals (such as Women's College Hospital) with unique historical legacies, were forced to amalgamate into large hospital networks.

The 1990s proved to be a difficult decade for research as well, as evidenced by cuts to the Medical Research Council of Canada (MRC), the federal granting agency responsible for coordinating taxpayer-supported medical research across the country. In response to the Paul Martin budget of 1995, the MRC's base budget was reduced by 13 per cent (from $267 to $237 million) over two years.[45] By 1998, the MRC had lost $31 million in annual funding in four years.[46] The slow decline of the proportion of medical research coming from public funds was neither sudden nor unnoticed. Indeed, the president of the MRC recognized in his annual reports the trend towards non-government-funded clinical research between the mid-1980s and mid-1990s. "Over the last decade," he acknowledged, "MRC's percentage of support of all health research funding in Canada has declined from 40 percent to 25 percent ... This means that 75 percent of all direct health research funding now comes from outside the federal government – from industry, provincial health research organizations, and the voluntary disease-specific organizations."[47] As Michael Bliss has well documented, the federal MRC conveniently turned to the promotion of "university-industry partnerships" as a means of bridging the difference. In an emerging climate of fiscal restraint, the president of MRC, Dr. Henry Friesen, oversaw publication of *Investing in Canada's Health: A Strategic Plan for the Medical Research Council of Canada*, which heralded the trend towards formation of strategic partnerships with "virtually anyone interested in injecting dollars and energy into health research."[48] New alliances with private industry and non-profits provided crucial sources of funding, such as a 1993 agreement with the Pharmaceutical Manufacturers Association of Canada, which the MRC president hoped would "generate $200 million worth of industry-sponsored, MRC peer-reviewed research in five years."[49]

The combined blow of reduced funding for both health care and medical research and the advent of hospital restructuring affected individual hospitals in different ways. Although large groupings of medical institutions in Toronto would emerge – the Toronto General Hospital, Princess Margaret, Toronto Western, and Toronto Rehab came together as the University Health Network – The Hospital for Sick Children managed to avoid the wave of forced amalgamations due to its unique status as the only children's hospital in the metropolis. However, restructuring did accelerate plans for the outsourcing of certain programs. The Health Services Restructuring

Commission, which amalgamated and closed hospitals across the province, nominated SickKids to assume a leadership role in a new Child Health Network that was to "coordinate and enhance services for children across Metro [Toronto]."[50] Certain clinical care programs were relocated to community-based hospitals, where they would continue to be overseen by hospital-based directors.[51]

One of the targeted programs was the thalassemia and sickle-cell disease (SCD) program at the hospital, which had expanded rapidly in the new Atrium hospital. Indeed, from 1986 to 1998, the patient load of the lead clinician, Nancy Olivieri, had trebled from 150 to 450 patients (100 patients with thalassemia and 350 with sickle-cell disease), a reflection, in part, of the waves of Southern European, Middle Eastern, and African-Caribbean immigrants to the Metro Toronto area. The sickle-cell disease program (but not the thalassemia program) was designated in 1995 as "one of several programs to be decentralized (or 'satellited') to regional hospitals." Both clinics had been part of one joint haemoglobinopathy program (established in 1988), of which Olivieri was the head. Nancy Olivieri had long felt a lack of support for her program within the hospital; hospital administrators, by contrast, felt that Olivieri was unable to accept that, in a climate of diminishing institutional resources, some programs would need to be closed, reorganized, or decentralized. As relations soured in the early 1990s, the chief of paediatrics, Robert Haslam, initiated an investigation into Olivieri's work and relations in the department of paediatrics. As Miriam Shuchman summarized in her book *The Drug Trial*, "She [Olivieri] thought her bosses could be investigating her as a way of retaliating for her efforts to get the resources she deserved."[52] By contrast, Olivieri's superiors believed that she was not accepting the new fiscal reality of hospital funding, nor fully appreciating the limits of program resources. In May 1996, the hospital informed Olivieri that they were going to continue with their plan to decentralize or "satellite" the SCD program.[53]

In October 1996, Olivieri was presented with the ultimatum that if she was "unable to cooperate" with the decision, another individual would be asked to direct the program.[54] Olivieri later referred to this as an initial attempt to remove her as program head. As a sympathetic reporter retold it, "A decision was taken to move Olivieri's sickle-cell anemia clinic several kilometres away to a hospital in suburban Scarborough. When the scientist protested against the removal of the clinic from a teaching and research hospital, the job of overseeing the move was taken away from her."[55] The fight over resources and the situation of the patients became conflated, and thus inflamed, over time, with the scientific disputes arising over the efficacy and side effects of an experimental thalassemia drug – L1.[56]

L1

Thalassemia patients are treated with blood transfusions, which lead to iron overload in their bodies. Iron-chelation (removal) therapy was needed to address this effect. The drug deferoxamine was the standard iron chelating therapy, but was intrusive, needing to "be administered by subcutaneous infusion, driven by a pump ... for many hours, several days every week." Moreover, the drug had "several known toxic side-effects."[57] This treatment restricted patients' schedules and had unpleasant effects. Patient adherence to the treatment dropped among adolescents and young adults, with hazardous or fatal results. In search of an alternative, Olivieri learned of "an experimental iron-chelation drug" that could be taken orally, a distinct advantage over the existing drug.[58] In 1988, Health Canada approved a protocol to test the new drug. Soon thereafter, Olivieri began enrolling patients at The Hospital for Sick Children in a preliminary trial. Over the next few years, she partnered with Gideon Koren, the director of the division of clinical pharmacology and toxicology, on a Medical Research Council of Canada (MRC) grant, to conduct a so-called "compassionate use" study of L1. In order to develop L1 for therapeutic use, additional clinical trials for efficacy and safety were required. In 1991, Olivieri applied unsuccessfully for another MRC grant, with one reviewer apparently advising her to "collaborate with a drug company and reapply for a grant under the MRC's university industry program[.]"[59] In March 1993, the pharmaceutical company possessing the patent, Ciba-Geigy, dropped work on L1 and gave up patent, presumably as it saw no profitable future for the drug.[60]

Without ongoing MRC funding for L1, Olivieri and Koren approached Apotex, one of the largest generic drug manufacturers in North America, for external funding. The company agreed, in 1993, to fund a three-year randomized trial, known as "LA-01," comparing L1 with deferoxamine, the standard drug used in this patient group for three decades. The contract contained a one-year post-trial confidentiality clause for data produced during this trial. The Hospital for Sick Children's Research Ethics Board approved the study protocol, apparently without any knowledge of the confidentiality clause that was part of the contract. At the time, before the strict formalization of externally funded research at university-based hospitals, confidentiality clauses were not unheard of, nor was the system of researchers signing independent protocols. In April 1995, the team published an article in the prestigious *New England Journal of Medicine*, suggesting positive findings from the initial clinical trials. A few months later, Olivieri signed a contract with Apotex to act as consultant for a further, one-year international acute toxicity (safety) trial (LA-02). This consulting contract also contained "a three-year post-termination publication ban" and involved no patients based at SickKids.[61]

In October 1995, after complaints from the research team about the need for more administrative support to analyse the results, Apotex agreed to support data management in order to study possible reasons for apparent lack of efficacy of L1. A third contract pertaining to long-term trials of L1, "LA-03," was signed by Olivieri; an important aspect of the new contract was that it contained no confidentiality restriction at all. Sometime between late 1995 and early 1996, Nancy Olivieri discovered what she believed was "loss of sustained efficacy of the drug" during her analysis of the data of the patient cohort of the long-term trial. Apotex saw no reason to "raise red flags" over a perceived loss of efficacy and disagreed with Olivieri's interpretation of the data. They also questioned Olivieri's insistence that she would need to inform patients before further validation.[62] The Research Ethics Board of the hospital, by contrast, affirmed her need to inform patients involved in the trials after she formally reported the loss of efficacy in March of 1996. They instructed her to modify consent forms and advise other physicians who were using L1 as part of the compassionate use program. In May of 1996, Olivieri complied and modified the consent forms, submitting them to the hospital's Research Ethics Board and to Apotex for approval. At this point, Apotex terminated the clinical trial and ended Olivieri's consulting contract. Further, according to a later Canadian Association of University Teachers report, the company warned of "legal consequences to Dr. Olivieri should she inform patients or anyone else of the risk."[63] In such an environment, Olivieri and Koren, responding to what they perceived as thinly veiled threats of lawsuits, informed the hospital and university that they had sought legal advice and contacted the Canadian Medical Protective Association (CMPA), the national body responsible for the legal protection of licensed medical practitioners.[64]

From this point onwards, the scientific dispute, complicated by the long-standing clash over the future of the hospital's SCD program, cascaded into a dizzying array of accusations, counter-accusations, and lawsuits that would poison the atmosphere in the hospital for many years to come. One aspect of the legal dispute was over the proprietorial dimensions of the medical data itself: Who owned the information? Apotex certainly indicated that they considered the data produced by the trial to be proprietorial. By contrast, the legal stance defending Olivieri and Koren was based on the fact that the last contract contained no confidentiality restriction. Since a clause stated that the contract "supplant[ed] any other previous agreement on this cohort of patients," a later report argued that it legally invalidated the "confidentiality clauses" of the earlier LA-01 and LA-02 contracts.[65] Legal positions intersected, of course, with principles of academic freedom, since one of the purposes of confidentiality agreements was, after all, to control the release of ambiguous or unpromising scientific results. With lawyers now fully involved, Olivieri informed the hospital in July 1996 that her team intended to report data despite what Apotex were claiming were contractual restrictions. The hospital took the position that the conflict was a scientific controversy and that the peer-review process was best equipped to decide the issue; it encouraged Dr. Olivieri to proceed with her plan to submit her data to the American Society of Haematology. Caught in the middle were the thalassemia patients themselves, whose access to L1 was jeopardized by the trial's sudden termination. The then dean of medicine, Dr. Arnold Aberman, mediated an agreement between Olivieri and Apotex whereby some patients could continue to receive the drug through Health Canada's Emergency Drug Release Program. However, the drug supply "remained irregular into early 1997."[66]

In the winter of 1996–7, Olivieri became aware of studies suggesting liver fibrosis in animal models (the animals were receiving "an iron chelator" that was similar, in terms of chemical composition, to L1). She obtained patient biopsies and initiated pathological examination, leading to the identification of a second risk of the drug L1.[67] In early 1997, she informed her patients of the second potential risk of progressive liver damage. By this time, Gideon Koren and Nancy Olivieri, who had both worked together on the L1 trials, had become estranged and ceased collaborative work. Koren asserted that he disagreed with the scientific conclusions drawn by Olivieri and believed "that there was no risk of loss of sustained efficacy of its drug." According to the *Olivieri Report* (sponsored by the Canadian Association of University Teachers), Koren "re-analysed data from the terminated L1 trials and published findings that the drug was effective and safe" without disclosing Apotex's support, Olivieri's identification of risks, or her role in generating the data. The report further contended that Apotex used Koren's work "to counter Dr. Olivieri's adverse findings on its drug."[68] In the opinion of the hospital's Naimark review (see below), Olivieri had neglected to "share her findings suggesting liver toxicity of L1" with Koren before presenting on it.[69] Shuchman reports that Koren "was hurt" by this exclusion, particularly because he had been acting as the intermediary with Apotex to supply her patients with L1. When he learned of her findings through a third party, he informed her that he would cease to collaborate with her. The *Olivieri Report* authors maintain that she informed Koren of the risk on the same day that she informed patients.[70]

As the controversy began to engulf the hospital in 1998, attempts to stem the tide of recrimination achieved little. Now every move, every initiative of either side, was challenged for its authenticity and motive. Supporters of Olivieri circulated a petition in August 1998 asking University of Toronto Vice-President Heather Munroe-Blum and the hospital's Research Institute director to have the hospital "undertake an external independent review of the Olivieri/Apotex issue." The director of the hospital's Research Institute, Dr. Manuel Buchwald, held an open forum for Research Institute staff. A group that became known as the "Gang of Four" (a rather odd and somewhat unfortunate reference to political leaders in China's Cultural Revolution) formed the bridgehead of support for Olivieri. Other researchers wrote letters of support for the administration. Meanwhile, within the scientific realm, Olivieri's findings of loss of efficacy were published in the *New England Journal of Medicine* in August 1998, alongside an unusual editorial advising caution in drawing conclusions. Later that month, acknowledging the media coverage and the hospital petition, The Hospital for Sick Children announced an external review of its policies and procedures by Arnold Naimark, then director of the Centre for the Advancement of Medicine and president emeritus at the University of Manitoba. It began its investigations in September 1998 and reported in December, making its findings available through the hospital's website, intranet, and library. Notably, the two sides were unable to reach an agreement about the size or composition of this review panel; as a consequence, Olivieri and her supporters refused to participate.[71]

Following the completion of the Naimark Review report, the hospital trustees directed the Medical Advisory Committee to review the Naimark Report's allegation that Olivieri did not report adverse effects to its Research

Ethics Board in appropriate fashion and continued using L1 after finding a second risk. In January 1999, in a decisive move, the chief of paediatrics chaired a meeting that removed Olivieri from her post as head of the haemo-globinopathy program (apparently over the objections of the president of the University of Toronto). Subsequently, the hospital president, Michael Strofolino, issued letters directing Olivieri's supporters not to speak to the media. Two weeks later, they reversed themselves through a deal brokered by University of Toronto President Robert Prichard, Dr. David Nathan of Harvard University, and Sir David Weatherall, the prominent British scientist who had come to Olivieri's support. By this time, the issue had become a major debate about the academic freedom (or not) of clinical researchers.[72]

Facing mounting costs for legal support and the media campaign, Olivieri and the so-called Gang of Four sought aid from the University of Toronto Faculty Association, which led to the intervention of the Canadian Association of University Teachers (CAUT), the national umbrella organization advocating on behalf of university professors and academic staff. The CAUT had long identified clinical professors as a dangerous anomaly of researchers working in a university environment but without the traditional protection of tenure. In January 1999, the University of Toronto Faculty Association filed a grievance on behalf of Olivieri and three of her supporters (Gallie, Durie, and Chan) in response to the alleged violation of their "academic freedom" through the "gag order" imposed by Strofolino at the time of Olivieri's removal as head of the haemoglobinopathy program.[73] By February 1999, a complicated settlement was agreed between Olivieri, The Hospital for Sick Children, and the University of Toronto.

If the hospital had hoped that the settlement of February 1999 would put the affair to rest, they would be disappointed. By this time, the very public nature of the dispute had reached beyond Toronto and, indeed, beyond the Canadian medical community. The sheer size of the University of Toronto, the reputation of The Hospital for Sick Children, and its location in one of the largest and most influential cities in North America engendered significant international media coverage. For the CAUT, the situation of Nancy Olivieri became a cause célèbre. In October 1999, the CAUT Academic Freedom and Tenure Committee appointed its own independent committee of inquiry, which would deliver a report known later as the Olivieri Report. In a December 1999, in an interview with *60 Minutes*, the flagship investigative program of CBS, Apotex CEO Barry Sherman opined that Olivieri was "nuts," which prompted Olivieri to sue him for libel. Apotex then counter-sued for $10 million in the Ontario Superior Court, claiming that "her statements about its employees and products were defamatory."[74] Senior administrative officers of the hospital sued the university's Grievance Review Panel, the UFTA, Olivieri (and her supporters) in the Ontario Superior Court. Shortly after this, with the support of the UFTA, Olivieri and three of her supporters sought a court injunction to block an agreement about provincial payments to The Hospital for Sick Children that had been negotiated by the hospital, the Ontario Medical Association, and the provincial ministry of health. Any formal reporting of the affair

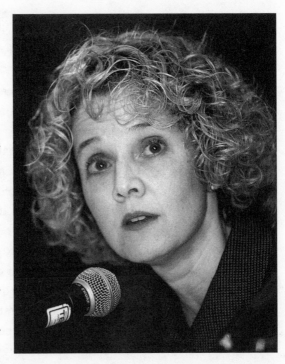

14.3 The case of the research scientist Nancy Olivieri became a cause célèbre in the English-speaking academic world. The issues arising from the protection (or lack thereof) of clinician researchers would lead to a fundamental reorganization of research ethics in Canada.

seemed to engender more lawsuits. According to Shuchman, Olivieri even brought a libel suit against various entities, including CBC television and the *National Post*.[75]

The increasingly litigious affair took a bizarre twist during the Naimark Review investigation when the media and Hospital for Sick Children staff began to receive anonymous letters attacking Drs. Olivieri, Durie, Gallie, and Chan. During 1999, Olivieri and her supporters privately funded investigations that yielded DNA evidence identifying none other than Gideon Koren as the author. The story broke to the media in December 1999 and Koren, after initially denying authorship, ultimately confessed. He stepped down from three of his posts at the hospital and university and was subject to disciplinary action in April 2000.[76] Revelations of "forgery and misrepresentation" by Koren emerged as the hospital's "poison pen probe" was poised to begin.[77] Olivieri's lawyers sought "to broaden" the investigation to include these allegations because he had been a core informant for the Naimark and other reviews.[78] The hospital had hired its own investigator, who was experienced in workplace harassment, but Olivieri's supporters did not trust the process and viewed the long wait time before action as evidence of "further mistreatment." The investigator, who released her report after Olivieri and her supporters had leaked the news about Koren, recommended mediation, announcing that "both sides were responsible for the delays she'd encountered."[79]

Ultimately Gideon Koren was charged by University of Toronto and the College of Physicians and Surgeons of Ontario with misconduct and was reprimanded for "conduct unbecoming a physician."[80] Much to the surprise of the media, Koren was not dismissed from the hospital. Rather, he had to pay back to the hospital the cost of the investigation, lost his chair in child health research, was removed from his position in University of Toronto's Interdepartmental Division of Clinical Pharmacology, and was suspended for six months.[81] He retired in June 2015, amidst a new scandal at the MotherRisk Hair Testing Laboratory that he had founded.[82] In 2000, another Research Institute senior scientist, Sergio Grinstein, the University of Toronto Pitblado Chair in cell biology, "admitted sending an anonymous note ... to Michele Brill-Edwards," an Olivieri supporter. She reported the "intimidating" note, received in July 1999, to David Naylor, the new dean of medicine.[83] Meanwhile, the hospital's Medical Advisory Committee review process dragged on. In April 2000, the Medical Advisory Committee of the hospital recommended that the trustees refer Olivieri to the College of Physicians and Surgeons of Ontario (CPSO), the provincial regulatory body, for "concerns" that she had allegedly not alerted the Research Ethics Board to the harmful side effects of L1. This charge was dismissed by the CPSO in December 2001.[84]

Ultimately, in 2002, a new mediation process led to a new settlement between Olivieri, The Hospital for Sick Children, and the University of Toronto. "The settlement that has been reached is comprehensive and will resolve all outstanding litigation and arbitrations pending between the parties," the *National Post* reported from the joint statement by Dr. Olivieri, the hospital, and the university.[85] The *Globe and Mail* indicated that both sides claimed a victory of sorts: Olivieri and her supporters "[saw] the settlement as a vindication of their position," whereas the vice-president of The Hospital for Sick Children, Alan Goldbloom, stated that the hospital viewed it "as a settlement without any victory or finger-pointing for any one side."[86] Following the settlement, Nancy Olivieri took a sabbatical to pursue master's degree in medical ethics and law at King's College (2003). Upon her return, she moved to the Toronto General Research Institute (TGRI) Cancer Clinical Research Unit (CCRU), Princess Margaret Cancer Centre as a research scientist.[87]

Conclusions

By the middle of the 1990s, the media excitement arising from multiple genetic discoveries helped propel a transnational collaboration to map and sequence the entire human genome. The subsequent Human Genome Project was characterized as "the largest and most expensive scientific study since the Apollo project and the race to send a human to the moon."[88] Underpinning the hype around the mapping of the human genome was an implicit link between scientific discovery and therapeutic transformation. Once the genome had been mapped, "gene therapy" – a theoretical process whereby one could insert a "functional" gene in a host in order to replace or control a "defective" one – would provide the bridge to new and life-changing clinical advances. Scientists believed in good faith in such a link. As Ron Worton and Margaret Thompson, two of the most senior geneticists at The Hospital for Sick Children, opined in a scientific article in 1988, "The ultimate prospect of alleviation [of Duchenne muscular dystrophy] is not yet within reach, but the pace of discovery makes us hopeful that it is no longer totally beyond our grasp."[89]

But clinical advances arising directly from this genetic research proved to be more elusive than many had predicted. Yes, the discovery of the cystic fibrosis gene helped transform scientific understanding of the disease and assisted with earlier detection, but in the minds of some researchers looking back two decades, it soon became "an object lesson in how difficult it is, and how long it takes, to convert genetic knowledge into treatments."[90] The initial goal of developing gene therapy was pursued to little avail, and advances in treatment were held up, in the case of cystic fibrosis, by "lack of a complete understanding of how the CFTR protein leads to the disease."[91] As one researcher recalled,

> I think nobody knew how hard it was. Nobody knew where this gene would be expressed. It turns out like in your lungs, it's in one little cell there that lines your lungs. Well, how do we get a gene in there? Nobody had any idea! How do we fix it? I don't know! ... we didn't know. We didn't know near as much about lung biology ... We didn't

even know about the development of the lung or the biology of the lung to even know ... I realized like, how could we even dream about gene therapy when we didn't even know what regulates genes and we didn't know how to get the gene in there?[92]

With gene-therapy research ongoing, the main practical application of new knowledge became improved genetic counselling and diagnosis. As team member Jack Riordan cleverly summed up, "The disease [CF] has contributed much more to science than science has contributed to the disease."[93]

If the challenges of translating laboratory science into clinical implications turned out to be a lesson in humility, the Olivieri affair shattered the sometimes caricatured world of objective and dispassionate scientific research. Scientific laboratories – within and without medical science – vary enormously in size, purpose, longevity, and character. Some nurture deep personal and professional relationships, sometimes even amorous entanglements. Others disintegrate or reconstitute themselves, due to the termination of funding, the exodus of key researchers, a lack of institutional support, or differences of intellectual opinion. Ultimately, science may make claims to objectivity, but can never avow to being depersonalized. Quite the contrary. Entire careers are made (and unmade) based upon the success of grants and the interpretation of results. In extreme cases, when the stakes are high, extraordinary behaviour occurs, including the falsification or suppression of results, the portrayal of other's research as one's own, and interpersonal harassment and intimidation.

The Olivieri controversy revealed how the scientific endeavour could go badly wrong. It deeply embarrassed both The Hospital for Sick Children and the University of Toronto. It permanently reshaped careers and left long-lasting enmities. Few could doubt, however, that the issues arising from this sad chapter in the hospital carried with them national, and indeed, international ramifications. In Canada, the federal Tri-Council funding agencies (the Social Sciences and Humanities Research Council, Natural Sciences and Engineering Research Council, and Medical Research Council) worked together to strengthen the protocols and culture around research ethics, creating a national ethics policy at the height of the dispute at the hospital, one that was to apply to *all* researchers engaged in research involving human subjects (in contradistinction to research involving animals). The Tri-Council mandated, among other things, permanent research ethics boards at universities across the country as well as strongly encouraging boards at any medical or quasi-medical institutions to do the same. In the wake of the Olivieri affair, many hospitals across the country followed suit, by clarifying and strengthening their ethics procedures. Unsurprisingly, at The Hospital for Sick Children itself, the chair of the Research Ethics Board was transformed from a voluntary position to a paid, half-time appointment.[94]

What the national Tri-Council could not regulate as easily was the ever-changing relationship between for-profit companies (primarily, but not solely, pharmaceutical businesses) and health-care practitioners working in public-sector health-care institutions. What voluntary, or compulsory, obligation should individual researchers have to disclose real or potential conflicts of interests in their talks, to their patients, to research audiences, or in professional journals? What role, if any, should "Big Pharma" play in the medical education of undergraduate and postgraduate medical students, and at professional society meetings? Should data generated by the involvement of patients in a public hospital system be proprietorial (and thus private) if the clinical trial itself was funded by a private company? Do physician-researchers (who are technically self-employed professionals) have the right to "academic freedom" in the same manner as full-time university-based academics, such as sociologists, philosophers and, for that matter, historians? To be sure, these debates existed before the events of the late 1990s, but they were given greater urgency in light of The Hospital for Sick Children and University of Toronto's own troubles. Many of these questions remain unresolved, not because of a lack of reflection, but due to the ambiguous position of university-affiliated research hospitals.

Stung by criticism that the University of Toronto had abandoned Olivieri and denied her rights to academic freedom, leading figures attempted to clarify the relationship of what had become Canada's largest and most powerful medical research establishment with its affiliated teaching hospitals. The university had initially constructed an argument that teaching hospitals were at arm's length from university regulations. Although this might have been true in a narrow technical way, it had more than a whiff of an argument arising from expediency. Following the entente between Olivieri and the hospital in January 1999, the University of Toronto began to develop policies concerning academic freedom and the ethical conduct of research for its affiliated (non-tenured) researchers at eight medical institutions. The university attempted to walk the fine line of giving researchers the protection of academic expression without recognizing them as tenure-stream faculty members in the same way as non-clinical members of the university. The university established a new affiliation agreement with the teaching hospitals which "protects [a] researcher's rights to disclose safety concerns to research subjects, forbids research sponsors from suppressing research results, limits publication delays to six months, and proposes a dispute resolution mechanism."[95] This policy "harmonization" was completed in March 2001.[96]

Sadly, hopes within the University of Toronto community that these issues had been put to rest were shattered when, only weeks later, the University of Toronto medical research community once again became engulfed by a new scandal, involving the psychiatrist David Healy and the University of Toronto–affiliated Centre for Addiction and Mental Health (CAMH). Healy, who had been recently hired to take up a senior position at CAMH, had his letter of offer rescinded after he voiced what were then deemed to be "unconventional" views of the relationship between a certain class of anti-depressants (SSRIS) and suicidal impulses. The situation involved potential side-effects of a class of drugs being increasingly used on children (in this case, adolescents), a major pharmaceutical company and donor to the University of Toronto (Eli Lilly), and another University of Toronto–affiliated teaching hospital. It soon became directly associated, at least in the minds of the general public, with the as-yet unsettled Olivieri/Apotex dispute. In the words of one bioethics commentator, "No discussion of academic freedom, research integrity, and patient safety could begin with a more disquieting pair of case studies than those of Nancy Olivieri and David Healy."[97]

By the end of the 1990s, The Hospital for Sick Children had endured a roller-coaster decade of great scientific successes as well as gut-wrenching controversy. Many of the thousands of employees felt an increasing sense of distress that the daily work of caring for thousands sick children had been crowded out under the bright lights of the Canadian media establishment. Even those involved in the cystic fibrosis gene research felt a resentment towards the media that they felt had overhyped the scientific discovery and unnecessarily exaggerated the therapeutic benefits of the laboratory work. Many at the hospital talked in medical terms, and in no purposeful sense of irony, of the need to "heal" the institution. As the Naimark Report observed, "The controversy ha[d] taken an enormous toll on professional relationships in the Hospital and beyond. Collegiality, friendship, civil discourse, trust and common courtesy have all been victims of the controversy."[98] Even the *Journal of Medical Ethics* symposium on bio-ethics in 2004 had a contribution subtitled "Moving Beyond the Olivieri/Apotex Affair."[99]

When the Krever Commission delivered its report, the tainted blood scandal was considered to be the worst disaster in public health adminis-tration/oversight in Canadian history. Over 1,000 people had been infected with HIV-tainted blood, another 30,000 with hepatitis C. Within this scan-dal, The Hospital for Sick Children was considered the flagship in terms of notifying former patients, despite the inevitable anxiety that this would merely lead to multiple lawsuits. In terms of patient therapies, unlike the growing frustration over gene therapies, the turning point for paediatric AIDS care emerged in the mid-1990s, as a new generation of retrovirals increased life expectancy. By the turn of the twenty-first century, the gen-eration of Canadian children with tainted blood had become a chapter in the hospital's history, with the reported 70 children in the HIV/AIDS Com-prehensive Care Clinic mostly infected perinatally. As Stanley Read recalled in 2013, "Children born with HIV since 1996 ... are all living well with their HIV and we have had no deaths since that time."[100] Eventually, control over the national blood supply was taken away from the Red Cross, and a new agency – Canadian Blood Services – began its life in a renovated building in downtown Toronto, none other than 67 College Street, the former Victoria Hospital for Sick Children.

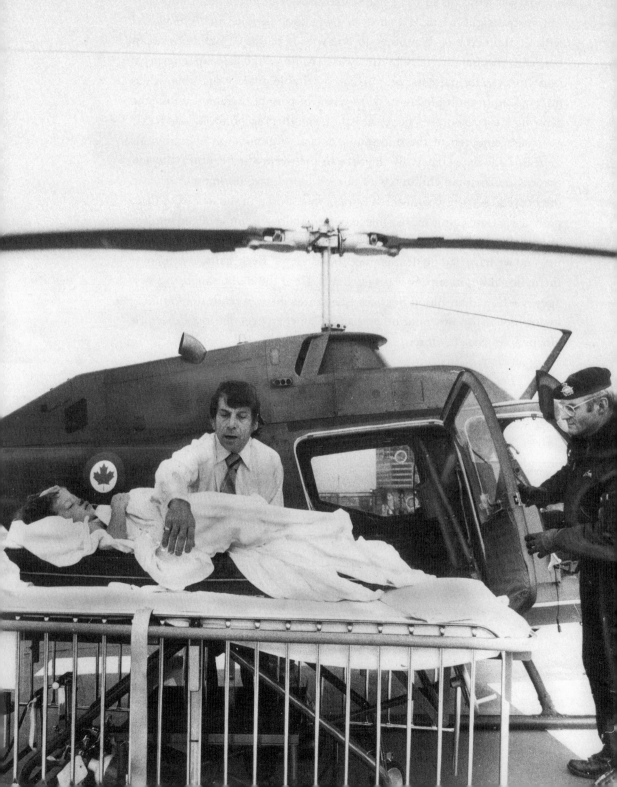

FIFTEEN

A Hospital without Walls

Once somebody caught something and it spread in the whole school like wildfire, and they would just more or less, we had to live out whatever it is that we caught, whether it's measles, mumps, sores, bedbugs, all that kind of stuff, we just had to live with it ... We used to have a matron that sort of acted as a nurse as well. So a medical doctor we never saw.[1]

Roger Cromarty, former Sioux Lookout residential school
student, *The Survivors Speak*, 2015

Sioux Lookout Zone

Sioux Lookout is a remote town in Ontario, a community 200 kilometres northwest of Thunder Bay. For most of the twentieth century, it was a mining and railway community of a few thousand people, a predominantly European settler population amidst communities of the Cree and Ojibwa First Nations. The rise and fall of fortunes in the nearby mines sustained the local economy, assisted by indirect commerce associated with the Canadian National Railway as well as the growing popularity of seasonal fishing and recreational activities. The district had its own residential school – Pelican Lake – opened in 1926 about ten kilometres west of the town and run by the Anglican Church of Canada. Ojibwa, Cree, and Swampy Cree children were relocated from reserves in the surrounding 680,000 square kilometres in what was part of a

15.1 Three-year-old patient Steven Wilson arrives at the SickKids rooftop heliport on a Canadian Armed Forces helicopter piloted by Major Jack Jackman.

national, multi-generational project of forced assimilation. Medical attention, as the quotation above highlights, was minimal. As one later medical report acknowledged, as Ontario was rolling out universal health insurance in the late 1960s, there was only one doctor and one dentist for 10,000 to 12,000 Cree and Ojibwa scattered among twenty-four communities.[2] In many key social, cultural, and epidemiological aspects, Sioux Lookout reflected the common dynamics of Indigenous communities in the near North throughout twentieth-century Canada.

The British North America Act of 1867 designated "Indian Affairs" as a federal, rather than provincial, responsibility. The numbered treaties of the 1870s and 1880s, which would divide and subdivide what are now Northwestern Ontario and the provinces of Manitoba and Saskatchewan, constituted agreements between Indigenous peoples and the British Crown (and the new Dominion government), not with provincial governments. One of Ottawa's principal duties was the provision of medical attention to "status Indians," an exception (along with the armed forces) to the general rule that provinces were responsible for health care in post-Confederation Canada. The federal government, however, was neither able nor, it seems, particularly willing to engage in the direct provision of medical services for Indigenous populations. When it was organized at all, health care tended to be administered on an ad hoc basis by provincial health departments upon the request of the federal government. From time to time, the federal government would be forced into action, but usually in reaction to a particular crisis that it could not ignore. For example, in response to the very high mortality rates (particularly from tuberculosis) among Indigenous populations in the 1930s and 1940s, Ottawa established a series of "Indian Hospitals," racially segregated medical institutions that were often indistinguishable from, or were indeed appendages to, the residential schools themselves.[3]

Sioux Lookout's own seventy-bed sanatorium was built in 1949 in response to epidemic tuberculosis in northern First Nations communities. In 1951, the town's only general hospital was rebuilt as the forty-bed Sioux Lookout General Hospital, though this medical institution was intended primarily for non-Indigenous townspeople. This decades-long racial separation of hospital services was an ongoing source of tension and bore no little resemblance to the segregated schools and hospitals of the American South at the same time. By the early 1970s, however, the "Indian Hospital" (the former sanatorium) began to accept "non-Indians" from the town and changed its name to the "Zone Hospital."[4] Still, the disparities of health outcomes were evident to any informed observer. Nearly one-quarter of deaths in the Sioux Lookout district were of children under the age of five (compared to a mere 3 per cent in Canada as a whole). Death rates were three times higher than the national average for those aged five to fourteen. Infant mortality among Indigenous children, though significantly reduced in the post-war period, hovered around three times the national rate.[5]

It was in this social context that the then chief of paediatrics of The Hospital for Sick Children, Harry Bain, wrote to the federal government, offering to provide health-care services for Northern communities. According to one account, Bain, a self-described "man of the North," was on a fishing trip near Sioux Lookout in the late 1960s when he read a local newspaper article about starvation and malnutrition on local reserves.[6] Bain, who had been raised by a lumberman near North Bay, used his considerable influence to establish an outreach program for Northern Ontario, serving as director of the initiative long after his term as chief of paediatrics had expired. Indeed, in the year after the completion of his administrative duties at The Hospital for Sick Children, Bain moved to Sioux Lookout with his wife and two of his youngest children for a sabbatical year to oversee the program more directly.[7]

The Canadian Paediatric Society, using the terminology of the time, organized an Indian and Eskimo Child Health Committee in the late 1960s, while university paediatric departments and voluntary associations initiated health programs in various Aboriginal communities. The dominant approach then was to twin medical schools with particular communities (which were often dubbed health-care "zones"), such as Moose Factory Zone (Queen's University), Baffin Zone (McGill University), and Keewatin Zone (University of Manitoba). The universities of Alberta, Calgary, Laval, Dalhousie, and Memorial similarly answered the call for support in their respective provinces. In most cases, the universities were responsible for recruiting personnel, paediatricians directed the programs, and the Department of National Health and Welfare in Ottawa provided funding. The motivation was not solely the result of "awakening" to the public health challenges of First Nations communities. These programs met the changing educational needs of medical schools, which sought to provide students with more training in community health and non-hospital-based services.

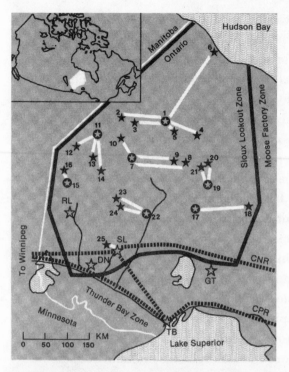

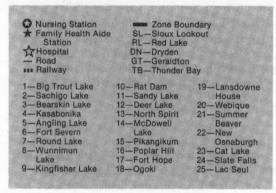

15.2 The growing challenge of providing medical care to Indigenous peoples in Canada prompted the creation of large health care "zones" in the 1970s. This contemporary map shows the extraordinary size of the Sioux Lookout Zone, with its scattered First Nations communities.

In the revealing language of the time, a contemporary commentator explained, "It is to be hoped that some of the unfulfilled needs of medical education may be met through contact with the native Canadian, who in turn will benefit from contact with the 'centre of excellence.'"[8]

Run by The Hospital for Sick Children on behalf of the Medical Services Branch of the Department of Health and Welfare, the Sioux Lookout initiative aimed to improve health-care services in the Sioux Lookout Zone, a huge tract of land in Northwestern Ontario (nearly one-third of the province) extending from Lake Superior to the Hudson Bay, a geographical land mass equivalent to half of the size of France. According to contemporary figures, there were between 10,000 and 15,000 "status Indians" in the Zone.[9] The town of Sioux Lookout itself consisted of about 2,500 people, nearly all of whom were non-Aboriginal.[10] Of the Sioux Lookout Zone's two dozen First Nations communities, only three were accessible by road. Indeed, most of the communities were north of the Canadian National Railway junction and could be reached only by plane or canoe. Inclement weather and organizational issues often delayed or precluded transportation for medical reasons. Indeed, when the Sioux Lookout Project began, nursing stations were connected only via radio.[11] The project was overseen by a Zone director, assistant director, several full-time family physicians, seven nursing stations designed to be staffed by two to five nurses each, and community health aides in twenty communities. "Community health aides" – Indigenous workers supervised remotely by nurses – ran medical clinics and overnight facilities in the twenty smaller communities without nursing stations.[12]

Bain hoped to establish a permanent physician presence in the Sioux Lookout area and sought to recruit family doctors to serve for at least a year. Children composed 30 to 40 per cent of the anticipated caseload, and upper-year paediatric residents were enlisted to provide rotating care. Hospital for Sick Children physicians, post-graduate students, and residents flew in for a week or more each month to act as specialist consultants. Student nurses fulfilled four-week rotations, four nurses at a time, at the Sioux Lookout Hospital. The departments of dentistry and psychiatry also provided personnel and training.[13] In 1972, Bain and the then project director, Gary Goldthorpe, announced that the approach had proved to be a workable system of health-care delivery that could potentially serve as a model for other "underdoctored" areas of the country. Understaffing and shortages of health-care providers, however, continued to be chronic problems. Nurses delivered primary care and bore an immensely heavy workload. Lack of preparation, burnout, stress, and separation from family and friends contributed to a high turnover rate. By the late 1970s, it proved so difficult to staff the remote nursing stations that some were simply closed. In June 1978, after nearly a decade of the system being in operation, ten of the thirteen full-time nursing positions were vacant, and during the two decades following the initiation of the project in 1969, the maximum number of physicians never exceeded seven, even though there was funding for at least ten.[14] Despite or perhaps because of its ambitious goals, the Zone system of providing comprehensive paediatric care to remote populations revealed the challenges and limitations of the most well-intentioned outreach as well as the stubborn persistence of health inequalities among children within Canada.

Horses to Helicopters

The distance between health-care providers and recipients in remote communities thus formed a major impediment to health-care delivery and access in the Sioux Lookout Zone. About half of the 10,000 First Nations people lived in "fly-in" locations north of the Canadian National Railway line.[15]

Periodically, acute cases would be airlifted to Dryden, Winnipeg, Thunder Bay, or – more rarely – Toronto. As The Hospital Sick Children's role as a tertiary care centre expanded with universal health care, and as terrestrial transportation into the downtown core became more difficult, new methods were needed to reach the centralized technology of the hospital. This problem was addressed, in the most urgent cases, by the hospital's roof-top heliport, part of the $20-million Elm Street Wing addition, completed in 1972. As part of the provincial funding for the new wing, it was agreed that the helipad was intended to serve adult as well as paediatric emergency cases. Of course, permitting helicopters to take treacherous flights into densely populated urban areas during sometimes inclement Canadian weather carried the risk of possible catastrophe. As a consequence, strict flight paths were delineated, and six hospital staff members were even trained to fight potential rooftop fires. The airborne network was captured in a contemporary film, *Horses to Helicopters*, which celebrated the new era of emergency transportation on the centenary of the hospital's foundation.

The heliport was first employed on 22 August 1972. Jennifer Lynn Smith, a newborn girl suffering from diaphragmatic hernia, was flown by plane from Thunder Bay to Toronto's Pearson Airport and from there by helicopter "over evening traffic" to The Hospital for Sick Children.[16] The second and third flights transported two Georgian Bay adult scuba divers with "the bends" who were treated next door at the Toronto General Hospital. Initially, there was no dedicated helicopter; patients were flown by the Canadian Armed Forces or by a private helicopter company. However, in October, 1977, the Ministry of Health initiated an air ambulance service based at Buttonville Airport, in Markham, north of the city. The service was intended for emergency cases that could not be transferred to Toronto hospitals within an hour due to weather or distance, and made use of landing pads at Sunnybrook Hospital as well as The Hospital for Sick Children. Unsurprisingly, with Sioux Lookout twinned with The Hospital for Sick Children and the University of Toronto, Indigenous and non-Indigenous children figured in the emergency flights. Transportation log books from the Sioux Lookout Hospital showed that from 1976–7, children under age fifteen composed 21 per cent of all emergency flights, though these figures also included all flights to Dryden, Thunder Bay, Winnipeg, and Toronto.[17]

From 1977 through the mid-1980s, over 500 flights transported patients to the rooftop. In 1980, after a contest among the hospital's patients, the

helicopter was named Bandage, a moniker that was perhaps a bit too under-
stated, considering the drama that would attend the sighting of the
helicopter overhead in the Toronto skyline.[18] Half of the patients who landed
on the hospital helipad were treated at SickKids; the other half were adults
whose ultimate destination was usually Sunnybrook Hospital or the Toronto
General Hospital. Usage substantially increased in the 1990s: there were
551 landings, for example, during the year 1994 alone. In subsequent decades,
the explosion of high-rise building projects in the city of Toronto reduced
the number of available flight paths to the hospital's helipad. Indeed, one
of the dozens of factors involved in the planning of the hospital's new
twenty-one-storey research tower (completed in 2013) was protecting the
integrity of one of the helicopter flight paths through what had become an
incredibly dense downtown core of ever-taller condominium buildings.[19]

The helicopters were used both to transport patients to Toronto as well
as to fly Hospital for Sick Children specialists out to rural and remote areas.
Within this ever-expanding system of outreach, the Neonatal Transport
Team figured prominently.[20] The team was created in response to a study
that indicated that improved care before and during transportation could
improve health outcomes for neonates. In 1996, the team transported 649
infants by ambulance, helicopter, or airplane to the special unit, "giving a
high level of intensive care along the way."[21] Remarkably, only one patient
out of 3,000 transported in the four years leading up to 1997 had died during
transport.[22] Transportation by helicopter was enormously expensive and
did not necessarily provide a reasonable approach for the 99 per cent of
paediatric patients who may have benefited from the expertise of The Hospital for Sick Children. The hospital needed to find a new way to bring the
expertise of the institution to children and families, rather than bringing
everyone to the crowded downtown core of Toronto.

Telemedicine

The centralization of medical expertise in large, technologically dependent
institutions attached to urban research universities created enormous disparities of medical practice and knowledge that were hard to overcome. The
very downtown core of Toronto was bursting with prestigious medical institutions literally side by side – Toronto General, SickKids, Princess Margaret,
Mount Sinai, Women's College. By contrast, other parts of the country,
such as Sioux Lookout, suffered from medical isolation. Although projects

initiated by hospitals such as SickKids attempted to overcome the chronic lack of health-care practitioners by integrating post-graduate training, these projects were often short-lived and rarely yielded graduates who returned to set up practice permanently. As a consequence, information technology represented one imperfect means to overcome disparities in health-care delivery. Early telemedicine projects began in various North American locations in the 1970s. The University of Toronto and the University of Western Ontario (UWO), for example, began experimenting with different telemedicine technologies in 1974, determining that "a relatively inexpensive video system (slow scan)" was as effective as hands-free telephone, black-and-white television, and colour television.[23] In October 1976, investigators began using a Canadian-American satellite, Hermes. UWO researchers carried out a five-month experiment connecting London's University Hospital, Moose Factory General Hospital, and a James Bay nursing station through satellite connection "for medical consultations, data transmission (for example, ECGs, X-rays, heart sounds) and some continuing education."[24]

As technology advanced, new opportunities presented themselves. In 1976–7, for example, the University of Toronto and the University of Waterloo experimented with audio-visual telemedicine, using existing telephone lines to transmit slow-scan (freeze-frame) video. The system connected the nursing stations, the Sioux Lookout Zone Hospital, The Hospital for Sick Children, and Sunnybrook Medical Centre for emergency consultations and continuing medical education for health-care providers and program directors. Other regional communications included rentals of trail radios to individuals in the bush and the local media (Wawatay), which provided regional health information. In theory, telemedicine could avoid unnecessary patient transportations, hasten necessary transfers, and improve patient care not just by improving access to health-care providers but also by enabling communication with families. Patients who were taken far from home and immersed in foreign surroundings often suffered from loneliness and isolation.[25] The clinical effectiveness was constrained by technological factors that would be resolved, in part, by the advent of the Internet in the 1990s.

Telemedicine (later known as Telehealth) commenced formally at Sick-Kids in 1996. It began life as a "collaborative pilot project" between Sudbury Regional Hospital and Thunder Bay Regional Hospital. In 1998, the program was folded into a larger initiative dubbed the NORTH (the Northern Ontario Remote Telecommunications Health) Network.[26] The Telemedicine

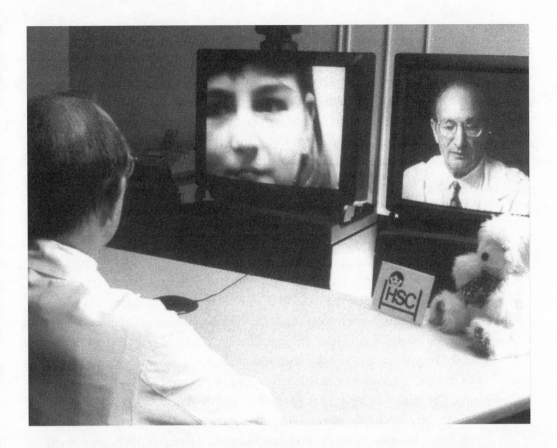

Clinic in Thunder Bay, for example, hosted an inter-active video link between SickKids and Health Sciences North, enabling physicians to examine and potentially diagnose at a distance. In the year 1995 alone, 161 patients from the Sault Ste. Marie area and 133 from Thunder Bay had been treated at The Hospital for Sick Children. Families in Thunder Bay

could thus substitute telemedicine consultations for disruptive, time-consuming, and expensive trips to Toronto that were sixteen hours by car. It is noteworthy that the pilot project began with $100,000 in private funds and no direct funding from the Ontario Ministry of Health or the federal government.[27]

When he stepped down as surgeon-in-chief in 1994, Robert Filler became the first head of the Telehealth initiative at SickKids. He successfully lobbied the provincial ministry of health to encourage use of the clinic in Thunder Bay. In the first three years of telemedicine, practitioners in twenty-six specialties participated in 452 video consultations, half of which were routine follow-up, one-quarter initial consultations, 11 per cent clinical trials, 9 per cent pre-op assessment, and 7 per cent post-op assessments.[28] What appeared, at first, to verge on science fiction became clinical reality. An electronic stethoscope enabled physicians to hear a patient's breath and heartbeat, while "a special telescope with a video camera" peered into throats and ears. The program emerged as one of Canada's first and most wide-ranging telehealth programs.[29] Specific initiatives to improve services to Northern populations included the Ontario Telemedicine for Retinopathy of Prematurity project, begun in 2009 by a hospital ophthalmologist to enable screening of premature newborns in Sudbury and Barrie without "lengthy and potentially dangerous trips" to Toronto.[30]

Digitizing medical expertise and clinical practice transformed patient care and the boundaries of the hospital itself. As personal computers invaded the offices, corridors, and research labs of major medical institutions in the 1990s, a discussion about the circulation of medical information in general, and the patient record in particular, began to emerge organically. Touted by politicians and administrators as the great panacea for health-care efficiency and accuracy, electronic records often represented an elusive nirvana. The logic was seductive. Essential medical information would follow patients between departments of large hospitals, and indeed between hospitals and community, thereby eliminating thousands of duplicate tests, providing immediate medical histories for more efficient decision-making, as well as reducing medical mistakes through human error involved in interpreting handwritten notes. Electronic patient records would therefore be more efficient, cheaper, safer, and more accurate. However, the realization of an effective system of electronic patient records, one responsive to the growing cultural sensitivity towards the protection of health-care data, would prove to be more challenging than many first thought.

The origins of a comprehensive system of e-health records at The Hospital for Sick Children lay in the controversial restructuring and amalgamation of Toronto hospitals during the cost-cutting years of the mid-1990s. The Metropolitan Toronto and District Health Council recommended the establishment of a Child Health Network for the Greater Toronto Area. The provincial government quickly accepted the recommendation and, through its Health Services Restructuring Commission (as mentioned in the last chapter) directed the establishment of such a network as well as four other regional child health networks in the province. Officials and clinicians from SickKids and all the other hospitals in the Toronto

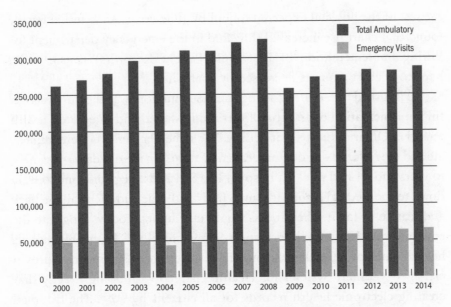

Chart 15.1 Patient visits to SickKids, 2000–14 (ambulatory and emergency)

region soon realized that an electronic enabler was required if they were to share the data, information, and knowledge that would be the lifeblood of the new network. SickKids began to research possible software products with which it could construct a shared and integrated health record. Even at the outset, it was looking for a software application that eventually might be able to serve not only the hospital's own patients, but, potentially, the paediatric population of the entire province. The hospital team ultimately adopted an IBM application called Health Data Network (HDN).[31]

The provincial government embraced this nascent electronic network, seeing it as an early experiment that held the promise of a pan-provincial vision for e-health. The Electronic Child Health Network (eCHN) was launched in 1999, billed as Canada's "first integrated electronic health record solution."[32] By 2001, the database encompassed over 80,000 children;[33] by 2004, 204,317 patients and 26 hospitals; by 2009 the system eclipsed 1,000,000 patients and 100 institutional sites.[34] All patient charts in The Hospital for Sick Children, from May 2000 onwards, were entered into the system. The electronic gathering of medical data gathered steam and affected every aspect of hospital operations. The emergency department was the first to begin using an electronic patient chart (EPC) in January 2004; cardiology, ENT, general surgery, orthopaedics and communication disorders followed suit in May, research departments in September, with the rest of the hospital expected to join by June 2005. An external review found that chart use increased threefold in the emergency department following implementation of Electronic Patient Record(s) (EPR), while hard-copy chart requests decreased by nearly half.[35]

As it turned out, eCHN, costing some $60 million, was the only successful implementation of an actual functioning shared and integrated health record in Ontario during that decade. For some, the benefits were immediate and tangible. As one doctor recalled in 2009, "In the old days – meaning 10 years ago – I had to call a hospital like SickKids, beg someone to walk down to the medical records room to find a kid's file and then call me back and read it, or fax it. The process would take hours. Today, I log into the computer and I have the information on my screen[.]"[36] Electronic records held so much promise that the provincial government set up a new provincial agency, Smart Systems for Health, charged with doing exactly that, creating electronic health records for all citizens by 2015. The troubled agency was reborn in 2008 as eHealth Ontario, under the directorship of neurosurgeon and former University Health Network (Toronto General) CEO Alan Hudson.

The ease of transfer of patient records was, of course, the greatest advantage of e-health records, but also its Achilles heel. In 2007, a laptop holding health information for almost 3,000 patients was stolen from the trunk of a doctor's car. The hospital was subsequently ordered to encrypt information and institute stricter policies against the removal of patient files.[37] Less than two months later, a SickKids physician lost an external hard drive containing over 3,000 records at Toronto Pearson International Airport.[38] Meanwhile the eHealth Ontario initiative came tumbling down amidst accusations of conflicts of interest, exorbitant consultants' fees, and an inability of key players to work together.[39] These incidents came amidst a new wave of privacy and freedom of information laws that greatly restricted the circulation of health records. An unresolved tension thus emerged in the first decade of the twenty-first century between the internal logic of electronic patient records that were personalized and portable, and increasing concerns over privacy and data sharing.

Notwithstanding the many challenges involved in rolling comprehensive electronic record systems out beyond individual institutions, the advent and evolution of the electronic age transformed the very nature of the medical encounter as well as the visual work environment of the hospital itself. Large computer screens began to populate the hospital, organizing and updating in real time, for example, the entire network of surgical theatres. The patient record became more interactive, with ever more sophisticated layers of knowledge. Even education was subtly transformed; the time-honoured tradition of rounding and questions (whereby a student doctor or nurse was interrogated and forced to answer skill-testing questions) was being supplanted by trainees carrying tablets and smartphones. Searching for up-to-date medical information or clinical protocols became normative, an acknowledgment that no health-care practitioner could keep abreast of the infinitely expanding world of medical knowledge and practice. Checking and double-checking for practice guidelines became a sign of good professional practice. These profound changes in information technology transformed both clinical practice and the very nature of the "hospital," challenging the boundaries of physical structures (and their medical cultures) and the geographical constraints of patient care and medical expertise.

Conclusions

In January 1988, five men from Sandy Lake, a remote community near the Ontario-Manitoba border, went on a two-day hunger strike to "draw attention to years of worsening health care and deteriorating relations between First Nations Communities and the Medical Services Branch (Health and Welfare Canada)."[40] In response, the Medical Services Branch of the federal government and the Nishnawbe Aski Nation convened the Scott-McKay-Bain Health Panel, which issued a report and recommendations in March 1989. The panel held hearings with local communities and stakeholders in the Sioux Lookout Zone, in Ottawa, in Thunder Bay, and in Toronto. Panel members observed that both the range and quality of health-care services had improved dramatically since the Sioux Lookout Zone project had begun in the late 1960s. At the same time, they concluded that "the people's health status seems to have reached a plateau – at a level lower than that of non-native Canadians."[41] Health indicators became entangled with governance issues. Over the course of the 1970s, the First Nations communities bristled at the exclusion of Indigenous people from participation in health-care planning and delivery. Moreover, they sensed a poor appreciation for non-Western healing practices.[42]

The situation in Sandy Lake reflected more broadly the limitations of the Sioux Lookout Zone project. While leading paediatricians were flying into (and out of) First Nation reserves, too little time had been spent on producing a capacity for health services within these communities. More fundamentally, so many of the chronic health-care challenges were rooted in social conditions that dated back generations. Poor housing and living environments (polluted groundwater, lack of water, and sewage systems) were compounded by the haunting legacy of residential schooling. In this respect, the Sioux Lookout initiative represented the limitations of purely medical interventions; there was, as it were, no "physician cure" for many of these problems. T. Kue Young, a medical anthropologist and a former general practitioner in the Zone, concluded, "The most significant health problems of these people will not diminish unless the deficiencies in housing, sanitation, nutrition and overall socioeconomic conditions are corrected."[43] Ultimately, the Chiefs and their Negotiating Unit agreed to create one regional hospital, joining the previously independent Sioux Lookout General Hospital and the First Nations Hospital (formerly known as the Indian Hospital).[44] Meanwhile, the chronic problem of flying into the near North from Toronto was indirectly addressed, in part, by the establishment in 2005 of a Northern Ontario School of Medicine (NOSM), based jointly in Thunder Bay and Sudbury. The first new medical school in Ontario since the late 1960s, NOSM was given direct responsibility for providing rural and remote medicine in the former Zone and for having medical students and post-graduate residents rotate through First Nations communities. In addition, they would stay in contact with the medical centres through Telehealth and satellite videoconferencing.[45]

The advent of electronic health records also proved to be a qualified success. In 2002, the Royal Commission on Health Care (the Romanow Commission) was one of several major national investigations seeking to ensure that Canada's health-care system would remain sustainable for the next generation. One of its much-publicized recommendations was the swift adoption of electronic health records for all Canadians.[46] Although defensible from an intellectual standpoint, such e-aspirations failed to fully appreciate the myriad technological and political challenges. Information technology changes constantly; it does not plateau, nor does it consolidate. Seemingly dominant software and infrastructure companies – such as the famous Canadian examples of Corel and Nortel – rise and fall dramatically. Software systems become the norm and then are suddenly displaced by newer, unanticipated platforms. Hospitals purchase different systems, stymying the sharing of records between major medical institutions. Coordination with community-based practitioners is often slow, particularly in remunerative systems where most doctors are effectively self-employed contractors. These challenges appeared in full fruition when Ontario attempted to develop an e-health system. In the end, it was riddled with delays and had little to show for an outlay of hundreds of millions of dollars between 2002 and 2007, ending in frustration and the resignation of key individuals.[47] Hospitals, fearful of misplaced patient records (and potential lawsuits) became even more sensitive to the sharing of health records, making it almost impossible to implement the extension of the impressive paediatric system, pioneered by SickKids, to the entire provincial health-care population, let alone across Canada.

There was no avoiding, however, the huge impact of the new electronic age of information. Telehealth expanded the reach of The Hospital for Sick Children's clinical expertise, first to the near North, and then (as the next chapter will demonstrate) around the world. With the advent of the Internet, powerful and influential medical institutions, like The Hospital for Sick Children, were in a position to use their considerable expertise for both humanitarian and revenue-generating opportunities. Unlike a previous generation, where a select few patients would be transported around the world to Toronto for life-saving medical interventions, the emphasis at The Hospital for Sick Children, as elsewhere, moved more and more towards using novel technologies to help build capacity in the home countries. As technologies became more reliable and the reach of the Internet became increasingly international, the global possibilities expanded accordingly. Individuals both within the hospital and without began to rethink the scope of the hospital and what many were convinced was the untapped and unparalleled level of health-care expertise within the staff. If the hospital's clinicians could reach near North, then why not Trinidad? And if Trinidad, why not Qatar?

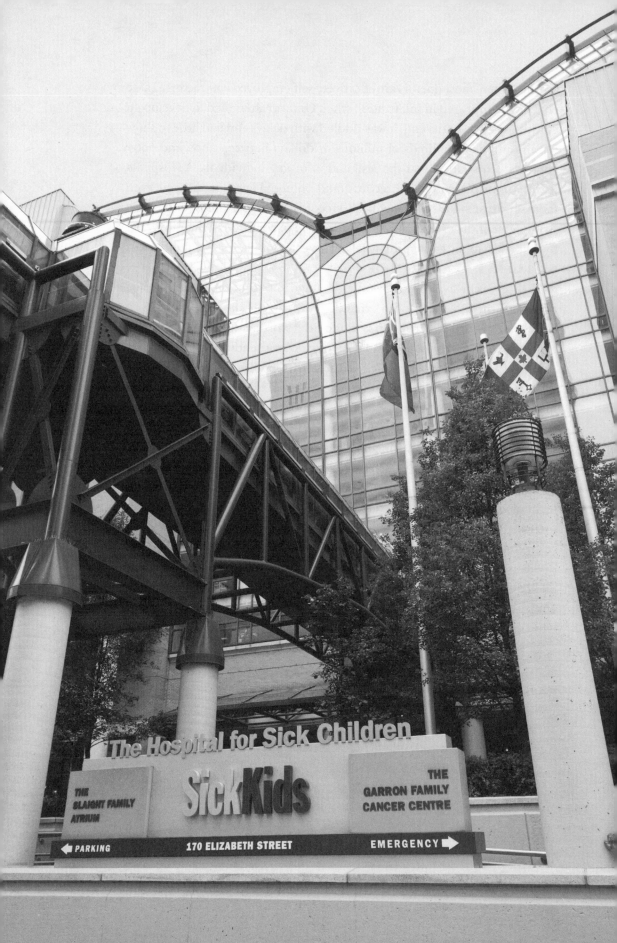

SIXTEEN

SickKids International

We look upon ourselves as a finishing school for pediatric medicine.[1]
Desmond Bohn, SickKids physician,
interview with the *Globe and Mail*, 2006

SickKids International

By the turn of the century, Toronto's Hospital for Sick Children had positioned itself as one of the pre-eminent children's hospitals in the world. However, most of its clinical work was still devoted to patients in the Greater Toronto Area, with concentric circles of therapeutic support for the province of Ontario, other Canadian provinces, and a handful of international patients. As the previous chapter has illustrated, the advent of the Internet and the political considerations of globalization widened the horizon of the hospital's activities. The growing global awareness increasingly drew The Hospital for Sick Children into international collaborations involving education, research, and clinical practice. Powerful, if not always reliable, videoconferencing enabled centres throughout Canada, and as far afield as Argentina and Israel, to participate in medical and nursing rounds from the 1990s onwards.[2] Meanwhile, new players entered the global paediatric scene, such as the Bill and Melinda Gates Foundation, which, with the deep pockets of one of the world's richest individuals, directed billions of dollars of research funding to solve global health scourges, many of which affected the world's most vulnerable children.

The first decade of the twenty-first century thus witnessed a cultural as well as a technological shift, a

16.1 The new Elizabeth Street facade of the expanded hospital. The entrance welcomed visitors to the soaring, light-filled atrium that reflected contemporary architectural trends of the 1990s.

new openness to begin to address, in a more comprehensive manner, global health priorities. Senior individuals at The Hospital for Sick Children recognized that the traditional research preoccupations no longer sufficed. One illustration of this new trend could be seen in the actions of Alvin Zipursky, then head of the Division of Haematology/Oncology at SickKids, who had garnered an international reputation for researching leukemias related to Down Syndrome. In 1999, he was appointed editor-in-chief of the medical journal *Pediatric Research*, the first Canadian to hold that position. During his time as editor, he observed that all of the abstracts he received seemed to be relevant primarily to the health needs of wealthier Western countries. In 2004, while attending the Pediatric Academic Societies' (PAS) annual meeting, the largest annual meeting of paediatric researchers in North America, he recalled that of 3,400 abstracts submitted for academic sessions, not one, to his mind, was particularly relevant to children in developing countries. This paralleled the observation, circulating at the time, that only 10 per cent of global health research resources were devoted to the health problems of the developing world, even though these countries were burdened with 90 per cent of the world's disease. It was clear that millions of children were dying annually from diseases that were entirely manageable in the West. Upon his retirement from regular clinical practice, Zipursky, together with Executive Director Margaret Manley, founded the Program for Global Pediatric Research in 2004, to address this asymmetry of research interest and direct paediatric research capacity towards improving the health of children in developing countries.

Zipursky's vision aligned with that of the new senior hospital administrators. The new president and CEO, Mary Jo Haddad, was the first woman to assume the highest administrative position in the hospital. Shortly after her appointment, she engaged in a re-visioning of the institution that prioritized these new global interconnections, resulting in the "Healthier Children: A Better World" initiative. One direct result of the rethinking of the hospital's priorities was to establish a new entity, SickKids International (SKI). SickKids International consolidated the international teaching, research, and clinical activities of the hospital which, as previous chapters have illustrated, had taken various, often uncoordinated, forms, from Tele-health to the Herbie Fund. By going global, the hospital was following trends of other leading health science centres in North America and responding to the new challenges of health care in the age of the Internet.[3]

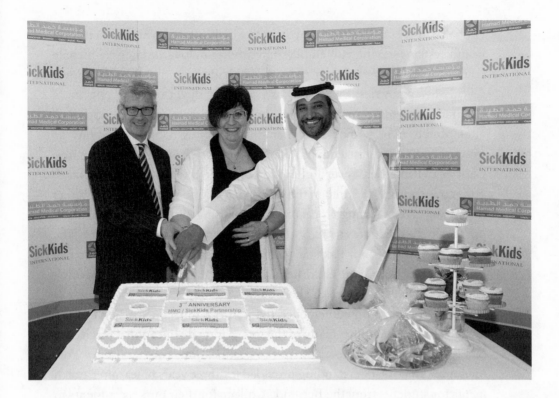

In practice, the advent of SickKids International was not just a reflection of the trend towards the globalization of health-care services. One of the senior physician-administrators acknowledged that SKI was also created, in part, as a "revenue-generating organization."[4] Indeed, an Ivey School of Business case study that examined the new administrative configuration of the hospital concluded that The Hospital for Sick Children "was anxious to find new ways to recover from an operating deficit caused by the aftershock of the [2003] SARS outbreak."[5] In 2011, the Institute of Public Administration of Canada even awarded SickKids a Gold Award in Innovative Management in acknowledgment of what it termed an "innovative business model" that was informing the strategic direction of SKI.[6] The hospital appears to have had some success in generating new revenue streams: from 2006 to 2010, international revenue grew dramatically from 2.1 per cent to 10.1 per cent of total non-governmental and non-research income.[7] Given this success, but also with a sensitivity to the optics of revenue-generating initiatives of a not-for-profit hospital, the SickKids trustees renewed and expanded SKI in 2011, absorbing the existing

16.2 The global reach of The Hospital for Sick Children was formalized, and encouraged, by the creation of SickKids International. Here, Chair of the Board of Trustees Robert Harding, President and CEO Mary Jo Haddad, and project director Dr. Abdullah Al Kaabi celebrate a partnership in Qatar.

Global Child Health Program (GCHP), which aimed to strengthen local health systems serving vulnerable communities in low- and middle-income countries. As of the summer of 2013, SKI had expanded to involve over seventy-five countries; SickKids was providing direct ongoing education and training to more than twenty countries.[8] Ultimately, the new approach attempted to remedy the issues arising from "flying in and flying out," as exemplified in the last chapter. Rather, one of the initiatives – the new Caribbean Pediatric Cancer and Blood program – highlighted that it wasn't "about transporting children in the Caribbean to Canada for care, but rather improving care ... through local capacity building and infrastructure development."[9] To illustrate the importance of this new strategic direction, the hospital recruited from Pakistan Zulfiqar Bhutta, an international star in maternal, newborn, and child health, as the Inaugural Robert Harding Chair in Global Child Health and Policy.

It was perhaps no coincidence that, with a nurse at the helm of the hospital for the first time, many of the international educational services of SickKids International focused on nurse education. For example, a 2013 Memorandum of Understanding provided for three years of learning attachments for students from the Bermuda College for their nursing students to participate in learning experiences at SickKids. By 2013, the International Learner Program had served eighty-two individuals from nineteen countries. Another major SKI initiative was the development and implementation of a pediatric nurse training program in Ghana with the goal of reducing child morbidity and mortality. The partnership was the brainchild of SickKids' Isaac Odame, a Ghanaian-born, British-educated paediatric hematologist.[10] "The major issue for me," Odame acknowledged, "is that, having left Ghana to work in Canada, I am always looking for opportunities where I could make a positive impact on Ghana ... I see it as a duty that I owe to my country and that's what inspires me."[11] Beginning in May 2011 with four-year funding from the Canadian International Development Agency (CIDA), a one-year certificate program in paediatric nursing was introduced for experienced general nurses. The intention was for graduates to carry on the paediatric specialization within the undergraduate nursing program at the University of Ghana.[12]

By 2010, scores of countries were participating in exchanges and SickKids learning outreach initiatives. The hospital Foundation, through yet another global initiative – HealthyKids International (HKI) – sponsored fellows from India, Rwanda, China, Guyana, and Kenya. Local organizations in Canada also got involved in sponsorship. In 2009–10, the Indo-Canada Chamber of Commerce, for example, initiated a Fellowship program "to brin[g] medical professionals from India to Canada to train at SickKids."[13] HKI received $5 million in support from the Indian Government. Ever mindful of a previous generation of Indian medical practitioners, some of whom left the sub-continent for training in the West only to settle permanently, this HKI scheme emphasized that Indian fellows would return home to contribute to their own nation's health infrastructure.[14]

The global challenges of pediatric health were manifold and did not always default to the headline-grabbing field of infectious diseases. One area – childhood nutrition – remained an almost intractable problem in many developing countries. In 1996, UNICEF issued a challenge to devise "a viable and reproducible solution to the problem of micronutrient malnutrition" experienced by an estimated 750 million children (as well as pregnant and lactating women) in developing countries.[15] It was in this context that SickKids paediatrician and nutritionist Stanley Zlotkin conceived of Sprinkles, a tasteless powder containing ferrous fumarate, iron, zinc, folic acid, and Vitamins A, C, and D that can be added to any meal. Zlotkin himself acted as the product's advocate globally, and, by 2009, 4 million children had benefited from the product.[16] Sprinkles have been "supplied on a cost-recovery basis for non-commercial distribution" at an initial cost of about $0.03 per sachet, achieving "unsurpassed" declines in anemia rates in places as remote as Mongolia.[17] By 2014, the various micronutrient powders could be found in over sixty countries, affecting as many as 20 million children.[18]

Internationalizing efforts also manifested themselves in formal transnational relationships. The first such partnership was formed with Hamad Medical Corporation, the largest public health-care provider for the state of Qatar. Joint agreements to provide advanced medical training for cash-rich, but infrastructure-poor, states of the Persian Gulf dated back at least to the 1970s, when universities in Canada and the United States provided undergraduate and postgraduate training for Saudi medical students. By the early twenty-first century, many of the Gulf states and principalities began to cease outsourcing their medical education and to construct their own comprehensive physical and human resource infrastructures. Thus, in February 2010, with consultants from Bloorview Kids Rehab hospital, SickKids began a five-year agreement to advise on the development of a new children's hospital in Doha, the capital of Qatar. SickKids personnel (from nurse practitioners to the library director) were responsible for providing expertise in clinical services, education, and research.[19] As with some of SKI's other partnerships, the staff of Hamad Medical Corporation would participate in exchanges with SickKids. By 2013, for example, over 700 nurses from Qatar had completed The Hospital for Sick Children's Paediatric Nursing Education Program. SKI's role went beyond the new hospital itself; SickKids experts also acted as expert consultants to the Qatari government for the formation of national strategies in disparate areas from paediatric oncology to child psychiatry.[20]

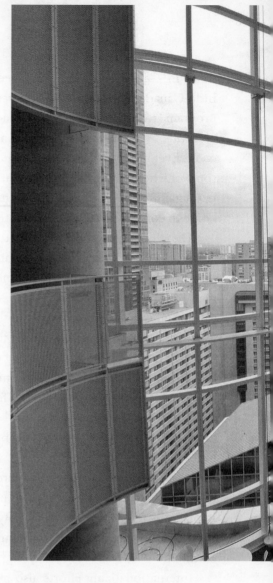

The Research Cathedral

Underpinning many of these global initiatives was the ever-growing pre-eminence of research at the hospital. Although research had always situated itself alongside clinical practice, by the early twenty-first century SickKids had solidified its position as one of the leading paediatric research centres in the world. Bouncing back from the lean years of the 1990s, the hospital reported over $150 million of research activity by 2010, 20 per cent of which derived from the SickKids Foundation to fund research projects under the auspices of the Research Institute.[21] However, research groups were distributed in various permanent and rented spaces in the downtown Toronto core. With the support of the successful hospital Foundation, administrators looked to consolidate the research labs that hitherto had operated in different locations.

Conceiving of the first major extension of the hospital since the famous Atrium, the vision for a new research tower received $75 million from the

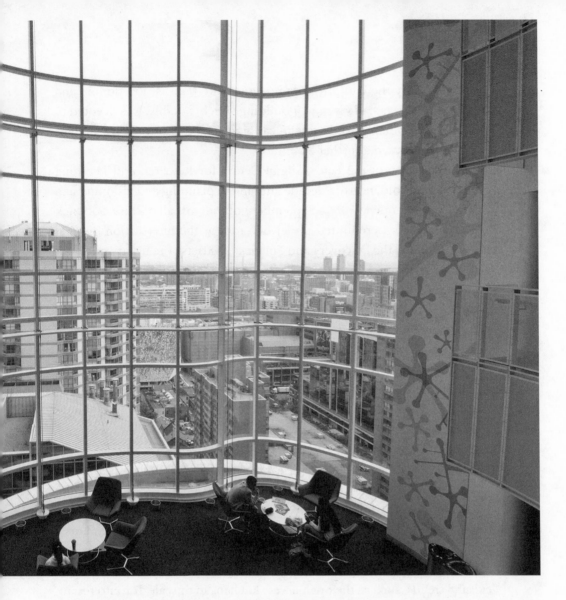

provincial government and $91 million from the Canada Foundation for Innovation (the federal government's program to fund substantial research infrastructure projects). To fund the balance, the hospital successfully offered $200 million 40-year Series A Senior Unsecured Debentures, backed by the financial resources of the hospital's Foundation.[22] Tim Hockey (then president and CEO of TD Canada Trust) led the Foundation's $200-million fundraising campaign and organized a "cabinet" of philanthropists who would "look for people who would want naming opportunities ... as small as a brick all the way to the building itself."[23] In March 2012, the Hospital announced that Peter Gilgan (founder of Mattamy Homes) had agreed to donate

16.3 The Gilgan Tower – variously referred to as a "research cathedral" and a "highrise laboratory" – with its dramatic sightlines and open concept illustrates the centrality of research to The Hospital for Sick Children.

$40 million. By the end of the campaign, more than 13,000 donors and corporate partners had given to a building which, notably, was devoted to research rather than directly to clinical practice. Staff and the researchers themselves donated a further $5 million.[24]

Construction of the Peter Gilgan Centre for Research and Learning began in May 2010, nearly a decade after initial planning and visioning had begun. When it opened on 17 September 2013, almost all of the 2,000 Sick-Kids researchers were united under one roof at the intersection of what Toronto dubbed the Discovery and Financial districts. The twenty-one-floor building, atop a parking garage, had seventeen floors of laboratory space, constituting the largest child health research tower in the world. The bottom floors were dedicated to administration and learning spaces, including a 250-person auditorium. The layout of the so-called "highrise laboratory" space proved innovative, almost trendy. The guiding principle was to break down the post-war pattern of enclosed offices and labs, and open up the entire building to "free-flowing communities of researchers." Hospital leadership undertook to bring scientists out of silos and into a single tower designed to maximize interaction, "cross-pollination" of ideas, and "impromptu collaboration."[25] Laboratory space itself was designed to be flexible, where different kinds of researchers were deliberately mixed. Each of six research divisions (the so-called "neighbourhoods") occupied multiple floors, sharing communal, three-floor atria. Prominent central staircases were placed to create "connectivity." The design inspired many metaphors — from the "research cathedral"[26] to the "research aquarium," to the "vertical city."[27] In design terms, the visibility of research reflected other social and cultural trends, such as the open-access kitchens in upscale Toronto restaurants. A major buzzword was "visibility"; project architects "sought to demystify the role of medical research by bringing it to street level" with a transparent, multilevel lobby.[28] The manager of construction observed, only semi-jokingly, that the height of the structure was purposively chosen to be sufficiently tall to loom over Toronto City Hall.[29]

Conclusions

By the second decade of the twenty-first century, The Hospital for Sick Children had engaged in complicated international research protocols, welcomed fellows arriving from all parts of the world for specialist training, and refined systems for global health outreach. Many of these trends had been presaged, of course, by the Internet and telehealth initiatives of the 1990s. Telehealth expanded the reach of The Hospital for Sick Children's clinical expertise, first to the near North and then around the world. Unlike a previous generation, where a select few lucky patients would be transported around the world to Toronto for life-saving medical interventions, the emphasis at The Hospital for Sick Children moved more and more towards using novel technologies to help build capacity in home countries.

Research was inextricably linked to the internationalizing of the hospital's activities. The research tower now physically and symbolically *towers* over the old hospital structure, and opens up, coincidentally, onto Bay Street, the symbolic avenue of finance and power in Canada's largest city. Indeed, the state-of-the-art facilities were purposefully touted as key to attracting leading researchers from around the world. By the time of the construction, there were over 300 international fellows from forty-eight countries in training, 30 per cent of whom came from developing countries.[30] The global influence built on a growing tradition to train leading clinicians from around the world. Dr. Harold J. Hoffman, who joined the staff in 1964 and rose to Chief of Neurosurgery at the hospital, estimated that he had trained 120 international fellows in addition to the 200 Canadian neurosurgery residents by the time he retired.[31] As Dr. Desmond Bohn (chief of critical care medicine), who himself had been involved in training and supervising more than two hundred critical care specialists from thirty different countries, memorably concluded: "We look upon ourselves as a finishing school for pediatric medicine."[32]

The quaint reference to a Swiss boarding school aside, The Hospital for Sick Children had evolved into a medical juggernaut on multiple clinical, administrative, and research levels: by 2010, over 15,000 inpatient visits every year, and 100,000 patient days; close to 7,000 inpatient surgeries and 5,000 day surgeries; clinic visits approaching 250,000 per year, dwarfing the mere 130,000 diagnostic visits; a hospital of over 3,000 staff, with 600 medical and dental part-time and full-time consultants; and a research institute staff somewhere between 1,000 and 2,000 employees. In some respects, the hospital had morphed into an institution the size and diversity of which, in many key respects, resembled an international non-governmental organization, one based in Toronto but with far-reaching global influences and partnerships.

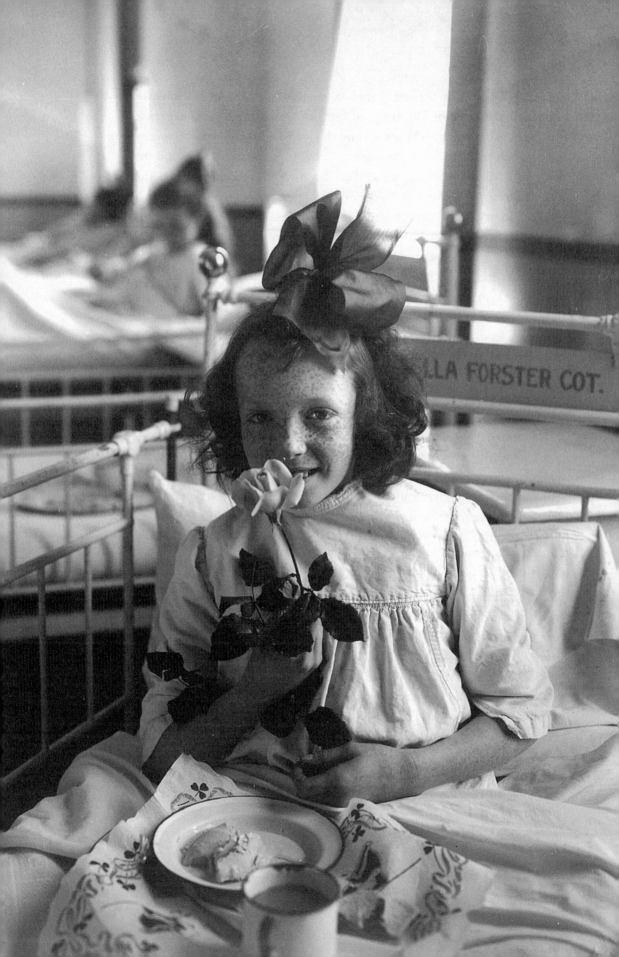

Epilogue

Dear Madam,

 Will you kindly accept the coins enclosed, as a contribution to the Hospital for sick children. Practically they are of small value, but events with which they are associated have invested them with peculiar preciousness in the estimation of the writer and his family. They once belonged to a dear child who accumulated them during six weeks of great suffering, caused by a sad accident and ending in her death.

 Hitherto we have preserved them for her sake, feeling that we could not devote them to any common purpose. But now, and equally for her sake, we beg to transfer them to you, as the most suitable disposition that can be made of them, and henceforward we shall doubtless find greater satisfaction in connecting the memory of our beloved child, with the valued institution under your charge, than with a few pieces of money laid idly by. That the divine blessing may continually rest upon the Hospital, its inmates and promoters, is the prayer of

 Yours most truly.[1]

[Anonymous], 1876

A Peculiar Preciousness

When I left Canada to complete my postgraduate studies in England, I fell unexpectedly into the orbit of the history of medicine, and the munificence of the Wellcome Trust, then the largest charitable foundation in the world. Unbeknownst to me before I arrived,

E.1 Medical charity necessitated a symbiotic relationship between hospitals and their communities. Here, a patient poses for a St Patrick's Day photograph; the named cot just behind her reminds the viewer of the financial support needed for the hospital's success.

the Wellcome Trust administered a vast network of biomedical research units that were funded by the bequest of Henry Wellcome, an early twentieth-century British drug retailer whose empire would morph into Burroughs-Wellcome, one of the large pharmaceutical companies of the twentieth century. Henry Wellcome was fascinated by the history of medicine and ensured that part of his massive estate would fund a Wellcome Institute for the History of Medicine on Euston Road in London. Many young doctoral students benefited, as I did, from the generous financial support and vibrant intellectual communities that had formed in Britain around the various Wellcome Units.

During my formative training years in the 1990s, the paterfamilias of the Wellcome Institute was a larger-than-life figure named Roy Porter, who almost single-handedly placed the history of medicine on the map in terms of academic scholarship and popular interest. It is hard to describe the impact that he had on the intellectual lives of historians of all shades in Britain; the fact that he published over 100 books and edited volumes, however, gives some quantitative indication of his industry and his influence. Porter was, by training, a social historian of eighteenth-century England, what historians refer to as the Georgian period (after the series of King Georges, the third of whom happened to lose the American colonies before he lost his own mind). During the years of my doctoral work at Oxford, I read one of Porter's earliest and most influential essays on the rise of the Georgian infirmary. He examined, in particular, what he termed the "Gift Relation," a theme that I mentioned in the very first chapter of this book. His question was simple: Why did people give to medical hospital charities? Certainly, the principal answer was that they wanted to "do good." But of course, unpacking what that actually meant led him, and subsequent researchers, to dig deeper into the complex psychological and social terrain of medical giving. How did successful generations define the "public good"? Why medical institutions rather than other charities?

I reflect on Porter's essay in the epilogue to this book, for it is clear (as the opening quotation conveys) that the relationship between the public and children's hospitals remains powerful, even if motivations of giving often remain complicated. Toronto's own Hospital for Sick Children began life as a modest project in a rented (and somewhat dingy) house, surviving on requests for donated, often used, goods. No contribution was too small, and all were dutifully enumerated in the first annual reports. Indeed, one could even conclude that the more modest offerings were given the greater spiritual meaning by the early lady visitors. Not soon thereafter, the hospital – if the rented houses merited that name – was co-opted by a newspaper magnate who, in an unusual form of benevolent dictatorship, completely transformed the small charity and bankrolled the new College Street institution. John Ross Robertson's personal donations and political influence would ensure that the Toronto hospital would quickly rise to prominence as a major medical institution in North America. As the twentieth century progressed, the public became increasingly implicated in support of the institution, most notably in the annual Christmas appeal. As the University Avenue hospital took shape, communities were engaged in an even more comprehensive manner. The long line-ups of thousands of citizens that marked the opening of 555 University Avenue spoke not only to a curiosity of the new medical institution, but to something much more profound – a sense of pride in, and part ownership of, the hospital. Changing cultural and social trends framed the act of giving, as demonstrated by the telethons of the 1980s; by the 1990s, SickKids even had its own television programming. And yet there was always something broader at play, a collective enterprise of giving that appealed to rich and poor, to individuals of different religions and backgrounds, *because* it was a shared civic project.

One might have assumed (as many American institutions now fear) that the advent of "socialized medicine" in the 1950s and 1960s would fracture this benevolent impulse, the fragile, yet all-important relationship between the public and the hospital. Surely, the funding by the state and the meddling of "bureaucrats" would undermine this long tradition of support? But nothing of the kind happened. The investment, financial and emotional, increased yet further. Donations, small and large continued to flood in to the hospital. Even during the very difficult years of the 1990s, when public debt in Canada reached record highs, public support for The Hospital for Sick Children never seemed to wane. In the mid-1990s, The Hospital for Sick Children Foundation (HSCF) launched an $82-million campaign, Help Make Sick Kids Better. The campaign was novel in that it sought to raise funds not for "bricks and mortar," but to bolster research and attract top scientists through endowed chairs and centres.[2] Chairs started at $2 million and were named for "an outstanding health-care professional" or the benefactor him- or herself.[3] The campaign initially aimed to establish fourteen chairs, but by March 1998, it proved so popular that organizers decided to raise the number of chairs to twenty-five. These included the Women's Auxiliary Chair in Neonatology, the Anne and Max Tanenbaum Chair in

Molecular Medicine, and the Robert M. Filler Chair in Paediatric Surgery. The campaign ultimately raised $85.8 million for research and education.[4]

Indeed, by the 1990s, million-dollar gifts were becoming almost commonplace. On the day the campaign was launched, SickKids announced its largest-ever family gift of $5 million. The gift established the Arthur and Sonia Labatt Brain Tumour Research Centre and was followed up one decade later with $30 million to establish the multi-site Labatt Family Heart Centre and support the Brain Tumour Research Centre. The Gerrard Wing was renamed the Roy C. Hill Wing after a $5-million donation from the charitable foundation for cancer care. Meanwhile, the hospital received its largest planned gift of $12.2 million from the Macarthur family in 1999, and a gift of $3.5 million from Mitchell Goldhar.[5] Magnanimous donations from influential businessmen could sometimes carry with them uncomfortable associations. Close on the heels of the first Labatt gift came a $5-million donation to the hospital through the Black Family Foundation and the newly launched *National Post*. The Black name soon bedecked the Elm Wing, and remained there even after the former lord had been imprisoned in the United States.

Of course, The Hospital for Sick Children was not alone in relishing the new era of mega-philanthropy. In 1993 Peter and Melanie Munk announced a gift of $5 million for Toronto General Hospital's Cardiac Centre, repeating the act sevenfold in 2006 with a donation of $37 million (and an additional $18 million in 2011). At the time, the 2006 gift was "the largest single donation to a hospital in Canadian history."[6] It didn't remain so for long, as Joseph and Wolf Lebovic soon gave $50 million for a new wing at Mt. Sinai, alongside a $25-million donation from Larry and Judy Tanenbaum. Donations on this scale, referred to as "transformational gifts," also boosted St. Michael's Hospital, which received two individual gifts of $25 million in 2005. Donations continued to spiral upward. In 2010, The Hospital for Sick Children received a $30-million donation from the Garron family for the Garron Family Cancer Centre, including two Chairs in Childhood Cancer. A $40-million donation for the Peter Gilgan Centre for Research and Learning became the largest gift to a paediatric hospital in Canadian history.[7]

The staggering size of these substantial donations might easily distract attention from the thousands of smaller donations that have taken many forms, from the "peculiar preciousness" of a father's small donation in memoriam through to the thousands of pledges during the telethons of the

1980s. Giving back to the hospital has taken important non-monetary forms, as witnessed by the lady visitors of the 1870s, the Women's Auxiliary of the 1950s, and the thousands of SickKids "champions" who presently assist in scores of annual fundraising events. They speak to a common social mission, which has its roots in Georgian traditions of philanthropic giving but has evolved and adapted to modern Canadian society, to changing epidemiological realities and technological innovations, and to the growing awareness of the inequalities of health that exist within Canada, and between Canada and the world. Currently, over 1,680 volunteers devote their time and energy to the Foundation, with members of the community holding more than 1,000 events annually in support of the Foundation and the hospital. In the most recently reported year, beginning 1 April 2014 and ending 31 March 2015, nearly 232,000 donors contributed to the Foundation.[8]

The history of The Hospital for Sick Children is much more than a series of medical discoveries and changing clinical interventions of the most prominent medical institution in the country. The hospital has also acted as a prism, reflecting diverse social practices and cultural preoccupations of the time period and society in which it operated. Beyond its notable discoveries, setbacks, and indeed tragedies outlined in this book, The Hospital for Sick Children is retained with deep affection in the hearts of generations of Canadians. Indeed, former patients often self-identify, with pride, as "SickKids kids." Many of the major and minor benefactors listed above have been affected deeply, and directly, by the actions of hospital medical staff, administrators, and volunteers. Their contributions to the hospital, large and small, thus speak to their own gift relation with this famous medical institution. In some key respects, then it may still be considered, to borrow the words of one of the earliest Victorian annual reports, not just a hospital, but rather the "sweetest of all charities."

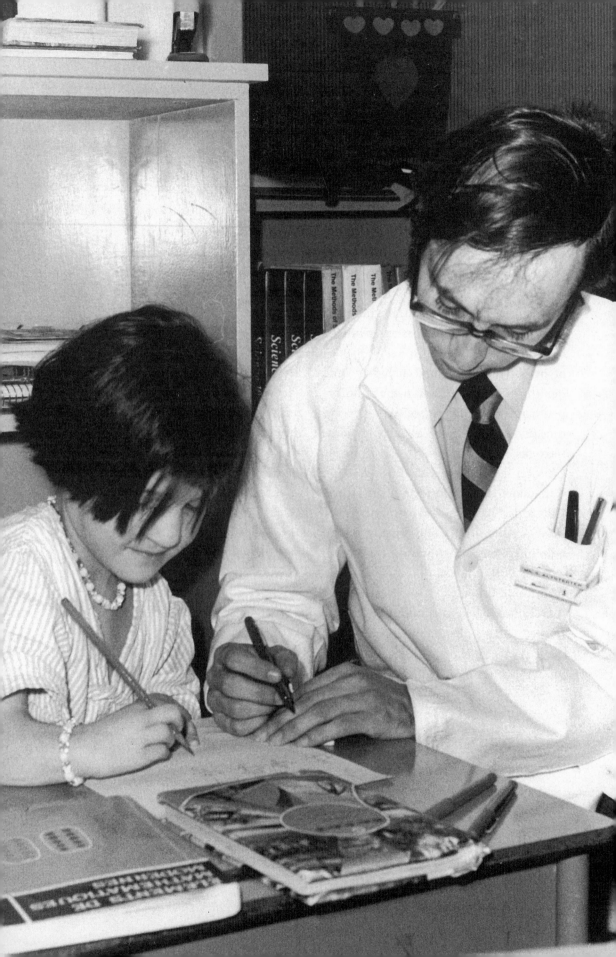

Further Reading

Any work of historical scholarship owes a debt of gratitude to the contributions of a previous generation of researchers. As even a brief review of the hundreds of references will confirm, this history of The Hospital for Sick Children draws on a wealth of journal articles, chapters, books, and edited volumes which intersect with not only the history of SickKids itself, but also a host of cross-cutting themes, such as the history of medical professionalization, the history of nursing, the history of public health, the history of childhood, the history of surgery, and the history of Medicare. This scholarship attests to the remarkable depth and breadth of scholarship in the history of health and medicine in Canada, only a few principal works of which can be discussed in this brief section of further reading.

The Hospital for Sick Children possesses many narratives of its own past. Indeed, self-described "histories" of the hospital were written as early as 1881, including *The Hospital for Sick Children Toronto. Established March 23rd, 1875. A Retrospect* (Toronto, 1881); *The Hospital for Sick Children, College Street, Toronto The Lakeside Home for Little Children, The Convalescent Branch of the Hospital on Gibraltar Point, Toronto Island. History of These Institutions* (Toronto, 1891); *The Story of the Lakeside Home for Little Children, the Summer Home of the Patients of the Hospital for Sick Children, Toronto, Situated at the Point Park, Toronto Island, with Sixty Engravings* (Toronto, 1893); Miss Josephine Kane, *The History of the Hospital for Sick Children, College Street, Toronto, Ontario, Canada, and The Lakeside Home for Little Children, Summer Branch of the Hospital Toronto Island* (Toronto: Hospital for Sick Children, rev. to 1918); and J. Stuart Crawford, *A History of the Hospital for Sick Children 1918 to 1958* (unpublished, HSC Archives, 1959). Many of these are digitized and available online. In 1974, on the occasion of the centenary of the first organizing committee meetings, the journalist Max Braithwaite authored a popular monograph, *Sick Kids: The Story of the Hospital for Sick Children in Toronto* (Toronto: McClelland and Stewart, 1974), in which fourteen eras are told through the vignettes of fourteen individual patients. Although out of print, it is still available in libraries and constitutes a vivid remembrance of childhood sickness in the past. More recently, an arresting photo history of the hospital, *A History of Healing: The Hospital for Sick Children* (Toronto: The Hospital for Sick Children, 2010), showcases the remarkable iconographic collection of the hospital, juxtaposing historical and contemporary scenes of hospital life and clinical care.

Unsurprisingly, given the importance of the hospital, there have been numerous master's theses and doctoral dissertations examining defined eras and themes of The Hospital for Sick Children. These include the following: Judith Young, "Attitudes and Practices Towards the Families of Inpatients at the Hospital for Sick Children, Toronto from 1935 to 1975" (PhD diss., University of Toronto, 1987); Christopher J. Rutty, "'A Grim Terror More Menacing, More Sinister Than Death Itself': Physicians, Poliomyelitis and the Popular Press in Early 20th-Century Ontario" (PhD diss., University of Western Ontario, 1990); Diane Gilday, "The Founding and the First Quarter Century of Management of the Hospital for Sick Children" (master's thesis, University of Toronto, 1991); and Noah Schiff, "'The Sweetest of All Charities': The Toronto Hospital for Sick Children's Medical and Public Appeal, 1875–1905," (master's thesis, University of Toronto, 1999); and Fiona Miller, "A Blueprint for Defining Health: Making Medical Genetics in Canada, c. 1935–1975" (PhD diss., York University, 2000).

In addition to these histories of the hospital itself, there are various published, unpublished, and partially completed histories of different departments and specialties, including extensive work on the history of nursing and the history of the paediatrics department: *Beyond the Dream: The Legacy of Nursing at SickKids*, DVD (Culver City, CA: Marcy and Marc Stone, MHS Productions, 2006); *100 Years: A Celebration of the Alumnae Association of the School of Nursing, The Hospital for Sick Children* (Toronto: The Alumnae Association, 2003); Hilda Rolstin, *The Hospital for Sick Children School of Nursing, Toronto* (Toronto, 1973); *Brief History of the School of Nursing, Hospital for Sick Children, Toronto, 1886–1936* (Toronto: Hospital for Sick Children, 1936); resources on the website of the Alumnae Association of the School of Nursing (http://hscnursingalumnae.org); and Hugh O'Brodovich, with the assistance of Elizabeth Uleryk, Susan Belanger, Daune MacGregor, and Michelle O'Brodovich, *Doctors Who Care for the Future: The History of Medical Care at Toronto's Hospital for Sick Children* (December 2008, unpublished manuscript, 248 pp., HSC Archives).

There are also several informal histories about clinical departments or subspecialties, including Alan W. Conn, Jeremy Sloan, Robert Creighton, and David Steward, "History of the Department of Anaesthesia, the Hospital for Sick Children," in Robert J. Byrick, Joan C. Bevan, and David J. McKnight, eds., *A Commemorative History of the Department of Anesthesia, University of Toronto* (Toronto: University of Toronto Department of Anaesthesia, 2004); A. Jea, M. Al-Otibi, J.T. Rutka, J.M. Drake, and P.B. Dirks, "The History of Neurosurgery at the Hospital for Sick Children in Toronto," *Neurosurgery* 61, no. 3 (2007): 612–24; David Kenny and David Wencer, "Dentistry at SickKids, Toronto," *Ontario Dentist* 91, no. 2 (2014): 14–19; D.J. Kenny, A.C. Dale, and D.G. Wencer, "John G.C. Adams: Father of Dental Public Health in Canada," *Journal of the History of Dentistry* 62, no. 2 (2014): 77–83; and Sanford H. Jackson, *The Development of Research: Research Institute of the Hospital for Sick Children, Toronto: Research Conducted by Members of the Staffs of the Hospital for Sick Children and Its Research Institute from 1919–1977* (Toronto: Hospital for Sick Children, 1977).

A small handful of biographies of some of the principal figures in the hospital's history have been published over the years, including studies of John Ross Robertson, Alan Brown, and William Mustard – two of which, coincidentally, feature the word "tyrant" in the title: Ron Poulton, *The Paper Tyrant: John Ross Robertson* (Toronto: Clarke, Irwin and Co., 1971); A.B. Kingsmill, *Dr. Alan Brown: Portrait of a Tyrant* (Markham, ON: Fitzhenry and Whiteside; Associated Medical Services, 1995); Medical Alumni Association, *Dr. Alan Brown. Brief Biography of the Physician-in-Chief of The Hospital for Sick Children, Comprised of Reminiscences of His Colleagues in the (Medical) Alumni Association and Family* (Toronto: HSC Archives); and Marilyn Dunlop, *Bill Mustard: Surgical Pioneer* (Toronto: Hannah Institute and Dundurn Press, 1989).

A substantial body of academic scholarship implicates The Hospital for Sick Children in some of the most important events in Canadian medical history. Edward Shorter, for example, has authored a monumental history of the University of Toronto Faculty of Medicine, *Partnership for Excellence: Medicine at the University of Toronto and Academic Hospitals* (Toronto: University of Toronto Press, 2013), one chapter of which discusses the role of The Hospital for Sick Children as the centre of academic paediatrics for the University of Toronto medical school. Heather MacDougall has written *Activists and Advocates: Toronto's Health Department 1883–1983* (Toronto: Dundurn Press, 1990), a history of the Toronto Department of Public Health, which worked closely with The Hospital for Sick Children in the early decades of municipal public health initiatives, particularly in the famous battle for pasteurized milk and the fight against infant mortality. There are, of course, landmark books by Michael Bliss, such as *The Discovery of Insulin* (Chicago: University of Chicago Press, 1982; 25th anniversary ed., 2007) and *Banting: A Biography* (Toronto: University of Toronto Press, 1984; 2nd ed. 1992), his award-winning biography of Frederick Banting, who was nominally in charge of the diabetes unit at the children's hospital in the 1920s and 1930s.

Historians, such as Aleck Ostry and Ian Mosby, have analysed nutritional research and paediatrics in early twentieth-century Canada, illuminating the "Vitamania" that pervaded early twentieth-century paediatrics as well as the failed attempt to reverse the generation-long decline in breastfeeding. For key works, see Tasnim Nathoo and Aleck Ostry, *The One Best Way?: Breastfeeding History, Politics, and Policy in Canada* (Kitchener-Waterloo: Wilfrid Laurier University Press, 2009); Aleck Ostry, *Nutrition Policy in Canada, 1870–1939* (Vancouver: University of British Columbia Press, 2011); and Ian Mosby, *Food Will Win the War: The Politics, Culture, and Science of Food on Canada's Home Front* (Vancouver: University of British Columbia Press, 2014). In addition, the architecture of the hospital has come under the microscope. Annmarie Adams has researched the architecture of children's hospitals – including the 1892 building – in Annmarie Adams and David Theodore, "Designing for 'the Little Convalescents': Children's Hospitals in Toronto and Montreal, 1875–2006," *Canadian Bulletin of Medical History/ Bulletin canadien d'histoire de la médecine* 19, no. 1 (2002): 201–43, and the famous Atrium built almost exactly one century later in Annmarie Adams, David Theodore, Ellie Goldenberg, Coralee McLaren, and Patricia McKeever, "Kids in the Atrium: Comparing Architectural Intentions and Children's Experiences in a Pediatric Hospital Lobby," *Social Science and Medicine* 70, no. 5 (2010): 658–67.

Complementing the history of hospitals and research into the history of paediatrics, there is now a robust literature on the history of children, childhood, and childrearing in Canada. Cynthia Comacchio has explored the role of childrearing and the state in the first decade of the twentieth century and has written extensively on "scientific motherhood," focusing, in large part, on Toronto in *Nations are Built of Babies: Saving Ontario's Mothers and Children, 1900–1940* (Montreal: McGill-Queen's University Press, 1993). The larger question of what different eras believed was the "right" way to parent is explored in Katherine Arnup, *Education for Motherhood: Advice for Mothers in Twentieth-Century Canada* (Toronto: University of Toronto Press, 1994). The psychological dimensions of childrearing have been pursued by Mona Gleason, whose book *Small Matters: Canadian Children in Sickness and Health, 1900–1940* (Montreal: McGill-Queen's University Press, 2013) features case studies of patients admitted to The Hospital for Sick Children in the interwar period. These scholars have built on the pioneering scholarship of Neil Sutherland and Joy Parr, who authored numerous works on the history of childhood in Canada, including Neil Sutherland, *Children in English-Canadian Society: Framing The Twentieth-Century Consensus* (Toronto: University of Toronto Press, 1976); Neil Sutherland, *Growing Up: Childhood in English Canada from the Great War to the Age of Television* (Toronto: University of Toronto Press, 1997); and Neil Sutherland, Jean Barman, and Linda L. Hale, *History of Canadian Childhood and Youth: A Bibliography* (Westport, CT: Greenwood Press, 1992). Some of the newer scholarship has appeared in two edited volumes that reflect the intersection of the history of childhood and medical history: Cheryl Warsh, ed., *Children's Health Issues in Historical Perspective* (Kitchener-Waterloo: Wilfrid Laurier University Press, 2005) and Cynthia Comacchio, Janet Golden, and George Weisz, eds., *Healing the World's Children: Child Health in International and Interdisciplinary Perspective* (Montreal: McGill-Queen's University Press, 2008). A subset of this literature intersects with the emerging field of disability studies, in which historians of health and medicine have begun to look at the historical context of how disability has been labelled, treated, and experienced. For example, see J.A. Ellis, "'Backward and Brilliant Children': A Social and Policy History of Disability, Childhood, and Education in Toronto's Special Education Classes, 1910 to 1945" (PhD diss., York University, 2011); and David Wright, *Downs: The History of a Disability* (Oxford: Oxford University Press, 2011).

Over the last two decades, the history of medical institutions has slowly begun to re-emerge, with at least a dozen major works on psychiatric institutions, examinations of tuberculosis sanatoria, and – with a renewed interest in Indigenous history – publications such as Maureen Lux's *Separate Beds: A History of Indian Hospitals in Canada* (Toronto: University of Toronto Press, 2016). For those interested in comparing SickKids to sister institutions in the country, one can enjoy Denyse Baillargeon's excellent *Naître, Vivre, Grandir: Sainte-Justine, 1907–2007* (Montreal: Boréal, 2007), a captivating history of the francophone children's hospital in Montreal, whose development – as well as its governance for more than two generations by an all-women's committee and its unionization of staff – stands in striking contrast to that of its sister institution in Toronto. An older but still influential work on the evolution of general hospitals in Ontario is David and Rosemary Gagan's prize-winning *For Patients of Moderate Means: A Social History of the Voluntary Public General Hospital in Canada, 1890–1950* (Montreal: McGill-Queen's University Press, 2002).

Notes

References have been grouped in the following manner: In endnotes with multiple citations, references for quotations or data will come first in the sequence. All others are listed in the order they appear/ are used in the text.

INTRODUCTION

1 J.T. Law, "H.S.C. Today and Tomorrow," in *Bulletin of The Hospital for Sick Children* 13, no. 4 (1964): 2–3.
2 Anonymous interview by author, participant 37, 15 January 2014.
3 J.T.H. Connor, "Review Essay/Revue Critique: Hospital History in Canada and the United States," *Canadian Bulletin of Medical History* 7, no. 1 (1990): 93–104. See J.T.H. Connor, *Doing Good: The Life of Toronto's General Hospital* (Toronto: University of Toronto Press, 2000). See also E.A. Heaman, "Review Essay/Note critique: Review of Christopher J. Rutty, *A Circle of Care*," *Canadian Bulletin of Medical History* 16, no. 1 (2012): 163–8.
4 Michael Bliss, *The Discovery of Insulin*, 2nd ed. (Chicago: University of Chicago Press, 2007); Michael Bliss, *Banting: A Biography*, 2nd ed. (Toronto: University of Toronto Press, 1992).
5 David Wright, *Mental Disability in Victorian England: The Earlswood Asylum, 1847–1901* (Oxford: Clarendon Press, 2001); David Wright, *Downs: The History of a Disability* (Oxford: Oxford University Press, 2011).

1 BETWEEN THE CRADLE AND THE GRAVE

1 Charles Dickens, *Our Mutual Friend* (New York: Modern Library Editions, 1992), 319.
2 The history of the transformation of childhood and the family over the modern period constitutes an important theme in modern social history. For classic works in this field, see Philippe Ariès, *Centuries of Childhood: A Social History of Family Life* (New York: Alfred A. Knopf, 1962); Peter Laslett with Richard Wall, eds., *Household and Family in Past Time* (Cambridge: Cambridge University Press, 1972); and Edward Shorter, *The Making of the Modern Family* (New York: Basic Books, 1975).
3 Robert Newsom, "Fictions of Childhood," in *The Cambridge Companion to Charles Dickens*, ed. John O. Jordan (Cambridge: Cambridge University Press, 2001), 93.
4 A.J. Carter, "A Christmas Carol: Charles Dickens and the Birth of Orthopaedics," *Journal of the Royal Society of Medicine* 86, no. 1 (1993): 46; Newsom, "Fictions of Childhood," 93; Jules Kosky, *Mutual Friends: Charles Dickens and Great Ormond Street Children's Hospital* (London: Weidenfeld and Nicolson, 1989), 12.

5 Stanley F. Wainapel, "Dickens and Disability," *Disability and Rehabilitation* 18, no. 12 (1996): 632; Martha Stoddard Holmes, *Fictions of Affliction: Physical Disability in Victorian Culture* (Ann Arbor: University of Michigan Press, 2004), 96–8, 197–200; Asa Briggs, *The Age of Improvement, 1783–1867* (London: Longmans, Green, 1975).

6 The Victorian diagnosis for a particular form of tuberculosis manifesting in inflammatory swelling of the lymph glands in the neck, armpit, and groin.

7 Civil registration in England and Wales dates from 1837; the "modern" census began in 1841.

8 Charles Dickens, "Between the Cradle and the Grave," *All the Year Round* 145 (1862): 454.

9 F. Barry Smith, *The People's Health, 1830–1910* (London: Croom Helm, 1979), 144–5.

10 Kosky, *Mutual Friends*, 149–64, 180.

11 The first cot was endowed in 1868, a novel act that had not apparently been performed before in London hospitals. Jules Kosky and Raymond J. Lunnon, *Great Ormond Street and the Story of Medicine* (London: The Hospitals for Sick Children, in association with Granta Editions, 1991), 23–9. Charles Dickens or Henry Morley (the authorship is contested), "Drooping Buds," *Household Words* 106 (1852): 45–8.

12 Kosky, *Mutual Friends*, 197–8, 200, 203, 219.

13 Katharina Boehm, "'A Place for More than the Healing of Bodily Sickness': Charles Dickens, the Social Mission of Nineteenth-Century Pediatrics, and the Great Ormond Street Hospital for Sick Children," *Victorian Review* 35, no. 1 (2009): 153–74, 154; "Between the Cradle and the Grave," 454–6; Dickens, *Our Mutual Friend*.

14 Andrea Tanner, "Choice and the Children's Hospital: Great Ormond Street Hospital Patients and Their Families 1855–1900," in *Medicine, Charity and Mutual Aid: The Consumption of Health in Britain, c.1550–1950*, ed. Anne Borsay and Peter Shapely (Burlington, VT: Ashgate Publishing Group, 2007), 138–9.

15 Kosky and Lunnon, *Great Ormond Street*, 16.

16 This quotation refers to the East London Children's Hospital. Charles Dickens, "A Small Star in the East," *All the Year Round,* no. 3 New Series (19 December 1868): 61–6, quotation 66.

17 Elizabeth M.R. Lomax, *Small and Special: The Development of Hospitals for Children in Victorian Britain* (London: Wellcome Institute for the History of Medicine, 1996), 13, 111.

18 Lomax, *Small and Special*, 36, 41–2; Tanner, "Choice and the Children's Hospital," 144–6; Jonathan Reinarz, "Investigating the 'Deserving' Poor: Charity and Voluntary Hospitals in Nineteenth-Century Birmingham," in *Medicine, Charity and Mutual Aid*, 119–32.

19 Joan Lane, *A Social History of Medicine: Health, Healing and Disease in England, 1750–1950* (New York: Routledge, 2001), 82–3.

20 Roy Porter, "The Gift Relation: Philanthropy and Provincial Hospitals in Eighteenth-Century England," in *The Hospital in History*, ed. Lindsay Granshaw and Roy Porter (New York: Routledge, 1989), 149–78.

21 Eduard Seidler, "An Historical Survey of Children's Hospitals," in *The Hospital in History*, ed. Granshaw and Porter, 184. The date of the founding of this dispensary is sometimes listed as 1767.

22 Norman Alvey, *Education by Election: Reed's School, Clapton and Watford* (St Albans: St Albans and Hertfordshire Architectural and Archaeological Society, 1990), 2–3.

23 J.A. Walker-Smith, "Children in Hospital," in *Western Medicine: An Illustrated History*, ed. Irvine Loudon (New York: Oxford University Press, 1997), 221–2.

24 Thomas Malthus, *Essay on the Principle of Population*, vol. 2 (1803; repr., Cambridge: Cambridge University Press, 1989), iii, as quoted in Jacalyn Duffin, *History of Medicine: A Scandalously Short Introduction*, 2nd ed. (Toronto: University of Toronto Press, 2010), 312.

25 Reinarz, "Investigating the 'Deserving' Poor," 119.

26 David Sloane, "'Not Designed Merely to Heal': Women Reformers and the Emergence of Children's Hospitals," *Journal of the Gilded Age and Progressive Era* 4, no. 4 (2005): 330–3.

27 Lomax, *Small and Special*, 33.

28 Clement A. Smith, *The Children's Hospital of Boston: "Built Better Than They Knew"* (Boston: Little, Brown and Company, 1983), 31–2.

29 Anne Digby, *Making a Medical Living: Doctors and Patients in the English Market for Medicine, 1720–1911* (Cambridge: Cambridge University Press, 2002).

30 M. Jeanne Peterson, *The Medical Profession in Mid-Victorian London* (Berkeley: University of California Press, 1978).

31 Anton Sebastien, *A Dictionary of the History of Medicine* (New York: Parthenon Publishing, 1999), 573.

32 As cited in Smith, *The People's Health*, 146.

33 Lisa Rosner, *Medical Education in the Age of Improvement: Edinburgh Students and Apprentices, 1760–1826* (Edinburgh: Edinburgh University Press, 1991).

34 See W.F. Bynum, *Science and the Practice of Medicine in the Nineteenth Century* (Cambridge: Cambridge University Press, 1994).

35 Janet Golden, "Children's Health: Caregivers and Sites of Care," in *Children and Youth in Sickness and in Health: A Historical Handbook and Guide*, ed. Janet Lynne Golden, Richard A. Meckel and Heather Monro Prescott (Westport, CT: Greenwood Press, 2004), 75–6. Andrea Tanner, "Too Many Mothers? Female Roles in a Metropolitan Victorian Children's Hospital," in *The Impact of Hospitals 300–2000*, ed. John Henderson, Peregrine Horden, and Alessandro Pastore (Oxford: Peter Lang, 2007), 136; Kosky and Lunnon, eds., "A Table of the First Children's Hospitals up to 1900," in *Great Ormond Street*, np. By one count, between 1850 and 1900, thirty-six specialist children's hospitals opened in the United Kingdom. Jonathan Gillis, "Taking a Medical History in Childhood Illness: Representations of Parents in Pediatric Texts since 1850," *Bulletin of the History of Medicine* 79, no. 3 (2005): 396.

36 D.G. Hamilton, *Hand in Hand: The Story of the Royal Alexandra Hospital for Children, Sydney* (Sydney: John Ferguson, 1979), 9; Samuel X. Radbill, "Hospitals and Pediatrics, 1776–1976," *Bulletin of the History of Medicine* 53, no. 2 (1979): 287–8.

37 As cited in Debórah Dwork, "Childhood," in the *Companion Encyclopedia of the History of Medicine*, vol. 2, ed. W.F. Bynum and Roy Porter (New York: Routledge, 1993), 1073; Golden, "Children's Health: Caregivers and Sites of Care," 75.

38 Quotation in Stoddard Holmes, *Fictions of Affliction*, 103; Laura C. Berry, *The Child, the State, and the Victorian Novel* (Charlottesville: Virginia University Press, 1999), 2–3.

39 Peter G. Jones, "Dickens' Literary Children: The Harry Swift Memorial Lecture, Adelaide 1971," *Australian Paediatric Journal* 8, no. 5 (972): 240.

40 Kosky, *Mutual Friends*, 187. One could also include a long list of other late-Victorian charities, including the London Invalid Children's Aid Association (1888), which offered material relief to "crippled children of the poor." See Carter, "A Christmas Carol," 46–7.

41 Letter from the secretary of The Hospital for Sick Children, 49, Great Ormond Street, Queen's Square, London, England, 12 January 1875, in *Annual Report of The Hospital for Sick Children January 1st 1880 – December 31st 1880* (Toronto: Hart and Rawlinson, 1881), 26. The Hospital for Sick Children Archives (hereafter HSC Archives).

42 Sloane, "'Not Designed Merely to Heal,'" 335–6; Hamilton, *Hand in Hand*, 12, 14.

2 THE SWEETEST OF ALL CHARITIES

1 Hospital for Sick Children, Annual Report (hereafter AR), 1887 (Toronto: Hart and Company, 1888), 9. HSC Archives.

2 "City News," *The Globe*, 26 January 1875, 4.

3 Advertisement, *The Globe*, 22 March 1875, 2; "City News," *The Globe*, 24 March 1875, 1.

4 AR 1887, 9.

5 "City News," *The Globe*, 24 March 1875, 1.

6 AR 1887, 9.

7 AR 1876, 7.

8   AR 1876, 13, 20.

9   "City News," *The Globe*, 26 January 1875, 4.

10 AR 1876, p 17.

11 Quotation from AR 1876, 13–14; J.S. Crawford, "The First Seventy-Five Years," *Bulletin of The Hospital for Sick Children* 13, no. 4 (1964), 7.

12 AR 1875–6, 4.

13 AR 1893, 7. This unattributed quotation – "But perhaps the 'sweetest of all charities,' as someone has well said, is the care of little, sick children" – was invoked repeatedly in the hospital's annual reports from 1891 onwards. It is also used in the title of a University of Toronto MA thesis on the early years of the hospital; see Noah Schiff, "The Sweetest of All Charities," unpublished master's thesis, Department of History, University of Toronto, 1999.

14 Joey Noble, "Class-ifying the Poor: Toronto Charities, 1850–80," *Studies in Political Economy* 2, no. 2 (1979): 113.

15 Lynne Marks, "Indigent Committees and Ladies Benevolent Societies: Intersections of Public and Private Poor Relief in Nineteenth Century Small Town Ontario," *Studies in Political Economy* 47 (1995): quotation 62; Andrew C. Holman, *A Sense of Their Duty: Middle-Class Formation in Victorian Ontario Towns* (Montreal: McGill-Queen's University Press, 2000), 103, 109–10; Stephen Speisman, "Munificent Parsons and Municipal Parsimony: Voluntary vs. Public Poor Relief in Nineteenth Century Toronto," in *A History of Ontario: Selected Readings*, ed. Michael J. Piva (Toronto: Copp Clark Pitman Ltd, 1988), 55, 63.

     Boards of health existed throughout the nineteenth century but tended to be temporary in nature, in response to specific epidemics. They would then be disbanded, much to the chagrin of public health reformers who advocated for a permanent department. For a history of the Toronto public health board, see Heather MacDougall, *Activists and Advocates: Toronto's Health Department, 1883–1983* (Toronto: Dundurn Press, 1990).

16 Not that all charitable activities were strictly limited to religious groups. During the second half of the century, disparate lay, union, and fraternal organizations – Oddfellows, labour unions, the Orange Order – also engaged in various initiatives to address poverty and other social ills. This complementary pattern of targeted philanthropy unfolded throughout North America. See Thomas Adam, *Buying Respectability: Philanthropy and Urban Society in Transnational Perspective, 1840s to 1930s* (Bloomington: Indiana University Press, 2009), chap. 5.

17 Paula Maurutto, *Governing Charities: Church and State in Toronto's Catholic Archdiocese, 1850–1950* (Montreal: McGill-Queen's University Press, 2003), 19–20; Carmen Nielson Varty, "The City and the Ladies: Politics, Religion and Female Benevolence in Mid-Nineteenth-Century Hamilton, Canada West," *Journal of Canadian Studies* 38, no. 2 (2004): 158–9.

18 Maurutto, *Governing Charities*, 21–7.

19 Non-conformity here is being used in the historical sense, denoting Protestant churches that refused to accept the religious rites of the Church of England after it split from Rome. Richard Allen, *The Social Passion: Religion and Social Reform in Canada, 1914–28* (Toronto: University of Toronto Press, 1971), 5, 15–16. For a general survey, see Nancy Christie and Michael Gauvreau, *Christian Churches and their Peoples, 1840–1965: A Social History of Religion in Canada* (Toronto: University of Toronto Press, 2010).

20 Joy Parr, "'Transplanting from Dens of Iniquity': Theology and Child Emigration," in *A Not Unreasonable Claim: Women and Reform in Canada, 1880s–1920s*, ed. Linda Kealey (Toronto: The Women's Press, 1979), 175–6; Linda Kealy, "Introduction," *A Not Unreasonable Claim*, 3.

21 Mariana Valverde, *The Age of Light, Soap, and Water: Moral Reform in English Canada, 1885–1925* (Toronto: McClelland and Stewart, 1991), 19.

22 Maurutto, *Governing Charities*, 27.

23 Kenneth L. Draper, "Redemptive Homes – Redeeming Choices: Saving the Social in Late-Victorian London, Ontario," in *Households of Faith: Family, Gender, and Community in Canada, 1760–1969*, ed. Nancy Christie (Montreal: McGill-Queen's University Press, 2002), 264–89.

24 Speisman, "Munificent Parsons and Municipal Parsimony," 56.

25 Quotation in Draper, "Redemptive Homes – Redeeming Choices," 274; Noble, "Class-ifying the Poor," 116–17; Valverde, *The Age of Light, Soap, and Water*, 159; Marks, "Indigent Committees and Ladies Benevolent Societies," 72.

26 Carmen Nielson Varty, "'A Career in Christian Charity': Women's Benevolence and the Public Sphere in a Mid-Nineteenth-Century Canadian City," *Women's History Review* 14, no. 2 (2005): 253; Tanner, "Too Many Mothers?" 143–4.

27 Quotation Judith Young, "A Divine Mission: Elizabeth McMaster and the Hospital for Sick Children, Toronto, 1875–92," *Canadian Bulletin of Medical History* 11 (1994): 74; Rector William J. Hockin, Memo: Baptism Register, St. Paul's Church 227 Bloor East, Toronto, HSC Archives; *Hart Family Diary, 1842–1966*, 3, HSC Archives.

28 Quotation Gina Feldberg, "Wyllie, Elizabeth Jennet," in *Dictionary of Canadian Biography*, vol. 13, University of Toronto/Université Laval, 2003–, http://www.biographi.ca/en/bio/wyllie_elizabeth_jennet_13E.html. Ontario Civil Registration from 1869 to 1927, Provincial Archives, microfilm MS 932 vol. 10, p. 222, http://homepages.rootsweb.ancestry.com/~maryc/tor70p2.htm.

29 Feldberg, "Wyllie, Elizabeth Jennet." Elizabeth later transferred to the Yorkville Baptist Church. Correspondence: Glenn Tomlinson, Church Archivist, Jarvis Street Baptist Church, to Judith Young, 7 January 1991, Elizabeth McMaster Subject File, HSC Archives; In collaboration, "McMaster, William," in *Dictionary of Canadian Biography*, vol. 11, University of Toronto/Université Laval, 2003–, http://www.biographi.ca/en/bio/mcmaster_william_11E.html.

30 Young, "A Divine Mission," 75.

31 Annual reports of the HSC; Feldberg, "Wyllie, Elizabeth Jennet."

32 AR 1877, 6; Ladies Committee, Hospital for Sick Children. Rules finally passed by the Committee 11 December 1878.

33 See John R. Graham, "The Haven, 1878–1930: A Toronto Charity's Transition from a Religious to a Professional Ethos," *Social History* 25, no. 50 (1992): 286.

34 Ron Sawatsky, "Howland, William Holmes," in *Dictionary of Canadian Biography*, vol. 12, University of Toronto/Université Laval, 2003–, http://www.biographi.ca/en/bio/howland_william_holmes_12E.html; Graham, "The Haven," 286–7.

35 Mr. Henry O'Brien was a prominent lawyer later named trustee of the hospital. Ladies Committee minutes, 5 April 1878. He was also an advisory board member at the Haven, a noted Anglican philanthropist, and a supporter of W.H. Howland. G. Mercer Adam, *Toronto, Old and New: A Memorial Volume, Historical, Descriptive and Pictorial, Designed to Mark the Hundredth Anniversary of the Passing of the Constitutional Act of 1791 ...* (Toronto: The Mail Printing Co., 1891), 97–8.

36 "The City and Vicinity," *Toronto World*, 10 August 1881, 4.

37 *The Globe*, 25 January 1881, 9.

38 "Hospital for Sick Children: On Beginning of Toronto Hospital," *The Globe*, 21 December 1874, 2.

39 AR 1876, 15, 21.

40 AR 1876, 10–11.

41 AR 1876, 13, 12, 8.

42 AR 1894, 32.

43 The addresses were, respectively, 21 Avenue Street (1875–6), 206 Seaton Street (1876–8), and 245 Elizabeth Street (1878–86). The address on Elizabeth Street would form part of the land that would be dedicated to the permanent hospital in 1892.

44 AR 1877, 8.

45 Ladies Committee minutes, 4 October 1878.

46 AR 1877, 6.

47 AR 1877, 6, 8–9.

48 Ladies Committee minutes, 6 July 1877 and 3 December 1879. In August 1878, individual lady visitors were listed for August, due to "the absence of so many Ladies from the City." Ladies Committee minutes, 2 August 1878.

49 Remarks of the chairman at the Opening and Dedicatory Services of the Hospital, in the Ladies Committee minutes, 6 June 1878.

50 Ladies Committee minutes, 6 July 1877; Ladies Committee minutes, 1 February 1878.

51 Ladies Committee minutes, 4 February 1879.

52 AR 1877, 8–9.

53 Josephine Kane, *The History of the Hospital for Sick Children College Street, Toronto, Ont., Canada and The Lakeside Home for Little Children, Revised to 1918* (Toronto, 1918), 9.

54 Connor, *Doing Good*, 31, 51–2.

55 Lisa Chilton, "Managing Migrants: Toronto, 1820–1880," *Canadian Historical Review* 92, no. 2 (2011): 241–6. See also Mark G. McGowan, *Death or Canada: The Irish Famine Migration to Toronto, 1847* (Toronto: Novalis, 2009).

56 Connor, *Doing Good*, 86.

57 Ibid., quotation 104, 90–4, 107.

58 James Moran, *Committed to the State Asylum: Insanity and Society in Nineteenth-Century Quebec and Ontario* (Montreal: McGill-Queen's University Press, 2000), 49 and passim; Cyril Greenland, "Madness and the Media, 1840s–1990s," in *The Provincial Asylum in Toronto: Reflections on Social and Architectural History*, ed. Edna Hudson (Toronto: Architectural Conservancy of Ontario, 2000), 3–4.

59 Geoffrey Reaume, *Remembrance of Patients Past: Patient Life at the Toronto Hospital for the Insane, 1870–1940* (Oxford: Oxford University Press, 2000), 3, 6.

60 Moran, *Committed to the State Asylum*, 84–6; Christine I.M. Johnston, "Joseph Workman: Asylum Superintendent," in *The Provincial Asylum in Toronto*, 130.

61 John Radford and Deborah C. Park, "'A Convenient Means of Riddance': Institutionalization of People Diagnosed as "Mentally Deficient in Ontario, 1876–1934," *Health and Canadian Society* 1, no. 2 (1993), 369–92; Thelma Wheatley, *"And Neither Have I Wings to Fly": Labelled and Locked up in Canada's Oldest Institution* (Toronto: Inanna Publications, 2013).

62 W.H. Irwin, *Robertson & Cook's Toronto City Directory for 1870* (Toronto: Daily Telegram Publishing House, 1870), xxii–xxiii, xxix; W.R. Brown, *Brown's Toronto General Directory* (Toronto: Maclear and Co., 1856), xiv; Kevin Siena, "Hospitals for the Excluded or Convalescent Homes?: Workhouses, Medicalization and the Poor Law in Long Eighteenth-Century London and Pre-Confederation Toronto," *Canadian Bulletin of Medical History* 27, no. 1 (2010): 14–15; John McCullagh, *A Legacy of Caring: A History of the Children's Aid Society of Toronto* (Toronto: Dundurn Group, 2002), 19.

63 See Jennifer Bonnell, *Reclaiming the Don: An Environmental History of Toronto's Don River Valley* (Toronto: University of Toronto Press, 2014), 86–7.

64 Charlotte Neff, "Government Approaches to Child Neglect and Mistreatment in Nineteenth-Century Ontario," *Social History* 41, no. 81 (2008): table 1, 196–7.

65 Connor, *Doing Good*, 60–1.

66 J.T.H. Connor, "Rosebrugh, Abner Mulholland," in *Dictionary of Canadian Biography*, vol. 14, University of Toronto/Université Laval, 2003–, http://www.biographi.ca/en/bio/rosebrugh_abner_mulholland_14E.html.

67 Canada Dominion Bureau of Statistics, Registration and Statistics Board, *First Report of the Secretary of the Board of Registration and Statistics on the Census of the Canadas for 1851–52*, vol 1: *Personal Census* (Quebec: John Lovell, 1853), 66; "Provincial Lying-in Hospital and Vaccine Institution," *British Colonist*, 20 September 1850, vol. 15, no. 74, 1; William Canniff, *The Medical Profession in Upper Canada, 1783–1850: An Historical Narrative, with Original Documents Relating to the Profession, Including Some Brief Biographies* (Toronto: William and Briggs, 1894), 214; Judith Young, "'Monthly' Nurses, 'Sick' Nurses, and Midwives in 19th-Century Toronto, 1830–1891," *Canadian Bulletin of Medical History* 21, no. 1 (2004): 301n68; Connor, *Doing Good*, 123.

68 Ovariotomy is the older term for the removal of one or both of the ovaries.

69 J.H. Elliott, "Osler's Class at the Toronto School of Medicine," *Canadian Medical Association Journal* (August 1942): 165; Henri Pilon, "Hodder, Edward Mulberry," in *Dictionary of Canadian*

Biography, vol. 10, University of Toronto/Université Laval, 2003–, http://www.biographi.ca/en/bio/hodder_edward_mulberry_10E.html.

70 Quotation from David R. Keane, "Aikins, William Thomas," in *Dictionary of Canadian Biography*, vol. 12, University of Toronto/Université Laval, 2003–, http://www.biographi.ca/en/bio/aikins_william_thomas_12E.html.

71 Martin L. Friedland, *The University of Toronto: A History*, 2nd ed. (Toronto: University of Toronto Press, 2013), 128–30; Keane, "Aikins, William Thomas"; Adam, *Toronto, Old and New*, 104.

72 William Cathcart, ed., *The Baptist Encyclopaedia*, rev. ed. (Philadelphia: Louis H. Everts, 1883), 1298.

73 Cathcart, *The Baptist Encyclopaedia*, 1292–3; Ladies Committee minutes, 3 October 1877 and 15 February 1884; board of trustees minutes, 19 October 1891, HSC Archives.

74 Terrie Romano, "Professional Identity and the Nineteenth-Century Ontario Medical Profession," *Social History* 28, no. 55 (1995): 77–98. See Constance Backhouse, "The Celebrated Abortion Trial of Dr. Emily Stowe, Toronto, 1879," *Canadian Bulletin of Medical History* 8, no. 3 (1991): 158–87.

75 "Hospital for Sick Children," *The Globe*, 21 December 1874, 2.

76 E. McMaster, letter to the editor, *The Globe*, 22 December 1874, 2.

77 AR 1900, 44.

78 In 1879 children up to age sixteen were admitted as both in- and outpatients. In 1880, the maximum age for all patients was again lowered to fourteen years. AR 1879, 3; AR 1880, 4, 7.

79 The girl was successfully treated by a surgical excision of the head of her thigh. AR 1876, 9.

80 AR 1881, 21.

81 AR 1876, 5. The gender imbalance was attributed to the number of boys admitted for accidents. In 1905, there were 25 per cent more boys than girls treated as outpatients. In 1908, 4,265 girls and 6,398 boys were seen; in 1913, 11,954 girls and 13,553 boys were treated. AR 1905, 9; AR 1908, 8. Ladies Committee minutes, 26 October 1876. Cameron also requested that the hospital expand to accommodate "female diseases," but this was denied for reasons of space and resources. Ladies Committee minutes, 19 December 1876.

82 In total, to date, 1,399 externs received treatment, compared with 228 inpatients. AR 1880, 10.

83 Quotation in *The Hospital for Sick Children Toronto. Established March 23rd, 1875. A Retrospect* (Toronto: Dudley and Burns, 1881), 11; AR 1880, 36.

84 "Hospital for Sick Children," *The Globe*, 12 February 1875, 3.

85 "Hospital for Sick Children," *The Globe*, 11 December 1875, 4. This scenario is retold in the *Globe*, 20 September 1876, 4.

86 AR 1876, 7–8.

87 Review of *The Ladies Home Cook Book*, *The Canadian Methodist Magazine* 5, no. 3 (1877): 286.

88 AR 1887, 9. Emphasis in original.

89 "Canadian News. Latest from Toronto," *Ottawa Free Press*, 12 February 1875, 1.

90 AR 1880, 10–11.

91 The figure reported for 1896 was $12,951.10 as part of a total revenue that year of $27,582.75 ($7,951.10 from the province and $5,000 from the city corporation). AR 1896, 21. See also Neff, "Government Approaches to Child Neglect," 198–9.

92 In the interim, a special children's ward was established in 1874 in the Montreal General Hospital, which served as a teaching unit for McGill University medical students. Jessie Body Scriver, *The Montreal Children's Hospital: Years of Growth* (Montreal: McGill Queen's University Press, 1979), 2, and chap.1.

93 Quotation Tanner, "Choice and the Children's Hospital: Great Ormond Street Hospital Patients and Their Families 1855–1900," in *Medicine, Charity and Mutual Aid: The Consumption of Health in Britain, c.1550–1950*, ed. Anne Borsay and Peter Shapely (Burlington, VT: Ashgate Publishing Group, 2007), 137–8; Sloane, "'Not Designed Merely to Heal': Women Reformers and the Emergence of Children's Hospitals," *Journal of the Gilded Age and Progressive Era* 4, no. 4 (2005): 336–9.

94 Janet Golden, "Children's Health: Caregivers and Sites of Care," in *Children and Youth in Sickness and in Health: A Historical Handbook and Guide*, ed. Janet Lynne Golden, Richard A. Meckel and Heather Monro Prescott (Westport, CT: Greenwood Press, 2004), 75.

95 Ladies Committee minutes, 4 October 1887.

3 THE PAPER TYRANT

1 S.R. Wells, *Phrenological Chart of J. Ross Robertson, Given at Fowler and Wells*, 10 January 1871; Archives of Ontario, Series F 1174–1, File 7, 1–7.

2 Minko Sotiron, "Robertson, John Ross," in *Dictionary of Canadian Biography*, vol. 14, University of Toronto/Université Laval, 2003–, http://www.biographi.ca/en/bio/robertson_john_ross_14E.html.

3 Sotiron, "Robertson, John Ross." See also Augustus Bridle, *Sons of Canada: Short Studies of Characteristic Canadians* (Toronto: J.M. Dent, 1916), 23.

4 Quoted in Sotiron, "Robertson, John Ross."

5 Sotiron, "Robertson, John Ross"; G.S. Kealey, *Toronto Workers Respond to Industrial Capitalism, 1867–1892* (1980; repr. Toronto: University of Toronto Press, 1991), 95, 128–34; *The Canadian Illustrated News* 5, no. 13 (1872): 198.

6 Sotiron, "Robertson, John Ross." See also Charles Pelham Mulvaney, *History of Toronto and County of York, Ontario: Containing a History of the City of Toronto and the County of York, Ontario*, vol. 1 (Toronto: C. Blackett Robinson Publisher, 1885), 328.

7 Ron Poulton, *The Paper Tyrant: John Ross Robertson of the Toronto Telegram* (Toronto: Clarke, Irwin and Company Limited, 1971), 13, quotation 189.

8 Henry James Morgan, *Canadian Men and Women of the Time: A Handbook of Canadian Biography of Living Characters*, 2nd ed. (Toronto: William Briggs, 1912), 952–3.

9 Poulton, *The Paper Tyrant*, 104.

10 Sotiron, "Robertson, John Ross."

11 Poulton, *The Paper Tyrant*, 13, 114, 116, 142–3.

12 Ladies Committee minutes (devotional meeting), 31 December 1891, HSC Archives.

13 Bridle, *Sons of Canada*, 24, 25, 27.

14 Ontario's first tuberculosis sanatorium, for example, opened in Bracebridge, in 1896.

15 Seidler, "An Historical Survey of Children's Hospitals," in Granshaw and Porter, ed., *The Hospital in History*, ed. Lindsay Granshaw and Roy Porter (New York: Routledge, 1989), 192.

16 Elizabeth M.R. Lomax, *Small and Special: The Development of Hospitals for Children in Victorian Britain* (London: Wellcome Institute for the History of Medicine, 1996), 12; Samuel Whitford, secretary of The Hospital for Sick Children, 49, Great Ormond Street, to the Ladies Committee, 12 January 1875, repr. in AR 1880, 26; Clement A. Smith, *The Children's Hospital of Boston: "Built Better Than They Knew"* (Boston: Little, Brown and Company, 1983), 96, 99–100.

17 Records indicate that a Mrs. R. of Barrie accommodated children in her home for short stays between 1877 and 1880, when she returned to England. AR 1878, 16; AR 1880, 13, 18–9; AR 1882, 14–15.

18 AR 1882, 13.

19 It is notable that, in the early descriptions of the Island Home, it was often referred to as "Mrs. McMaster's Island Home." See "A Benevolent Enterprise – Mrs. S. F. Macmaster's Island Home for Sick Children," *Toronto World*, 20 February 1883, 2; Mrs. S.F. McMaster, "The Hospital for Sick Children," circular reprinted in *Weekly Sentinel Review* (Woodstock, ON), 10 July 1885, 2; *The Story of the Lakeside Home for Little Children with Sixty Engravings* (Toronto: 1893), 21; *The Lakeside Home for Little Children: The Convalescent Branch of The Hospital for Sick Children on the Island, Opposite Toronto* (Toronto: 1886), 4–5.

20 Josephine Kane, *The History of the Hospital for Sick Children College Street, Toronto, Ont, Canada and The Lakeside Home for Little Children, Revised to 1918* (Toronto, 1918), 21, 26, 59.

21 "The Lakeside Home is all that the wealthy could want," Appeal Booklet (1923) 16,
    972.46.24b, HSC Archives; *Story of the Lakeside Home*, 19, 34, 60.

22 *The Hospital for Sick Children, College Street, Toronto; The Lakeside Home for Little Children, The*
    Convalescent Branch of the Hospital on Gibraltar Point, Toronto Island: History of These Institutions,
    Toronto, Canada (Toronto: 1891), 37.

23 John Ross Robertson to the Ladies Committee secretary, 3 July 1883, reprinted in AR 1883, 31;
    This was included as a condition of the Agreement Re: Island Property between John Ross
    Robertson and The Hospital for Sick Children, Administered by Kerr, Macdonald Davidson
    and Paterson (6 July 1891), 2–3. Lakeside Home Subject File, HSC Archives.

24 Ladies Committee minutes 6 February 1885, 29. It is difficult to determine whether or not
    this was strictly enforced.

25 A 1906 advertisement referred to Hanlan's point as "Canada's Coney Island." Mike Filey,
    Trillium and Toronto Island: The Centennial Celebration (Toronto: Dundurn Press, 2010), 46.

26 The turn of phrase is from AR 1911, back cover.

27 AR 1886, 16; *The Lakeside Home for Little Children* (1886), 9; Appeal Booklet (1904), 0972-046
    series, HSC Archives; Appeal Booklet (1914), 0972-046 series, HSC Archives.

28 *Story of the Lakeside Home*, 42.

29 AR 1927, 20.

30 Appeal Booklet (1915) 6, 972.46.16e HSC Archives; AR 1910, 4: "'Going to The Lakeside' is the
    subject of talk from the beginning of April – The youngsters all look forward to it."

31 *Story of the Lakeside Home*, 35.

32 W.E. Gallie Surgical Report in AR 1922, 29; AR 1887, 16; *Story of the Lakeside Home*, 33; AR 1921, 29.

33 Appeal Booklet (1909), 17. 972.46.10a, HSC Archives. In 1925, the superintendent enthused
    that "the bright sunshine and cool lake breezes transformed, in many cases, these children
    into brown-skinned sturdy youngsters" (AR 1925, 20).

34 AR 1883, 12, 14.

35 Braithwaite, *Sick Kids*, 31.

36 Kane, *History of the Hospital for Sick Children*, 21.

37 Ibid., 46.

38 *Story of the Lakeside Home*, 70.

39 "Island Home Caretaker Retires after 46 Years," *Evening Telegram*, 3 April 1946, Lakeside
    Home File Folder, HSC Archives.

40 Ladies Committee minutes, 10 July 1885.

41 Appeal Booklet (1906), 14. 792.46.7d, HSC Archives.

42 Appeal Booklet (1907), 12. 972.46.8b, HSC Archives.

43 Appeal Booklet (1904), 36. 972.46.5b, HSC Archives.

44 Appeal Booklet (1906), 14. 792.46.7b, HSC Archives.

45 Sea Breeze "competed for tourists with Coney Island's nearby amusement venue, Luna
    Park." Meghan Crnic and Cynthia Connolly, "'They Can't Help Getting Well Here': Seaside
    Hospitals for Children in the United States: 1872–1917," *The Journal of the History of Childhood*
    and Youth 2, no. 2 (2009): 222. In 1893, 100 attendees of the thirteenth annual meeting of the
    Ontario Medical Association to the Lakeside Home were escorted to the island by John Ross
    Robertson and given a tour of the Lakeside Home. "Doctors at the Island," *Daily Globe*, 23
    June 1893, 8; *Story of the Lakeside Home*, 71.

46 Ladies Committee minutes (business meeting), 15 June 1894. See also AR 1886, 14.

47 Kane, *History of the Hospital for Sick Children*, 24–5, 59; *The Hospital for Sick Children, Toronto*
    Description and Opening of the New Residence for Nurses of the Institution Erected by Mr. J. Ross
    Robertson, and Presented to the Trustees 5th Feb., 1907 (Toronto, n.d.), 27; *The Hospital for Sick*
    Children, College Street, Toronto, 48; "Lakeside Home Burned in Early Morning Fire," *The*
    Globe, 22 April 1915, 1; "Lakeside Home Loss Placed at $100,000," *The Globe*, 23 April 1915, 7;
    "Lakeside Home, Luckily Empty, is Burned Down," *Toronto Daily Star*, 22 April 1915, 3. The

home remained closed during the First World War and then reopened for another decade, until its function was transferred permanently to Thistletown in 1928.

48 Andrea Tanner, "Too Many Mothers? Female Roles in a Metropolitan Victorian Children's Hospital," in *The Impact of Hospitals 300–2000*, ed. John Henderson, Peregrine Horden, and Alessandro Pastore (Oxford: Peter Lang, 2007), 142–50.

49 D.G. Hamilton, *Hand in Hand: The Story of the Royal Alexandra Hospital for Children, Sydney* (Sydney: John Ferguson, 1979), 20.

50 Reportedly, "the walls began to crumble to pieces." Kane, *History of the Hospital for Sick Children*, 24–5.

51 Ladies' Committee minutes (special meeting), 27 September 1886, AR 1886, 10.

52 Hilda Rolstin, *History of the School of Nursing, the Hospital for Sick Children* (Toronto, 1972), quotation 4, 3.

53 Rolstin, *History of the School of Nursing*, 5–6 (image of certificate).

54 Alumnae Association of the School of Nursing, *100 Years: A Celebration of the Alumnae Association of the School of Nursing The Hospital for Sick Children 1903–2003* (Toronto, 2003), 65. The first medal was awarded in 1891. *Nursing School Register of Candidates Accepted and Graduated from the School 1886–1906* (HSC Archives).

55 AR 1888, 11; Rolstin, *History of the School of Nursing*, 6.

56 AR 1889, 18.

57 Ibid.

58 This passage described McMaster's decision to train as a nurse. AR 1889, 16.

59 Minutes of the board of trustees, 5 December 1891, 26–7.

60 Ibid., 29–31.

61 Ibid., 31.

62 Ibid., 33.

63 Emphasis in original. Ladies Committee minutes (devotional meeting), 11 December 1891; AR 1891–2, 11–12.

64 Lease agreement between the Corporation of the City of Toronto and The Hospital for Sick Children, 7 August 1891, Kerr Macdonald Davidson and Patterson, HSC Archives (Lakeside Home File Folder).

65 Minutes of the board of trustees, 22 April 1892, 40.

66 Rolstin, *History of the School of Nursing*, 13–14.

67 Minutes of the board of trustees, 27 June 1893, 97.

68 A few applicants came from Detroit, Tacoma, and Montreal. Applicants were primarily Presbyterian, Methodist, Anglican, or Baptist, with a few Plymouth Brethren, Quaker, Church of Christ, and Congregational. *Nursing School Register of Candidates Accepted and Graduated from the School 1886–1906* (HSC Archives).

69 AR 1896, 26. Two nurses had no occupation listed.

70 Minutes of the board of trustees, 30 October 1896, 210–11, quotation 210.

71 "An Act to regulate public aid to Charitable Institutions" (The Charity Aid Act), *Statutes of the Province of Ontario, 1874*, 37 Vict., ch. 33.

72 Charity Aid Act, 1874, c. 3, my emphasis.

73 R.B. Splane, *Social Welfare in Ontario 1791–1893: A Study of Public Welfare Administration* (Toronto: University of Toronto, 1965), 60.

74 J.W. Langmuir, *Thirteenth Annual Report of the Inspector of Asylums, Prisons and Public Charities for the Province of Ontario for the Year ending 30th September, 1880* (Toronto, 1881), 12; Charity Aid Act, 1874, c. 4.

75 Charity Aid Act, 1874, c. 12. A second inspector was added in 1881. Langmuir retired in 1882 and went on to found Homewood Asylum. Peter Oliver, "John Woodburn Langmuir," *Dictionary of Canadian Biography*, vol. 14, http://www.biographi.ca/009004-119.01-e.php?&id_nbr=7511&terms=grant.

76 Ibid., c. 13.

77 Ibid., c. 10–11.

78 Ibid., c. 14.

79 J.W. Langmuir, *Twelfth Annual Report of the Inspector of Asylums, Prisons and Public Charities for the Province of Ontario for the Year ending 30th September, 1879. Sessional Papers* No. 8 (Toronto, 1880), 219–20.

80 By 1881, the Toronto General Hospital had moved all older, chronic cases to other institutions. Cheryl DesRoches, "Everyone in Their Place: The Formation of Institutional Care for the Elderly in Nineteenth-Century Ontario," *Journal of the Canadian Historical Association* 15, no. 1 (2004): 67–8.

81 Inspector of Hospitals and Charities R.W. Bruce Smith to John Ross Robertson, 23 June 1909, *Record of Inspector's Visits to Hospital for Sick Children* (972.50.14), Box 133, HSC Archives; Copy of an Order in Council approved by His Honour the Lieutenant Governor, the 31st day of March A.D. 1896, *Record of Inspector's Visits to Hospital for Sick Children* (972.50.14), Box 133, HSC Archives.

82 T.F. Chamberlain, *Twenty-ninth Annual Report of the Inspector of Prisons and Public Charities of the Province of Ontario for the Year Ending 30 September 1898. Sessional Papers* No. 14 (Toronto, 1899), 10.

83 AR 1881, 25.

84 Langmuir suggested that HSC be reclassified as Schedule B "without solicitation on the part of the Hospital." J.W. Langmuir, *Fourteenth Annual Report of the Inspector of Prisons and Public Charities. Sessional Papers* No. 8 (Toronto, 1882), 301–2.

85 AR 1881, "Extracts from the Secretary's Diary," 8 March 1881, Inspector Langmuir to Hospital Secretary, 17–18. 4 February 1881, *Journals of the Legislative Assembly of the Province of Ontario from Jan. 13th, 1881, to March 4th, 1881 (Both Days Inclusive)*, vol. 14, 55.

86 Charity Aid Act, 1874, c. 3. The grant was increased in July 1883. AR 1883, 14.

87 AR 1878, 3.

88 AR 1881, 23, 25, 30.

89 AR 1884, 10; AR 1885, 11

90 AR 1893, 11.

91 AR 1880, 10.

92 AR 1893, 4.

93 Minutes, meeting of the trustees of the Hospital for Sick Children held on 25 November 1892 in the board room of the hospital, 71.

94 AR 1894, 16.

95 AR 1896, 32.

96 AR 1888, 6; AR 1900, 9

97 For example, AR 1900, 9.

98 AR 1894, 16.

99 *Masonic Voice Review* 76, no. 1 (1891): 63; Morgan, *Canadian Men and Women of the Time*, 952–3; "Press Club House Warming," *Grip* 30, no. 5 (1888): 4; Gene Allen, "News across the Border: Associated Press in Canada, 1894–1917," *Journalism History* 31, no. 4 (2006): 207. Allen claims that the CPA was "dominated by Robertson of the *Telegram*, and was seen as his personal vehicle rather than a genuine news-sharing organization." Posthumously, John Ross Robertson Public School, the John Ross Robertson School Athletic Association, and John Ross Robertson Lodge were all named in his honour. Jesse Edgar Middleton, *The Municipality of Toronto: A History*, vol. 3 (Toronto: The Dominion Publishing Company, 1923), 97, 104, 178, 374.

100 Sotiron, "Robertson, John Ross." See John Ross Robertson, *Robertson's Landmarks of Toronto*, 6 vols. (Toronto: J.R. Robertson, 1894–1914) and John Ross Robertson, *History of Freemasonry in Canada*, 2 vols., 2nd ed. (Toronto: George N. Morang and Co., 1900); John Ross Robertson, ed., *The Diary of Mrs. John Graves Simcoe* (Toronto: William Briggs, 1911); Mary F Williamson, "The Art Museum and the Public Library under a Single Roof: A Nineteenth-Century Ideal Pursued at the Toronto Public Library from 1883 to World War I," *Ontario History* 98, no. 2 (2006): 150, 156; "John Ross Robertson," *The Canada Lancet* 51, no. 11 (1918): 492–3.

101 Poulton, *The Paper Tyrant*, 177.

102 Bridle, *Sons of Canada*, 27.

103 Poulton, *The Paper Tyrant*, 68.

4 CLUB FEET AND CROOKED LIMBS

1 Appeal Booklet (1902), 10. 972.46.3a, HSC Archives.

2 Patient names in this chapter have been changed pursuant to research access.

3 *Hospital for Sick Children Clinical Records*, vol. 2, 1890–1, 178–9; Census of Canada, 1891, District No. 119, Toronto West.

4 The application of several pounds of weight to extend the angle of the limb while it was immobilized by a splint or sandbags.

5 *Hospital for Sick Children Clinical Records*, vol. 2 (1890–1), 178–9.

6 John Ross Robertson, "Round the World Hospitals" Album, HSC Archives.

7 For a detailed discussion of the impact of Scottish medical graduates throughout the British world, see M. Anne Crowther and Marguerite W. Dupree, *Medical Lives in the Age of Surgical Revolution* (Cambridge: Cambridge University Press, 2007).

8 The hospital at Garnethill was a mansion, converted by Architect James Sellars & Partner Campbell Douglas into a hospital and opened in 1882. Later a purpose-built hospital was opened at Yorkhill. Quotation from *The Hospital for Sick Children, College Street, Toronto; The Lakeside Home for Little Children, The Convalescent Branch of the Hospital on Gibraltar Point, Toronto Island: History of These Institutions, Toronto, Canada* (Toronto: 1891), 40–1; Edna Robertson, *The Yorkhill Story: The History of the Royal Hospital for Sick Children, Glasgow* (Glasgow: Yorkhill and Associated Hospitals Board of Management, 1972), 53. See also A. Lindsay Miller, "Memoir of Mr. James Sellars, Architect," *Proceedings of the Royal Philosophical Society of Glasgow,* 20 (Glasgow: John Smith and Son, 1888–9): 42–3.

9 Geoffrey N. Hunt, "The Hospital For Sick Children, College Street, Toronto, The Building and its Context" (12 April 1976), 5. Hospital 5th Subject File 1, HSC Archives.

10 AR 1889, 10. The building is still listed as 67 College Street.

11 Samuel Blake at the turning of the sod in September 1889, quoted in *The Hospital for Sick Children* (1891), 48.

12 AR 1891–2, 13. The new name was never adopted legally (purportedly for fear that it would interfere with bequests).

13 Marta O'Brien, "Toronto's Third City Hall," 9 June 2008, Heritage Toronto Blog (posted 6 January 2013), http://heritagetoronto.org/torontos-third-city-hall/. As was Lady Meredith House (a.k.a. "Ardvana," c. 1897) in Montreal, at the corner of Avenues Pine and Peel, which would be converted later into a nurses' residence for Royal Victoria Hospital. See "The Ontario Medical College for Women," Heritage Toronto Blog, posted 25 March 2013. http://heritagetoronto.org/the-ontario-medical-college-for-women/

14 *The Hospital for Sick Children* (1891), 58.

15 Annmarie Adams and David Theodore, "Designing for 'the Little Convalescents': Children's Hospitals in Toronto and Montreal, 1875–2006," *Canadian Bulletin for Medical History* 19 (2002): 206–7.

16 Schiff, "The Sweetest of All Charities," 118.

17 Adams and Theodore, "Designing for 'the Little Convalescents,'" 206.

18 *The Hospital for Sick Children* (1891), 57–8.

19 The hospital plans include the terms "air flow" and have arrows running down the hallways.

20 The hospital contains a remarkable collection of photographs dating from the early years of the hospital, many of which have been beautifully enlarged in what is now the University Avenue entrance of the Hospital (which was, in 1951, the entrance to the "new" hospital). For a selection of the most famous images of the hospital, its patients and staff, juxtaposed with

more contemporary photographs, see The Hospital for Sick Children, *A History of Healing: the Hospital for Sick Children* (Toronto: Hospital for Sick Children, 2010).

21 *The Hospital for Sick Children* (1891), 70.

22 Historical sources suggest a range of inpatient capacities. The original plans were drawn up for 100 patients, and that was revised to include "up to 160" though 140 was most often cited. AR 1889, 11. Other reports suggest a capacity of "nearly" 200 patients including the isolation and suspect wards, although only up to 150 were admitted. AR 1896, 7; AR 1901, 9.

23 Quotation in AR 1905, 52.

24 Minutes of the Board of Trustees, 16 March 1903. See also AR 1890, 21 and AR 1895, 35.The 1912 renovations relocated the laundry above the power building, separate from the main Hospital. In Kane, *History of the Hospital for Sick Children*, 62.

25 See AR 1890, 20–1; Kane, *History of the Hospital for Sick Children*, 31–3.

26 Trustee Minutes, 28 April 1893, 92.

27 Kane, *History of the Hospital for Sick Children*, quotation 45, 43.

28 AR 1896, 31.

29 AR 1905, 46.

30 In AR 1903, 46.

31 Our Correspondent, "Canada," *The Lancet* 140, no. 3592 (1890): 60.

32 *The Hospital for Sick Children* (1891), 64.

33 Martin S. Pernick, *A Calculus of Suffering: Pain, Professionalism, and Anesthesia in Nineteenth-Century America* (New York: Columbia University Press, 1985), 172–3.

34 A.R. Colón with P.A. Colón, *Nurturing Children: A History of Pediatrics* (London: Greenwood Press, 1999); Kosky and Lunnon, *Great Ormond Street*, 42–3.

35 See Thomas Schlich, "The Emergence of Modern Surgery," in Deborah Brunton, ed., *Medicine Transformed: Health, Disease and Society in Europe, 1800–1939* (Manchester: Manchester University Press, 2004), 61–91.

36 For Groves, see Emily Claydon and Vivian C McAlister, "The Life of John Wishart (1850–1926): Study of an Academic Surgical Career Prior to the Flexner Report," *World Journal of Surgery* 36, no. 3 (2012): 684. See also Michael Worboys, *Spreading Germs: Disease Theories and Medical Practice in Britain, 1865–1900* (London: Cambridge University Press, 2000).

37 Connor, *Doing Good*, 129; J.T.H. Connor, "Listerism Unmasked: Antisepsis and Asepsis in Victorian Anglo-Canada," *Journal of the History of Medicine and Allied Sciences*, 49 (1994): 214.

38 Ladies Committee minutes, 13 July 1877; Ladies Committee minutes, 3 October 1877; Ladies Committee minutes, 1 February 1878.

39 Thomas Schlich, "Negotiating Technologies in Surgery: the Controversy about Surgical Gloves in the 1890s," *Bulletin of the History of Medicine* 87 (2013): 170–97.

40 Health records indicate that nurses routinely dressed surgical incisions with antiseptics – boracic dressing/lint, boracic lotion injected/used for washing; sprinkling of Iodoform for disinfectant purposes; use of Iodoform gauze; as well as gauze soaked in perchloride; salicylic wool; bichloride gauze, perchloride of zinc. *Hospital for Sick Children Clinical Records*, vol. 2 (1890–1), HSC Archives.

41 John G. Raffensperger, with contributing specialists, *Children's Surgery: A Worldwide History* (London: McFarland & Company Inc., 2012), 99–101; Colón with Colón, *Nurturing Children*, 205.

42 Bladder stones were common as a result of poor diets. Kosky and Lunnon, *Great Ormond Street*, quotation, 15–16.

43 As quoted in Roger Cooter, *Surgery and Society in Peace and War: Orthopaedics and the Organization of Modern Medicine, 1880–1948* (London: The Macmillan Press Ltd., 1993), 11–12, 254n6.

44 Quotation in Ulrich Tröhler, "Surgery (Modern)," in the *Companion Encyclopedia of the History of Medicine*, edited by W.F. Bynum and Roy Porter, vol. 2 (New York: Routledge, 1993), 1012; Raffensperger, *Children's Surgery*, 104, 107; Cooter, *Surgery and Society*, 18, 19, 41; Leonard F. Peltier,

Orthopedics: A History and Iconography (San Francisco, CA: Norman Publishing, 1993), 177–83; John Dove, "Evolution of Spinal Surgery," in *The Evolution of Orthopaedic Surgery*, ed. Leslie Klenerman (London: Royal Society of Medicine Press Limited, 2002), 160.

45 De Forest Willard, *The Surgery of Childhood: Including Orthopedic Surgery* (Philadelphia: Lippincott, 1910); Raffensperger, *Children's Surgery*, 113

46 Edward Shorter, *Partnership for Excellence: Medicine at the University of Toronto and Academic Hospitals* (Toronto: University of Toronto, 2013), 36, 40–3, 151–2; AR 1893, 20–4; AR 1894, 25; AR 1897, 6.

47 There were only two children who did not conform to the general hospital rule of prohibiting admission of those under the age of two.

48 *Hospital for Sick Children Clinical Records Surgical* (1891–2), patient #182, 483–8. HSC Archives.

49 Census of Canada 1891, District No. 130 York East.

50 *Hospital for Sick Children Clinical Records*, vol. 2 (1890–1), patient #42, 361–8. HSC Archives.

51 *Hospital for Sick Children Clinical Records*, vol. 2 (1890–1), patient #3, 34–41.

52 "What the Surgeon Has Done," Appeal Booklet (1906), 12. 792.46.7b, HSC Archives.

53 The text was interspersed with before and after photographs of patients. 1905 HSC Appeal Pamphlet, 9. 972.46.6d, HSC Archives.

54 Trustee Minutes, 4 July 1894, 132–7.

55 Trustee Minutes, 4 July 1894, 132–8; AR 1889.

56 Alan Brown, "Toronto as a Paediatric Centre," *The Canadian Medical Monthly* 5, no. 6 (1920): 207.

57 Trohler, "Surgery (Modern)," 996.

58 For an overview of nurse training schools and the origins of professional nursing in Canada, see Kathryn McPherson, *Bedside Matters: The Transformation of Canadian Nursing, 1900–1990* (Toronto: University of Toronto Press, 2003), 18, 27–9.

59 "A New Profession for Women" *The Canadian Independent* 2, no. 3 (1883): 92

60 *The Canadian Practitioner* 11, no. 4 (1886): 124; "Montreal General Hospital Training School for Nurses" *Canada Medical and Surgical Journal* 9, no. 6 (1881): 381.

61 AR 1893, 10.

62 AR 1894, 37–8.

63 Alumnae Association of the School of Nursing, *100 Years: A Celebration of the Alumnae Association of the School of Nursing The Hospital for Sick Children 1903–2003* (Toronto, 2003), 37; "Louise C. Brent" (later Goodson), typed biography (1941 or 1942), HSC Archives; Rolstin, *History of the School of Nursing*, 15.

64 In 1900, massage therapy was added to the curriculum. AR, 1900, 47–8.

65 AR 1900, 47–8.

66 Ibid.

67 AR 1907, 10.

68 AR 1902, 15; AR 1907, 10; AR 1913, 3.

69 Leslie Klenerman, "Setting the Scene: The Start of Orthopaedic Surgery," in *The Evolution of Orthopaedic Surgery*, ed. Leslie Klenerman (London: Royal Society of Medicine Press Limited, 2002), 1–12.

70 Rolstin, *History of the School of Nursing*, 16.

71 Tröhler, "Surgery (Modern)," 1012.

72 Smith, *The Children's Hospital of Boston*, 67.

73 Cooter, *Surgery and Society*, 20.

74 *Hospital for Sick Children, Toronto, Description and Opening of the New Residence for Nurses of the Institution, Erected by Mr. J. Ross Robertson, and Presented to the Trustees 5th Feb., 1907* (Toronto, 1907), 21, 23, 25.

75 *Hospital for Sick Children, Toronto, Description and Opening of the New Residence for Nurses of the Institution, Erected by Mr. J. Ross Robertson, and Presented to the Trustees 5th Feb., 1907* (Toronto, 1907), 5–7, 29, 34.

76   McPherson, *Bedside Matters*, 29–32, quotation on 37.
77   Quotation Lomax, *Small and Special*, 6; Tanner, "Too Many Mothers?" 149.
78   "The Nurse – the gentle hand of that daughter of Eve that shows heroic womanhood as she watches the little ones in her charge"; "A good nurse is a Queen among women"; "The Faithful Workers" Appeal Booklet (1903), 4–5, 972.46.4, HSC Archives.
79   AR 1894, 39.
80   *Hospital for Sick Children Clinical Records*, vol. 2 (1890–1), patient #1, 1–10.
81   Cooter, *Surgery and Society*, 40–3, 265n51; John A. Fixsen, "Children's Orthopaedic Surgery," in *The Evolution of Orthopaedic Surgery*, ed. Leslie Klenerman (London: Royal Society of Medicine Press Limited, 2002), 150.
82   Cooter, *Surgery and Society*, 56.
83   Tröhler, "Surgery (Modern)," 996–7.
84   A petition from 400 U of T students. Trustees Minutes 16 March 1903, 68–70.
85   Josephine Kane, *History of the Hospital for Sick Children*, 62.
86   Appeal Booklet (1907), 20. 972.46.8c, HSC Archives.

5   MILK SEWAGE

1   Dr. Charles Hastings quoted in AR 1912, 15.
2   "A Day at the Out-Patients Department of the Hospital for Sick Children," *Evening Telegram*, 19 December 1914. Scrapbook 1908–14, 168. HSC Archives.
3   Hon. S.H. Blake, QC, quoted in *The Hospital for Sick Children, College Street, Toronto; the Lakeside Home for Little Children, the Convalescent Branch of the Hospital on Gibraltar Point, Toronto Island, History of These Institutions* (Toronto, 1891), 46. John D. Blackwell, "Blake, Samuel Hume," *Dictionary of Canadian Biography*, vol. 14 (1911–20) University of Toronto/Université Laval, 2003–, accessed 25 November 2015, www.biographi.ca/en/bio/blake_samuel_hume_14E.html.
4   Stephen A. Speisman, "St. John's Shtetl: The Ward in 1911," in *Gathering Place: People and Neighbourhoods of Toronto, 1834–1945*, ed. Robert F. Harney (Toronto: Multicultural History Society of Ontario, 1985), 107.
5   Christina Burr, *Spreading the Light: Work and Labour Reform in Late-Nineteenth-Century Toronto* (Toronto: University of Toronto Press, 1999), 158.
6   Lesley Marrus Barsky, *From Generation to Generation: A History of Toronto's Mount Sinai Hospital* (Toronto: McClelland and Stewart, 1998), 4.
7   Bureau of Municipal Research, "What is 'The Ward' Going to Do with Toronto?: A Report on Undesirable Living Conditions in One Section of the City of Toronto – 'The Ward' – Conditions Which Are Spreading Rapidly to Other Districts" (Toronto, 1918), 37.
8   Dr. Charles Hastings, *Report of the Medical Health Officer Dealing With the Recent Investigation of Slum Conditions in Toronto, Embodying Recommendations for the Amelioration of the Same* (Department of Public Health, Toronto, 1911), 7.
9   Speisman, "St. John's Shtetl," 108. See Stephen A. Speisman, *The Jews of Toronto: A History to 1937* (Toronto: McClelland and Stewart, 2005), 81–3, 119.
10   Speisman, "St. John's Shtetl," 109; Speisman, *The Jews of Toronto*, 120, passim 119–23. Speisman also remarks that it was well known at the time that Robertson's mentor, Goldwin Smith (who provided the start-up monies for *The Telegram*), espoused anti-Semitic opinions, 119.
11   J.R. Sandomirsky, "Toronto's Public Health Photography," *Archivaria* 10 (Summer 1980): 145–55.
12   In total, there were 11,645 people living on 142 acres, a population density of 82 persons per acre. Hastings, *Report of the Medical Officer of Health*, 6, 12, 22.
13   Bureau of Municipal Research, "What is 'The Ward' Going to do with Toronto?" 37.
14   AR 1905, 33; AR 1915, 6.
15   Of 5,277 inpatients in 1921, 1,300 were Jewish in 1921. The appeal asked, "Do you realize what would happen to our Jewish kiddies if the Hospital for Sick Children did not exist, or if it

were not absolutely non-sectarian? As Jewish citizens of Toronto we appeal to you on behalf of our Jewish children to show your appreciation by sending your contribution ..." "Do You Care?", *Canadian Jewish Review*, 16 December 1921, 10.

16 "The Outdoor" Songbook, Alumnae Association, HSC, 2nd Annual Dinner, 1928 (Nursing School Alumnae Association, File 1: Associations and Members), HSC Archives.

17 R.R. Gagan, "Mortality Patterns and Public Health in Hamilton, Canada, 1900–14," *Urban History Review* 17, no. 3 (1989): 164, 171; Risa Barkin and Ian Gentles, "Death in Victorian Toronto, 1850–1899," *Urban History Review* 19, no. 1 (1990): 20–1.

18 Michael J. Piva, *The Condition of the Working Class in Toronto – 1900–1921* (Ottawa: University of Ottawa Press, 1979), 123: "At the same time American cities managed to reduce their infant mortality rate – Rochester's rate in 1908 was only 86."

19 Quotation D. Ann Herring, "Introduction: Surviving the Early Years," in *Surviving the Early Years: Childhood Diseases in Hamilton at the Beginning of the Twentieth Century*, ed. D. Ann Herring (Hamilton, ON: McMaster University Faculty of Social Sciences, 2008), 2; R.R. Gagan, "Mortality Patterns and Public Health in Hamilton, Canada, 1900–14," *Urban History Review* 17, no. 3 (1989): 167–8.

20 Michael E. Mercier and Christopher G. Boone, "Infant Mortality in Ottawa, Canada, 1901: Assessing Cultural, Economic and Environmental Factors," *Journal of Historical Geography* 28, no. 4 (2002): 493–5; Rose A. Monachino, "Hot Town, Summer in the City: Childhood and Infant Diarrheal Death in Hamilton, 1901 to 1911," in *Surviving the Early Years: Childhood Diseases in Hamilton at the Beginning of the Twentieth Century*, ed. D. Ann Herring (Hamilton, ON: McMaster University Faculty of Social Sciences, 2008), 75–7.

21 R.A. Meckel, *Save the Babies: American Public Health Reform and the Prevention of Infant Mortality, 1850–1929* (Baltimore, MD: Johns Hopkins University Press, 1990), 42.

22 P. Thornton and S. Olson, "A Deadly Discrimination among Montreal Infants, 1860–1900," *Continuity and Change* 16, no. 1 (2001): 104–6.

23 Helen MacMurchy, *Infant Mortality: Second Special Report* (Toronto: L.K. Cameron, 1911), 42.

24 For comparative American research, see Gretchen A. Condran and Harold A. Lentzner, "Early Death: Mortality among Young Children in New York, Chicago and New Orleans," *Journal of Interdisciplinary History* 34, no. 3 (2004): 322–7. See also Rose A. Cheney, "Seasonal Aspects of Infant and Childhood Mortality: Philadelphia, 1865–1920," *The Journal of Interdisciplinary History* 14, no. 3 (1984): 561–84.

25 M. McInnis, "Canada's Population in the Twentieth Century," in Michael R. Haines and Richard H. Steckel, eds., *A Population History of North America* (Cambridge: Cambridge University Press, 2000), 568.

26 M. McInnis, "Infant Mortality in Late Nineteenth-Century Canada," in *Infant and Child Mortality in the Past*, ed. A. Bideau, B. Desjardins, and H. Perez Brignoli (Oxford: Clarendon Press, 1997), 266, 270; Michael E. Mercier, "The Social Geography of Childhood Mortality, Toronto, 1901: Patterns and Determinants," *Urban Geography* 27, no. 2 (2006): 145–6.

27 Cynthia Comacchio, *Nations Are Built of Babies: Saving Ontario's Mothers and Children, 1900–1940* (Montreal: McGill-Queen's University Press, 1993), 122.

28 MacDougall, *Activists and Advocates*, 97. For a parallel situation in Montreal, see Denyse Baillargeon, *Babies for the Nation: the Medicalization of Motherhood in Quebec 1910–1970*, trans. W Donald Wilson (Waterloo: Wilfrid Laurier University Press, 2009), 31 & passim.

29 John P. Court, "Introducing Darwinism to Toronto's Post-1887 Reconstituted Medical School," *CBMH* 28, no. 1 (2011): 199–200, 191–212.

30 Hoyes Lloyd, "How Toronto Controls Her Milk Supply," *The Public Health Journal* 5, no. 7 (July 1914).

31 E. Herbert Adams, MD, "The Prevention of Tuberculosis in Ontario," *Canadian Practitioner* 18, no. 9 (1893): 65.

32 "Pure Milk in Toronto and How to Obtain It," *Toronto Evening Telegram,* 15 October and 5 November, 1908, 27. Miscellaneous Pamphlets, HSC Archives.

33 "The Bitter Cry of Helpless Childhood Against the Cruel Ignorance and Murderous Greed of Those that Destroy It with Filthy Milk," *The Home Journal* 5, no. 6 (1908): 6–7; MacDougall, *Activists and Advocates*; Paul Adolphus Bator, "Saving Lives on the Wholesale Plan: Public Health Reform in the City of Toronto, 1900 to 1930," (PhD diss., University of Toronto, 1979), 140–4; Manfred J. Waserman, "Henry L Coit and the Certified Milk Movement in the Development of Modern Pediatrics," *Bulletin of the History of Medicine* 46, no. 4 (1972): 376.

34 This movement peaked in the first decade of the century, and was overtaken by the movement for pasteurized milk. Waserman, "Henry L Coit and the Certified Milk Movement," 362–71; Apple, *Mothers and Medicine,* 60.

35 See, inter alia, "For Pure Milk: The City Dairy Company Takes Important Action," *Toronto Star,* 12 January 1901, 2; Advertisement, *Toronto Star,* 30 October 1900, 7; "Pure Milk in Toronto and how to Obtain It," *Toronto Evening Telegram,* 15 October and 5 November, 1908, 27. Miscellaneous Pamphlets, HSC Archives. Certified milk cost 15 cents a quart in Toronto in 1909. "Diverse Opinions on Milk Question," *Mail and Empire,* 3 June 1909, Pasteurization Department Scrapbook, HSC Archives.

36 *Report of the Milk Commission, Appointed to Enquire into the Production, Care and Distribution of Milk 1909* (Toronto: L.K. Cameron, 1910), 129–30. See also "Sterilized Milk for the City's Sick Children," *The Evening Telegram,* 10 January 1908.

37 Waserman, "Henry L Coit and the Certified Milk Movement," 373.

38 Cathy Leigh James, "Gender, Class and Ethnicity in the Organization of Neighbourhood and Nation: The Role of Toronto's Settlement Houses in The Formation of the Canadian State, 1902 to 1914" (PhD diss, University of Toronto, 1997), 260.

39 Mrs. F.N.G. Starr, presumably the wife of the HSC surgeon, was a treasurer of the CHEA Milk Depot Committee. "Women's Meetings," *Toronto Star,* 10 March 1911, 10; "Funds Needed to Provide Clean Milk to Infants," *Toronto Star,* 28 Feb 1910, 1; "Pure Milk Fund," *Toronto Star,* 8 April 1910, 1.

40 "The C.H.E.A. Endorses Inspector McConvey," *Toronto Star,* 25 January 1911, 9.

41 Bator, "Saving Lives on the Wholesale Plan," 144; *Report of the Milk Commission, Appointed to Enquire into the production, Care and Distribution of Milk 1909* (Toronto: L.K. Cameron, 1910), 5, 18–20.

42 *Report of the Milk Commission,* 15.

43 *Report of the Milk Commission,* 19–20; "Pure Milk in Toronto and how to Obtain It," *Toronto Evening Telegram,* 15 October and 5 November 1908, 27–30. Miscellaneous Pamphlets, HSC Archives.

44 MacDougall, *Activists and Advocates,* 100–2; Editorial, "Resignation of Dr Sheard," *The Canadian Practitioner and Review* 35, no.11 (1910): 742–3; Bator, "Saving Lives on the Wholesale Plan," 149–50; see also editorial, "The New Medical Health Officer of Toronto," *The Canadian Practitioner and Review* 35, no. 11 (1910): 743–4.

45 "Pure Milk in Toronto and How to Obtain It," *Toronto Evening Telegram,* 15 October and 5 November, 1908, 27. Miscellaneous Pamphlets, HSC Archives.

46 "Saving the Children," *Toronto Star,* 10 June 1910, 8. See Dr. Helen MacMurchy, *Infant Mortality: Special Report* (Toronto: L.K. Cameron, 1910); Dr. Helen MacMurchy, *Infant Mortality: Second Special Report* (Toronto: L.K. Cameron, 1911); Dr. Helen MacMurchy, *Infant Mortality: Third Report* (Toronto: L.K. Cameron, 1912).

47 Bator, "Saving Lives on the Wholesale Plan," 154.

48 "Pure Milk in Toronto and how to Obtain It," *Toronto Evening Telegram,* 15 October and 5 November 1908, 27. Miscellaneous Pamphlets, HSC Archives.

49 "Urges Milk Plant – Nathan Straus Here in Interest of his Laboratory," unknown source, Pasteurization Department Scrapbook; Secretary of Nathan Straus Pasteurized

Milk Laboratory to John Ross Robertson, 8–12–1913, Pasteurization Department Scrapbook; Circular to Toronto Physicians, "Modified Milk Mixtures Formulae Prescribed by the Physicians of the Hospital," (Toronto: 1 March 1910), 1. Dairy Subject File; Miss Jean I. Hutt, "Recollections of the 'Dairy' in old H.S.C.," 3, Dairy Subject File; Hospital for Sick Children, "Pure Milk at the Hospital For Sick Children and How We Obtain It," Pasteurization Department Scrapbook. All in HSC Archives.

50 AR 1914, 10, 15.
51 AR 1925, 17.
52 AR 1913, 27; AR 1914, 10, 15; Mary Adelaide Snider, "The Hospital for Sick Children. A Description of its Pasteurization Plant and how Pasteurized Certified Milk is Supplied to Sick Babies of Toronto," Dairy Subject File, HSC Archives.
53 AR 1911, 18; " ... statistics from hospitals prove that the better quality of this food, the lower the death rate" (AR 1913, 1).
54 AR 1911, 18.
55 AR 1925, 17; Editorial, "Hospital for Sick Children," *The Canadian Practitioner and Review* 35, no. 5 (1910): 315; Mary Adelaide Snider, "A Story for the Mothers of Toronto. The Hospital for Sick Children: Its Milk, Pasteurizing Plant a Perfect Equipment," (1915), 10, Miscellaneous Pamphlets, HSC Archives.
56 In "How Babies are Cared for – A Wonderful Milk Plant – Over 2,000 Babies Cared for in 1916 by The Hospital for Sick Children," typed and edited in pencil, Pasteurization Department Scrapbook, HSC Archives, 1–2.
57 AR 1928, 21; Snider, "A Story for the Mothers of Toronto," (1915), 3, Miscellaneous Pamphlets, HSC Archives.
58 AR 1925, 17.
59 Marion Royce, *Eunice Dyke, Health Care Pioneer: From Pioneer Public Health Nurse to Advocate for the Aged* (Toronto: Dundurn Press, 1983), 46.
60 AR 1911, 9.
61 AR 1916, 9.
62 Mary Adelaide Snider, "One Day with the District Nurse," (January 1913) Miscellaneous Pamphlets, HSC Archives, 7; "Pure Milk at the Hospital For Sick Children and How We Obtain It"; "Death Roll of City Babies 145 out of 1000 recorded succumb before year old," *Toronto Star,* 11 July 1913, 1, 10; Hoyes Lloyd, "How Toronto Controls Her Milk Supply," *The Public Health Journal* 5, no. 7 (1914): 449–50.
63 AR 1916, 9.
64 AR 1912, 9.
65 James, "Gender, Class and Ethnicity," 260–2.
66 Neil Sutherland, *Children in English-Canadian Society: Framing the Twentieth-Century Consensus* (Waterloo: Wilfrid Laurier University Press, 2000), 65.
67 Bator, "Saving Lives on the Wholesale Plan," 127–9.
68 Gertrude E.S. Pringle, "A Progressive Profession for Girls," *Maclean's* (15 May 1922): 64, 67. At U of T, Lillian Massey instigated the establishment of a School of Domestic Science and Art (1896). Nutritional Sciences Department, "Department History," http://nutrisci.med.utoronto.ca/history.html; AR 1913, 9.
69 AR 1914, 4.
70 AR 1916, 10.
71 AR 1912, 9; Snider, "A Story for the Mothers of Toronto," (1915), 6, Miscellaneous Pamphlets, HSC Archives.
72 Hutt, "Recollections of the 'Dairy'"; AR 1905, 14; AR 1910, 10.
73 Alan Brown and Dr. George Campbell, "Infant Mortality," *Canadian Medical Association Journal* 4, no. 8 (1914): 696.

74 Brown, quoted by journal editor, preceding Alan Brown "Pasteurization of Milk and Infant Mortality Rates in Toronto, Vancouver, and Victoria," *British Medical Journal* 2 (31 July 1943): 133; AR 1921, 13.

75 N.E. McKinnon, "Mortality Reductions in Ontario, 1900–1942," *Canadian Journal of Public Health* 35, no. 12 (1944): 482–4.

76 John Walter-Smith, "Sir George Newman, Infant Diarrhoeal Mortality and the Paradox of Urbanism," *Medical History* 42, no. 3 (1998): 359; McInnis, "Canada's Population in the Twentieth Century," 569; Mercier, "The Social Geography of Childhood Mortality," passim.

77 AR 1929, 29.

78 Alan Brown and D.E. Robertson apparently appealed to the Liberal caucus about the pasteurization bill. "During the discussion of the Bill in caucus, a member rose from his chair and walked in front of the assembled group. He was a cripple with a hunched back, the result of tuberculosis of the spine." The man identified himself as a victim of "dirty milk," and the bill passed with no dissenting voters. Brink, "How Pasteurization of Milk Came to Ontario," 972–3; AR 1930, 26.

79 Connor, *Doing Good*, 187–8; Richard Dennis, "Private Landlords and Redevelopment: 'The Ward' in Toronto, 1890–1920," *Urban History Review* 24, no. 1 (1995): 21–35.

80 Quoted in Connor, *Doing Good*, 211.

81 "Every Friday," *Canadian Jewish Review* (12 March 1926): 12.

82 "Do You Care?" *Canadian Jewish Review* (16 December 1921): 10.

83 Rabbi Ferdinand M. Isserman, "Anti-Semitism in Hospitals," *Canadian Jewish Review* 8, no. 37 (1927): 1, 10 ; "Jews Back Isserman on Prejudice Charge," *Toronto Daily Star,* 15 July 1927, 24; "Anti-Semitism Seen in City Hospitals by Rabbi Isserman," *The Globe,* 15 July 1927, 13; "Isserman's Charge of Anti-Semitism Denied and Backed," *The Globe,* 16 July 1927, 15; Rabbi Ferdinand M. Isserman, "Discrimination – Conscious or Unconscious" *Canadian Jewish Review* 8, no. 39 (1927): 1, 17.

84 Arlene Chan, *The Chinese in Toronto from 1878: From Outside to Inside the Circle* (Toronto: Dundurn Press, 2011), 35–6, 104–6.

85 Comacchio, *Nations Are Built of Babies,* 120.

6 IRRADIATION

1 Harry J. Ebbs, "Alan Brown," The Alan Brown Memorial Week Lecture (March 1975), 16. Alan Brown Subject File, HSC Archives.

2 Dr. A.L. Chute, interview by Valerie Schatzker (Hannah Institute for the History of Medicine / AMS Medical Services, Inc., 1977), 13–14.

3 He continued, "Breast milk is best because it doesn't have to be warmed, you can take it on picnics, the cat can't get at it and it comes in such cute containers." The Hospital for Sick Children Alumni Association, *Dr. Alan Brown* (Toronto: Hospital for Sick Children in conjunction with University of Toronto Press, 1984), 35–6.

4 See, inter alia, Alan Brown, "The Ability of Mothers to Nurse their Infants," *Canadian Medical Association Journal* 7, no. 3 (1917): 247; Alan Brown, "The Prevention of Neonatal Mortality," *Canadian Medical Association Journal* 29, no. (1933): 267–8; Alan Brown, *The Normal Child: Its Care and Feeding* (Toronto: McClelland and Stewart, 1926), 78.

5 "Must Buy From Association City Dairy President Declares," *Telegram* (10 September 1920), Special Album #1, 83, HSC Archives.

6 Aleck Samuel Ostry, *Nutrition Policy in Canada, 1870–1939* (Vancouver: UBC Press, 2006), 37–8; Alan Brown, "Preventive Paediatrics and Its Relation to the General Practitioner," *Canadian Medical Association Journal* 24 (April 1931): 518–19.

7 Alan Brown, "The Ability of Mothers to Nurse their Infants," *Canadian Medical Association Journal* 7, no. 3 (1917): 244, 247.

8   Quoted without attribution in Brown, *The Normal Child*, 143–4; Aleck Ostry, "The Early Development of Nutrition Policy in Canada," in *Children's Health Issues in Historical Perspective*, ed. Cheryl Krasnick Warsh and Veronica Strong-Boag (Waterloo: Wilfrid Laurier University Press, 2005), 191–2.

9   Letter, Alan Brown to JRR (7-2-1916), Pasteurization Department Scrapbook, HSC Archives.

10 See, for example, AR 1917, 5.

11 AR 1924, 23. See also F.F. Tisdall, T.G.H. Drake, and A. Brown, "The Carbohydrate Metabolism of Infants with Diarrhea, Infections and Acute Intestinal Intoxication." With a note on the use of insulin (read at the third annual meeting of the Canadian Society for the Study of Diseases of Children, June 1925), *American Journal of Diseases of Children* 30, no. 6 (1925): 837–43.

12 AR 1924, 36–7; *First Annual Report of the Infants' Department – The Cubicle System* (1915): 14–15, Baby Ward Subject File, HSC Archives.

13 Alan Brown, "Frederick F. Tisdall," *Canadian Medical Association Journal* 64 (March 1951): 264–5.

14 T.G.H. Drake, "Frederick Fitzgerald Tisdall," *Journal of Nutrition* 56, no. 1 (1955): 6–7; AR 1929, 40–1; AR 1930, 38.

15 Medical Advisory Board (hereafter MAB) members include heads of services (Medical, Surgical, Ophthalmology, Otolaryngology); Trustees Minutes, Executive Meeting, 24 March 1925. For Summerfeldt, see MAB 22 December 1925; Ebbs, "100 Years of Lady Physicians," 10; Trustees Minutes, 10 February 1925; Trustees Minutes, 20 March 1925; Dr. Fayle of Dublin did not keep his appointment. MAB 29 September 1925; MAB 27 June 1927; MAB 24 February 1928.

16 Rima Apple, *Vitamania: Vitamins in American Culture* (New Brunswick, N.J.: Rutgers University Press, 1996).

17 Ian Mosby, "Making and Breaking Canada's Food Rules: Science, the State, and the Government of Nutrition, 1942–1949," 409–32, in *Edible Histories, Cultural Politics: Towards a Canadian Food History*, ed. Franca Iacovetta, Valerie J. Korinek, and Marlene Epp (Toronto: University of Toronto Press, 2012), 413.

18 Ostry, *Nutrition Policy*, 54, 91.

19 Peter Wilton, "Cod-Liver Oil, Vitamin D and the Fight Against Rickets," *Canadian Medical Association Journal* 152, no. 9 (1995): 1516.

20 Kumaravel Rajakumar, "Vitamin D, Cod-Liver Oil, Sunlight, and Rickets: A Historical Perspective" *Pediatrics* 112, no. 2 (2003): e132–e135, quotations e133. See also Daniel Freund, *American Sunshine: Diseases of Darkness and the Quest for Natural Light* (Chicago: The University of Chicago Press, 2012), 38–40.

21 Ostry, *Nutrition Policy*, 54–5.

22 Alan Brown and Frederick F. Tisdall, *Common Procedures in the Practice of Paediatrics*, 3rd ed. (Toronto: McClelland and Stewart, 1939), 62.

23 Trustees Minutes, 12 October 1926 (HSC Archives).

24 Trustees Minutes, 7 June 1927. The trustees recorded a $1,000 donation to the PRF from Pilkington Brothers Ltd, "as a mark of appreciation for the work of the Research Department in connection with the therapeutic properties of glass." Trustees Minutes, 1 December 1931.

25 Brown and Tisdall, *Common Procedures* (1936), 62. See F.F. Tisdall and A. Brown, "An Address on the Seasonal Variation of the Antirachitic Effect of Sunshine and its Effect on Resistance to Disease," *American Journal of Diseases of Children* 17, no. 12 (1927): 1425–9; See also F.F. Tisdall and A. Brown, "Relation of the Altitude of the Sun to Its Antirachitic Effect, *Journal of the American Medical Association* 92, no. 11 (1929): 860.

26 Drake, Tisdall, Brown, "The Incorporation of Vitamins in Bread," *Canadian Medical Association Journal* 24 (February 1931): 210–11.

27 Brown and Tisdall, *Common Procedures* (1939), 62.

28 Trustees Minutes, 26 October 1926 and 8 March 1927.

29 Mark Collar, "The Pablum Connection," *The City*, 17 December 1978, 120. See Professor
    J. Ross Cavers, "The Origins of Pablum," 1988, General file on the invention of Pablum,
    Guelph McLaughlin Archives.

30 F.F. Tisdall, T.G.H. Drake, P. Summerfeldt, and A. Brown, "A New Whole Wheat Irradiated
    Biscuit Containing Vitamins and Mineral Elements," *Canadian Medical Association Journal* 22,
    no. 2 (1930): 170.

31 "Sun-Wheat Biscuits," (Report on Departmental History, circa 1930), 1. Pablum Subject File,
    HSC Archives; Rima D. Apple, "Patenting University Research: Harry Steenbock and the
    Wisconsin Alumni Research Foundation," *Isis* 80 (September 1989): 375–94.

32 "Sun-Wheat Biscuits," (Report on Departmental History, circa 1930), 5. Pablum Subject File,
    HSC Archives.

33 "Sun-Wheat Biscuits," 1. Pablum Subject File, HSC Archives.

34 Drake, Tisdall, and Brown were asked to resign shortly thereafter. "Sun-Wheat Biscuits," 5.
    Pablum Subject File, HSC Archives; Douglas Snedden (Executive Director) to E.H. Shuter
    (Hospital Secretary) Re: Paediatric Research Foundation of Toronto (1 March 1972), with
    two photocopied pages of expense ledger. Pablum Subject file, HSC Archives.

35 "Sun-Wheat Biscuits," 2. Pablum Subject File, HSC Archives. McCormick's was a biscuit
    and confectionary producer bought by George Weston Ltd in the 1940s. "McCormick
    Manufacturing Company," London Public Library, http://www.londonpubliclibrary.ca/
    research/local-history/historic-sites-committee/mccormick-manufacturing-company; Tisdall,
    Drake, Summerfeldt, and Brown, "A New Whole Wheat Irradiated Biscuit," 169–70.

36 Frederick Griffin, "Perfectly-Balanced Biscuit Tested by Toronto Doctors," *Toronto Daily Star*,
    15 January 1930, 1–2; A Dominion Stores Limited advertisement advised readers to "Watch
    for the New McCormick's Sun-Wheat Health Biscuit which will be on sale in all our stores
    shortly!" *Toronto Daily Star*, 23 January 1930, 8. On January 30, Loblaws announced that
    Sunwheat Biscuits were available, *Toronto Daily Star*, 30 January 1930, 11.

37 The next week, Loblaws announced that "We Owe Our Customers an Apology for not
    being able to meet the demand for McCormick's SUNWHEAT Biscuits Last Week. We can
    assure you that we will have a complete stock available from now on at all out Groceterias."
    The Globe, 7 February 1930, 3; "Vitamin Biscuits Extremely Popular," *Toronto Daily Star*, 13
    February 1930, 3; McCormick's Sunwheat Irradiated-Vitamin Biscuits, advertisement, *Toronto
    Daily Star*, 31 March 1931, 10.

38 McCormick's Sunwheat Biscuit Irradiated-Vitamin Biscuits, advertisement, *The Globe*, 27
    February 1930, 17.

39 Tisdall, Drake, Summerfeldt, and Brown, "A New Whole Wheat Irradiated Biscuit," 166–70;
    Drake, Tisdall, and Brown, "The Incorporation of Vitamins in Bread," 210–13; Frederick
    F. Tisdall, T.G.H. Drake, and Alan Brown, with the technical assistance of Elizabeth
    McNamara, "A New Cereal Mixture Containing Vitamins and Mineral Elements," *American
    Journal of Diseases of Children* 40, no. 4 (1930): 791–9; AR 1930, 38.

40 Quotation Drake, Tisdall, and Brown, "The Incorporation of Vitamins in Bread," 212. See
    Untitled Report on NRL Vitamin Research, ca. 1928–31, typed. Pablum Subject file, HSC
    Archives; "Sun-Wheat Biscuits," 2–3. Pablum Subject File, HSC Archives.

41 "Sun-Wheat Biscuits," 3. Pablum Subject File, HSC Archives. See "New Incorporations," *The
    Globe*, 20 September 1930, 24.

42 Brown and Tisdall, *Common Procedures* (1936), 80; "Anti-Rachitic Vitamin to be Baked into
    Bread," *The Science News-Letter*, 19, no. 519 (1931): 184, 03/08/2013 15:51, http://www.jstor.
    org/stable/3907349; Henderson, "Vitamin D in Foods," 643–4; "Million Reported Bid for
    Vitamin D Rights," *New York Times*, 13 February 1931, 21.

43 "Sun-Wheat Biscuits," 4. Pablum Subject File, HSC Archives; Marjorie Henderson, "Vitamin
    D in Foods," *The American Journal of Nursing* 32, no. 6 (1932): 643–4.

44 George Weston, Limited, Advertisement, Weston's Bread, *Toronto Daily Star*, 31 August 1931, 7; Ideal Bread Co, Advertisement, Vitos White Bread, "Mothers ... your children need sunshine vitamin D," *Toronto Daily Star*, 1 September 1931, 7; Vitos Bread Ad, *Montreal Gazette*, 3 September 1931, 11; Weston's Advertisement, *Toronto Daily Star*, 15 October 1931, 41.

45 Untitled Report on Department Research (circa 1931), 8. Pablum Subject File, HSC Archives.

46 Alan Brown and Frederick F. Tisdall, "The Effect of Vitamins and the Inorganic Elements on Growth and Resistance of Diseases in Children," *Annals of Internal Medicine* 7, no. 3 (1933): 348.

47 Alan Brown and Elizabeth Chant Robertson, "Essential Features Concerning the Proper Nutrition of the Infant and Child," *Canadian Medical Association Journal* 48, no. 4 (1943): 300.

48 "Nutrition in Bread" *Toronto Daily Star*, 30 September 1947, 6.

49 Apple, *Vitamania*, 20–6.

50 Ideal Bread Co., Vitos Bread Ad, "Important News of a Priceless Health-Source for Your Family (Particularly Your Children)," *The Globe*, 1 September 1931, 15.

51 Henderson, "Vitamin D in Foods," 343–4.

52 Ostry, *Nutrition Policy*, 61.

53 Untitled Report on Department Research (circa 1931), 8–9. Pablum Subject File, HSC Archives.

54 Bond Bread Advertisement, *New York Sun*, 13 April 1931, 19.

55 Brown and Tisdall, "The Effect of Vitamins and the Inorganic Elements," 349.

56 Tisdall, Drake, and Brown, "A New Cereal Mixture Containing Vitamins and Mineral Elements," 791–9; Brown and Tisdall, *Common Procedures* (1926), 66; Brown and Tisdall, "The Effect of Vitamins and the Inorganic Elements," 350.

57 Quotation in Alan Brown and Frederick F. Tisdall, *Common Procedures in the Practice of Paediatrics*, 4th ed., revised and expanded (Toronto: McClelland and Stewart, 1949), 69.

58 "Sun-Wheat Biscuits," (Report on Departmental History, circa 1930), 5. Pablum Subject File, HSC Archives.

59 "Inquiring Investor," *Wall Street Journal*, 12 April 1934, 8.

60 Mead Johnson Co, "Our History," www.meadjohnson.com/company/pages/our-history.aspx, accessed 15 July 2013; Brown and Tisdall, *Common Procedures*, 1st ed. (1926), 24–5.

61 Nina Drake, "Tisdall, Drake, Brown, Pablum," 1984; I.D.A. Drug Stores, advertisement, *Toronto Daily Star*, 17 January 1934, 16; G. Tamblyn, Limited, advertisement, *Toronto Daily Star*, 4 April 1934, 9.

62 Mead Johnson & Co., advertisement, "Exploitation of the Medical Profession" *Harvard Medical Alumni Bulletin* 12, no. 1 (1937).

63 See Michael Bliss, *The History of the Discovery of Insulin*, 25th anniversary ed. (Chicago: University of Chicago Press, 2013).

64 R.P.T. Davenport-Hines and Judy Slinn, *Glaxo: A History to 1962* (New York: Cambridge University Press, 1992), 84.

65 Davenport-Hines and Slinn, *Glaxo: A History to 1962*, 85.

66 I.D.A. Drug Stores, advertisement, *Toronto Daily Star*, 15 August 1951, 9; IDA, *Toronto Daily Star*, 14 August 1951, 5.

67 Mark Collar "The Pablum Connection," *The City*, 17 December 1978, 18.

68 "Pablum, Milk and Formula, Regular Scientific Baby Food, Are Fed Barbara, 4 ½ -Month-Old Gibbon At Washington Zoo," *Toronto Daily Star*, 26 February 1945, 15; H.A. Johnson, "Notes on the Continuous Rearing of aëdes Aegypti in the Laboratory," *Public Health Reports* 52, no. 35 (1939): 1177–9; Harold Schlosberg, Marie Castaldi Duncan, and Betty Horenstein Daitch, "Mating Behavior of Two Live-Bearing Fish, Xiphophorus hellerii and Platypoecilus maculatus," *Physiological Zoology* 22, no. 2 (1949): 148–61; M.A. Ghani and Harvey L. Sweetman, "Ecological Studies of the Book Louse, Liposcelis Divinatorius (Mull.)," *Ecology* 32, no. 2 (1951): 230–44.

69 "Zoo Gets Pandas; Debut Is Formal," *New York Times*, 31 December 1941, 19.

70 Trustees Minutes, 24 November 1931: Tisdall sent letters proposing investigations into "the effect of diet on the condition and development of teeth in children" and "the effects of diet

on the mental development of children. Full details of the proposed investigations are covered in the letters of November 23rd addressed to the superintendent, Mr. Bower, by Dr. Tisdall." The next week, representatives of the trustees to the PRF attended a meeting; "the chief item of business considered at that meeting was the appropriation of a fund of $5,000.00 from the funds of the Foundation, for Research, into the effect of diet on children's teeth." Trustees Minutes, 1 December 1931.

71 Trustees Minutes, 14 September 1931. "Sun-Wheat Biscuits," 5. Pablum Subject File, HSC Archives.

72 HSC Superintendent Bower to PRF, Memorandum of Procedure approved by trustees, Trustees Minutes, 14 May 1931.

73 Trustees Minutes, 24 November 1931: Tisdall sent letters proposing investigations into "the effect of diet on the condition and development of teeth in children" and "the effects of diet on the mental development of children. Full details of the proposed investigations are covered in the letters of November 23 addressed to the superintendent, Mr. Bower, by Dr. Tisdall." The next week, representatives of the trustees to the PRF attended a meeting; "the chief item of business considered at that meeting was the appropriation of a fund of $5,000.00 from the funds of the Foundation, for Research, into the effect of diet on children's teeth." Trustees Minutes, 1 December 1931.

74 J.H.W. Bower, "Research Work at the Hospital for Sick Children," 26 October 1953, appended to photocopy of Tisdall, Drake, and Brown, "A New Cereal Mixture Containing Vitamins." Pablum Subject file, HSC Archives.

75 The trustees approved Brown's request for "permission to equip the present Chapel into a Laboratory, the cost of same to be paid for by Sir Joseph Flavelle," Trustees Minutes, 16 March 1920, 110.

76 AR 1930, 38–9.

77 Trustees Minutes, 8 November 1932.

78 Trustees Minutes, 15 January 1935, Appended, Superintendent to Dr. A Primrose, Chairman, PRF of Toronto. HSC Archives.

79 Bower, "Research Work at the Hospital for Sick Children."

80 Executive Director Douglas E. Snedden to Hospital Secretary E.H. Shuter, 1 March 1972. Pablum Subject File, HSC Archives.

81 "Baby Food Developer Leaves $312,494," *Toronto Daily Star*, 19 February 1960, 43.

82 Front Cover, *The City*, 17 December 1978. Pablum Subject File, HSC Archives.

83 James Fitzgerald alludes to the uses of horses for diphtheria toxin research as early as 1913. See J. Fitzgerald, *What Disturbs Our Blood: A Son's Quest to Redeem the Past* (Toronto: Random House, 2010), 236–7; Elizabeth Chant Robertson and John Ross, "Increased Resistance of Rachitic Rats Fed Irradiated Food," *Experimental Biology and Medicine* 27 (June 1930): 999–1002; "Elizabeth Chant-Robertson worked on nutrition studies with the nursery school children as subjects," in Mary L. Northway, letter to the editor, "William Emmet Blatz," *Canadian Medical Association Journal* 123 (5 July 1980): 15.

84 Tisdall, Drake, and Brown, "A New Cereal Mixture," 798.

85 Frederick Banting sent his son to one of the nursery schools involved in the studies. See Northway, "William Emmet Blatz," 15; Brown and Chant Robertson, "Essential Features Concerning the Proper Nutrition," 300; John R. Ross and P. Summerfeldt, "Haemoglobin of Normal Children and Certain Factors Influencing its Formation," *Canadian Medical Association Journal* 34, no. 2 (1936): 155–8.

86 Pearl Summerfeldt, "The Value of an Increased Supply of Vitamin B1 and Iron in the Diet of Children," *American Journal of Diseases of Children* 43, no. 2 (1932): 284–90.

87 P. Summerfeldt, F.F. Tisdall, and A. Brown, "The Curative Effects of Cereals and Biscuits on Experimental Anaemias," *Canadian Medical Association Journal* 26, no. 6 (1932): 66, http://www.ncbi.nlm.nih.gov/pmc/articles/PMC402381/pdf/canmedaj00119-0020.pdf.

88 Brown and Tisdall, "The Effect of Vitamins and the Inorganic Elements," 347.

89 Doris Monypenny, "The Early Introduction of Solid Foods in the Infant Diet," *Canadian Medical Association Journal* 42, no. 2 (1940): 137–40.

90 T.G.H. Drake, Frederick F. Tisdall, and Alan Brown, "Irradiated Evaporated Milk in the Prevention Of Rickets," *The Journal of Pediatrics* 8, no. 2 (1936): 161–5; Caulfield's Dairy Limited, advertisement, "Caulfields Announce Vitamin D Milk," *Toronto Daily Star*, 11 October 1934, 12.

91 F.F. Tisdall, T.G.H. Drake, A. Brown, "A Study of the Relative Antirachitic Value of Cod Liver Oil, Viosterol and Irradiated Milk," *Canadian Medical Association Journal* 31, no. 4 (1934): 368–76; Trustees Minutes, 3 October 1933.

92 T.G.H. Drake, "Comparison of the Antirachitic Effects on Human Beings of Vitamin D from Different Sources," *American Journal of Diseases of Children* 53, no. 3 (1937): 756. See also T.G.H. Drake, F.F. Tisdall, A. Brown, "The Antirachitic Value of Irradiated Yeast in Infants," *Journal of Nutrition* 12, no. 5 (1936): 528.

93 Angelia M. Courtney, "The Effect of Inadequate Diet on the Inorganic Salt Content of Mothers' Milk," *American Journal of Diseases of Children* 26, no. 6 (1923): 537.

94 E.C. Robertson, "Practical Methods of Supplying the Essential Vitamins of Childhood," *Canadian Medical Association Journal* 52 (May 1945): 494–8. http://www.ncbi.nlm.nih.gov/pmc/articles/PMC1581943/pdf/canmedaj00584-0144.pdf

95 Apple, *Vitamania*, 7.

96 Cynthia Comacchio, *Nations are Built of Babies: Saving Ontario's Mothers and Children, 1900–1940* (Montreal: McGill-Queen's University Press, 1993), 124. See also Tasnim Nathoo and Aleck Ostry, *The One Best Way?: Breastfeeding History, Politics, and Policy in Canada* (Waterloo: Wilfrid Laurier University Press, 2009), 77.

97 AR 1931, 41.

98 C.W. Penrose, "In Memory of Sunwheat Biscuit," *What's New* 16, no. 1 (1984): 17.

99 "Dr. P. Summerfeldt Is Bride of A.L. Rose" *Toronto Daily Star*, 4 June 1938, 25; Mary C. Williams, "Dr. P. Rose, Pablum Developer," *Sun Sentinel* (South Florida), 23 February 1994, accessed 14 October 2015, http://articles.sun-sentinel.com/1994-02-23/news/9402230041_1_pompano-beach-cereal-developer.

100 T.G.H. Drake, "Frederick Fitzgerald Tisdall," *Journal of Nutrition* 56, no. 1 (1955): 7–8.

101 The revelation of this, embedded in a scholarly history article, made national headlines in 2013. See Ian Mosby, "Administering Colonial Science: Nutrition Research and Human Biomedical Experimentation in Aboriginal Communities and Residential Schools, 1942–1952," *Histoire Sociale/Social History* 46, no. 91 (2013): 145–72.

102 Brown and Chant Robertson, "Essential Features Concerning the Proper Nutrition," 297.

103 Ostry, *Nutrition Policy*, Table 9.2, 91.

104 Gertrude E.S. Pringle, "A Progressive Profession for Girls," *Maclean's*, 15 May 1922), 64, 67.

105 "How Babies are Cared For," Pasteurization Department Scrapbook.

106 Graham Dutfield, *Intellectual Property Rights and the Life Science Industries Past, Present and Future*, 2nd ed. (New Jersey: World Scientific, 2009), 135.

107 Apple, *Vitamania*, 35–8; Marjorie Henderson, "Vitamin D in Foods," *The American Journal of Nursing* 32, no. 6 (1932): 643–4; "How Nature's Supply of Vitamin D, Ultra-violet Rays of Sunlight is Cut Off by Weather and Civilized Life," in Caulfield's Dairy Limited, advertisement, "Caulfields Announce Vitamin D Milk," *Toronto Daily Star*, 11 October 1934, 12.

7 IRON LUNGS

1 Alan Brown, "Preventive Paediatrics and its Relation to the General Practitioner," *Canadian Medical Association Journal* 24, no. 4 (1931): 518.

2 "Motor Car for District Nurse: $1,500," *John Ross Robertson Donation Ledger, 1883–1919*, 14, HSC Archives 972.50.6; AR 1912, 9; AR 1909, 9; AR 1913, 10. In 1911, Charters averaged 70 visits per week, or 3,657 total, to 700 patients (AR 1911, 9; AR 1912, 9).

3   Mary Adelaide Snider (special writer on the staff of the *Evening Telegram*), "One Day with the District Nurse," reprint from *Evening Telegram*, January 1913, 5–6. Dairy Subject File [also in Miscellaneous Pamphlets, item #972.57.1] HSC Archives. See also AR 1914, 10.

4   Snider, "One Day with the District Nurse."

5   Marion Royce, *Eunice Dyke, Health Care Pioneer: From Pioneer Public Health Nurse to Advocate for the Aged* (Toronto: Dundurn Press, 1983), 51, 53–4; Alan Brown, "Toronto as a Paediatric Centre," *Canadian Medical Monthly* 5, no. 6 (1920): 207.

6   Dr. Alan Brown, Report of the Physician-In-Chief, AR 1927, 25.

7   Alan Brown, "How the Children's Hospital Can Best Meet Community Needs," (Read at the 41st Convention of the American Hospital Association, Toronto, 25–9 September 1939), *Hospitals: The Journal of the American Hospital Association* 14 (1940): 45; Alan Brown, "The Relation of the Pediatrician to the Community," *Public Health Journal* 10, no. 2 (1919): 53.

8   Brown, "Toronto as a Paediatric Centre," 209.

9   Brown, "How the Children's Hospital Can Best Meet Community Needs," 45.

10 J.E. Bower to Mr. James W. Somers (City Clerk), 18 October 1941, Subject File Finances #1, HSC Archives.

11 AR 1923, 17. See Annual Reports for the 1910s–20s. Later clinics were added for immunization, habit, goitre, and orthodontia.

12 AR 1922, 5.

13 See, for example, AR 1923, 17, and AR 1922, 16–17.

14 See Cynthia R. Comacchio, *Nations are Built of Babies: Saving Ontario's Mothers and Children, 1900–1940* (Montreal: McGill-Queen's University Press, 1993), 148–9; Royce, *Eunice Dyke,* 53–4; AR 1927, 25.

15 See the editorial "Hospital Abuses," *Canadian Practitioner and Review* 46, no. 9 (1921): 280–1; see in response Letter to the Editor, A Subscriber, *Canadian Practitioner and Review* 46, no. 11 (1921): 363. The writer in the response complained of graduate nurses from " – – " recommending sickly babies to only one specialist (" – – "), the blanks implicitly being HSC and Brown. Also see letter to the editor, East End Practitioner, *Canadian Practitioner and Review* 46, no. 11 (1921): 363–4.

16 "Doctors' Review Makes Attack On the City Nurses," *Toronto Daily Star,* 6 October 1921. This article can be found in *Special Album,* 95, HSC Archives.

17 Brown, "The Relation of the Pediatrician," 51.

18 Ibid.

19 "Child Welfare in Toronto," editorial, *Canadian Practitioner and Review* 46, no. 9 (1921): 281.

20 As Heather MacDougall has demonstrated, a similar resentment and mistrust had emerged over school medical inspection in places such as New York and Montreal. MacDougall, *Activists and Advocates: Toronto's Health Department, 1883–1983* (Toronto: Dundurn Press, 1990), 164, 185–190. See also Kari Delhi, "'Health Scouts' for the State? School and Public Health Nurses in Early Twentieth-Century Toronto," *Historical Studies in Education* 2 (1990): 217–64, 251.

21 Letter to the Editor, East End Practitioner, *Canadian Practitioner and Review* 46, no. 11 (1921): 363–4.

22 AR 1916, 8.

23 On page 8, AR 1911 states: "Some days you can count about fifty baby carriages at the Elizabeth street door [sic], and some days over 200 patients in attendance, accompanied by about 150 adults – quite an army of youngsters, who require our aid." For statistics see AR 1911, 8; AR 1920, 4; AR 1921, 4; AR 1933, 28.

24 AR 1925, 33.

25 W.E. Gallie, Surgical Report, AR 1924, 27.

26 AR 1921, 5.

27 Ibid.

28 Marianne Fedunkiw, *Rockefeller Foundation Funding and Medical Education in Toronto, Montreal and Halifax* (Montreal: McGill-Queen's University Press, 2005), 38, 84.

29 Robert B. Kerr and Douglas Waugh, *Duncan Graham: Medical Reformer and Educator* (Toronto: Hannah Institute & Dundurn Press, 1989), 40–55, 81; *University of Toronto's President's Report for the Year Ended 30th June, 1920* (Toronto, 1921), 9.

30 Fedunkiw, *Rockefeller Foundation Funding*, 75–6.

31 AR 1919, 4.

32 I am grateful to David Martin for this insight.

33 AR 1920, 5.

34 *U of T Medical Bulletin* 1, no. 1 (1921): 2; Shorter, *Partnership for Excellence*, 44–5; MAB 13 March 1931; MAB 27 Feb 1920; *The Calendar of the University of Toronto Faculty of Medicine, 1920–1921* (Toronto: University of Toronto Press), 67, https://archive.org/stream/ calendarmed1920univ.

35 *University of Toronto Report of the Board of Governors for the Year Ended 30th June 1935* (Toronto, 1936), 226–7, 230–1; Dr. A.L. Chute, transcribed interview by Valerie Schatzker under the aegis of the Hannah Institute/AMS. The volumes are unpublished and stored in Archives, but there is a published index by Martina Hardwick: http://search.library.utoronto.ca/ details?3264110 (Hannah Institute for the History of Medicine / AMS Medical Services, Inc., 1977), 71; AR 1918, 18; AR 1920, 14; AR 1921, 10.

36 "The Teaching of Pediatrics," *British Medical Journal* 1, no. 3050 (1919): 747.

37 See *The Calendar of the University of Toronto Faculty of Medicine, 1920–1921* (Toronto: University of Toronto Press), 66–7, 70–1; Dr. J. Harry Ebbs interviewed by Valerie Schatzker, 20 February, 22 February, 27 February, and 6 March 1979 (Hannah Institute for the History of Medicine / Associated Medical Services, Inc.), 43. See also retirement speech of Vera Rose, in Cardiology Folder, Box 44, History of the Department of Paediatrics, HSC Archives.

38 "Rules Regarding the Admission of Patients to the Hospital for Sick Children, Toronto (1928)," as cited in The Hospital for Sick Children Alumni Association, *Dr Alan Brown* (Toronto: Hospital for Sick Children in conjunction with University of Toronto Press, 1984?), 20. Alan Brown Subject File, HSC Archives.

39 David Gagan, "For 'Patients of Moderate Means': The Transformation of Ontario's Public General Hospitals, 1880–1950," *Canadian Historical Review* 70, no. 2 (1989): 151–79.

40 Trustees Minutes, Executive Committee, 28 April 1925.

41 Trustees Minutes, 26 October 1926. Debts were also incurred by private patients at the Cottage Hospital. See Trustees Minutes, 26 March 1929.

42 Trustees Minutes, 29 June 1926.

43 Trustees Minutes, Executive Committee, 25 September 1923.

44 Trustees Minutes, Executive Committee, 18 December 1922.

45 Trustees Minutes, 8 February 1927.

46 Quotation Trustees Minutes, 14 July 1925. See also See Trustees Minutes, 2 April 1929, Trustees Minutes, 30 April 1923, Trustees Minutes, 1 September 1925.

47 Trustees Minutes, 12 May 1925. Trustees Minutes, Executive Committee, 8 September 1925.

48 Trustees Minutes, 18 August 1925. Records indicate that collectors called on the homes of at least fifteen of sixty-five cases written off as bad debts in August 1922. Trustees Minutes, 30 August 1922.

49 Trustees Minutes, 10 March 1925.

50 Trustees Minutes, 12 July 1921, 148.

51 One sibling was at the private Cottage Hospital, and the other at HSC. Trustees Minutes, 23 April 1929.

52 Trustees Minutes, 21 May 1929. In another case the board decided not to resort to court action to resolve an outstanding account of $87.50. Trustees Minutes, 27 November 1928.

53 David Gagan and Rosemary Gagan, *For Patients of Moderate Means: A Social History of the Voluntary Public General Hospital in Canada, 1890–1950* (Montreal: McGill-Queen's University Press, 2002), 56.

54 Trustees Minutes, 10 January 1922, 192; Trustees Minutes, Executive Committee, 30 August 1922; Trustees Minutes, Executive Committee, 18 August 1925.

55 Trustees Minutes, 10 January 1922, 192.

56 Trustees Minutes, 27 December 1927.

57 Trustees Minutes, 18 August 1925.

58 Trustees Minutes, 30 August 1922.

59 Trustees Minutes, Executive Committee, 30 August 1922.

60 Trustees Minutes, 20 April 1926.

61 For an example, see Trustees Minutes, 18 August 1925; Minutes list sixty-five cases to be written off as bad debts, including at least seven cases where a child died; "Account of child being put in quarantine after dischargeable, parents have refused payment"; Trustees Minutes, Executive Committee, 30 August 1922.

62 Trustees Minutes, 23 June 1903, 87–96, quotation 94.

63 Trustees Minutes, Executive Committee, 7 April 1924; Trustees Minutes, 24 October 1921, 23 May 1921, 13 August 1923, and 25 September 1923.

64 For examples see Trustees Minutes, 19 September 1921, 165; Trustees Minutes, 17 October 1921, 174; and 18 August 1926; Trustees Minutes, Executive Committee, 12 December 1921, 184; Trustees Minutes, 10 January 1922, 192.

65 Trustees Minutes, 10 February 1912, 426.

66 Trustees Minutes, 30 August 1922. See "An Act Respecting the Hospital for Sick Children," *Statutes of the Province of Ontario*, chap. 153, 12–13, George V (Assented to 26 May 1922), 916–17.

67 Trustees Minutes, 30 August 1922.

68 Trustees Minutes, 16 June 1930.

69 Ian Dowbiggin, "'Keeping this Young Country Sane': C.K. Clarke, Immigration Restriction, and Canadian Psychiatry, 1890–1925," *Canadian Historical Review* 76, no. 4 (1995): 598–627.

70 Trustees Minutes, 1 December 1930.

71 Sioux Lookout Sanatorium opened in 1949.

72 Trustees Minutes, 3 December 1929.

73 Plans to open up a private ward, which were strongly supported by Gallie/Brown following the abandonment of the Cottage Hospital scheme, were shelved in 1932 and not taken up again until 1934. Trustees Minutes, 22 February 1932 and 5 June 1934.

74 Trustees Minutes, 3 December 1929; Trustees Minutes, 14 March 1932, 7 March 1933, and 25 July 1933.

75 "The Hospital for Sick Children, Operating Cost, 1943–1946," Finances #1, Subject File, HSC Archives.

76 Bower was to consult with the superintendents of TGH and Western. Trustees Minutes, 11 April 1932; Trustees Minutes, 25 April 1932; Trustees Minutes, 15 November 1932.

77 Trustees Minutes, 7 February 1933.

78 Helen MacMurchy, "Paralysis: The New Epidemic," *Maclean's,* 1 November 1912, 109.

79 Christopher J. Rutty, "The History of Polio," *Health Heritage Services* (Originally prepared for Sanofi Pasteur in 2002), http://www.healthheritageresearch.com/Polio-Vaccine/PV-comHistory.html; Ontario Department of Health, *Report on Poliomyelitis in Ontario, 1937* (Toronto?: March 1938), 29, 57.

80 Joy Jaipaul, "In the Shadows: Poliomyelitis Epidemics and Nursing Care in Edmonton 1947–1955," *Alberta History* 53, no. 3 (2005): 3.

81 MacMurchy, "Paralysis," 111; Anne Hardy, "Poliomyelitis and the Neurologists: The View from England, 1896–1966," *Bulletin of the History of Medicine* 71, no. 2 (1997): 253.

82 Christopher Rutty, "'Do Something! ... Do Anything!': Poliomyelitis in Canada 1927–1962" (PhD diss., University of Toronto, 1995), 27.

83 Christopher J. Rutty, "The Middle-Class Plague: Epidemic Polio and the Canadian State, 1936–37," *Canadian Bulletin of Medical History* 13, no. 2 (1996): 277–314.

84 See M.R. Smallman-Raynor, A.D. Cliff, B. Trevelyan, C. Nettleton, and S. Sneddon, *Poliomyelitis: Emergence to Eradication* (New York: Oxford University Press, 2006), 81–9, quotation 84; Ontario Department of Health, *Report on Poliomyelitis*, 1.

85 MacMurchy, "Paralysis," 110.

86 Smallman-Raynor et al., *Poliomyelitis*, 178.

87 Ibid., 150.

88 The impact of the Spanish flu of 1918 has been well documented. For scholarship on the impact on Canadian communities, see Esyllt W. Jones, "Contact Across a Diseased Boundary: Urban Space and Social Interaction During Winnipeg's Influenza Epidemic, 1918–1919," *Journal of the Canadian Historical Association / Revue de la Société historique du Canada* 13, no. 1 (2002): 119–39; and Maureen Lux, "'The Bitter Flats': The 1918 Influenza Epidemic in Saskatchewan," *Saskatchewan History* 49, no. 1 (1997): 3–13.

89 Spinal taps often only served to confirm what was apparent to the naked eye, and "by the time this was done it was often too late." Researchers could not culture the virus outside of the human or animal body until 1949. Rutty, "'Do Something! ... Do Anything!,'" 32, 381–6.

90 Ontario's 1929 epidemic incurred 558 cases and 26 deaths, followed in 1930 by 671 cases and 71 deaths, mostly in Toronto. Rutty, "'Do Something! ... Do Anything!,'" 67; Ontario Department of Health, *Report on Poliomyelitis*, 4–5; M.L. Grimshaw, "Scientific Specialization and the Poliovirus Controversy in the Years before World War II," *Bulletin of the History of Medicine* 69, no. 1 (1995): 46–65; D.J. Wilson, "A Crippling Fear: Experiencing Polio in the Era of FDR," *Bulletin of the History of Medicine* 72, no. 3 (1998): 471.

91 Rutty, "'Do Something! ... Do Anything!,'" 41–4, 60–1, 69–75, 94–7; MacDougall, *Activists and Advocates*, 149.

92 Rutty, "'Do Something! ... Do Anything!,'" 97.

93 MacDougall, *Activists and Advocates*, 148–9; Rutty, "'Do Something! ... Do Anything!,'" 100.

94 Disturbingly, researchers correlated recent tonsillectomies with the onset of bulbar polio. Ontario Department of Health, *Report on Poliomyelitis*, 2, 4–5, 16, 24–5; MacDougall, *Activists and Advocates*, 149–50.

95 Rutty, "'Do Something! ... Do Anything!,'" 88, 100–13.

96 Ontario Department of Health, *Report on Poliomyelitis*, 1, 4–6, 15.

97 "Buy 'Iron Lung' to Help Victims Paralysis Rises," *Toronto Daily Star*, 25 August 1937; Frederick Edwards, "Iron Lungs," *Maclean's,* 15 January 1938, 12, 29–31; Rutty, "'Do Something! ... Do Anything!,'" 113–17.

98 Rutty, "'Do Something! ... Do Anything!,'" 115.

99 Ibid., 129.

100 Ibid., 120–3.

101 Jaipaul, "In the Shadows," 3.

102 Richard Carter estimated that, from 1938 to 1960, the NFIP spent "$315 million on medical, hospital, nursing, and rehabilitative care for 325,000 polio sufferers"; Wilson, "A Crippling Fear," 484.

103 Amy Fairchild, "The Polio Narratives: Dialogues with FDR," *Bulletin of the History of Medicine* 75, no. 3 (2001): 488–534.

104 Rutty, "'Do Something! ... Do Anything!,'" 100.

105 *University of Toronto Report of the Board of Governors for the Year Ended 30th June 1936* (Toronto: T.E. Bowman, 1937), 13.

106 J. Harry Ebbs, "The Canadian Paediatric Society: Its Early Years," *Canadian Medical Association Journal* 123, no. 12 (1980): 1235.

107 The Royal College of Physicians and Surgeons of Canada, "Historical Overview of Specialties Recognized by The Royal College of Physicians and Surgeons of Canada," http://www.royalcollege.ca/portal/page/portal/rc/common/documents/publications/historical_overview_of_recognized_specialties.pdf

108 Ontario Department of Health, *Report on Poliomyelitis in Ontario*, 46–7; Rutty, "'Do Something! ... Do Anything!,'" 116.

109 See Charles Webster, *The National Health Service: A Political History* (New York: Oxford University Press, 2002).

110 Rutty, "'Do Something! ... Do Anything!,'" 159.

111 Rutty, "The Middle-Class Plague," 279.

8 VISITING HOURS

1 W.H.R., "Out of the Iron Lung" (Toronto, written 28 May 1952), 6. Polio Subject File. 2006.416.018. HSC Archives.

2 J.D.M. Griffin, W.A. Hawke, and W. Wray Barraclough, "Mental Hygiene in an Orthopedic Hospital," *Journal of Pediatrics* 13, no. 1 (1938): 85.

3 Ibid.

4 Jean I. Masten, "Nursing Care in Poliomyelitis following Isolation Period," *The Canadian Nurse* 34, no. 5 (1938): 252.

5 AR 1938, 42.

6 Griffin, Hawke, and Barraclough, "Mental Hygiene in an Orthopedic Hospital," 82.

7 For a collection of essays on this topic, see *Permeable Walls: Historical Perspectives on Hospital and Asylum Visiting,* ed. Graham Mooney and Jonathan Reinarz (Amsterdam: Rodopi, 2009).

8 Training School Graduation Programme (1940), p 5, Nursing School Subject File #8 HSC Archives.

9 AR 1913, 6. Quotation from W.H.R., "Out of the Iron Lung," (28 May 1952), Polio Subject File, HSC Archives.

10 Bruce Lindsay, "Pariahs or Partners? Welcome and Unwelcome Visitors in the Jenny Lind Hospital for Sick Children, Norwich, 1900–50," in *Permeable Walls: Historical Perspectives on Hospital and Asylum Visiting,* ed. Graham Mooney and Jonathan Reinarz (Amsterdam: Rodopi, 2009), 121–2; Andrea Tanner, "Too Many Mothers? Female Roles in a Metropolitan Victorian Children's Hospital," in *The Impact of Hospitals 300–2000*, ed. John Henderson, Peregrine Horden, and Alessandro Pastore (Oxford: Peter Lang, 2007), 150.

11 Griffin, Hawke, and Barraclough, "Mental Hygiene in an Orthopedic Hospital," 76.

12 Andrea Tanner, "Choice and the Children's Hospital: Great Ormond Street Hospital Patients and their Families 1855–1900," in *Medicine, Charity and Mutual Aid: The Consumption of Health and Welfare in Britain, c. 1550–1950,* ed. Anne Borsay and Peter Shapely (Burlington, VT: Ashgate, 2007), 143.

13 For example Ladies Committee Minutes (LC), 1 June 1894.

14 Bruce Lindsay, "'A 2-Year-Old Goes to Hospital': A 50th Anniversary Reappraisal of the Impact of James Robertson's Film," *Journal of Child Health Care* 7, no. 1 (2003): 19.

15 Ladies Committee Minutes, 10 October 1877 and 7 December 1877; AR 1880, 5.

16 Ladies Committee Minutes, 4 May 1883.

17 Trustees Minutes, 4 July 1894, 143.

18 One example among many: "Miss Potts mentioned to the Trustees that Dr. Hannah desired to close the Hospital to all visitors, on account of infection, which was approved of by the Trustees, if Miss Potts saw fit," Trustees Minutes, 26 March 1921.

19 MAB 9 October 1922 and 18 June 1923; Trustees Minutes, Executive Committee, 27 June 1923.

20 Judith Young, "Changing Attitudes Towards Families of Hospitalized Children from 1935 to 1975: A Case Study," *Journal of Advanced Nursing* 17, no. 12 (1992): 1422.

21 Judith Young, "A 'Necessary Nuisance': Social Class and Parental Visiting Rights at Toronto's Hospital for Sick Children 1930–1970," in *Canadian Health Care and the State: A Century of Evolution,* ed. C. David Naylor (Montreal: McGill-Queen's University Press, 1992), 88, 102n62.

22 *Nurse Daily Journal,* 1911, 0985–005–005.

23 For example, "Johnny McFie continues very ill and his mother in attendance upon him" (Ladies Committee Minutes, 7 May 1880).

24 *Nurse Daily Journal,* 1909 (21 January 1909) Box 136. HSC Archives.

25 Coordinator of Infants Ward to Judith Young, Letter re: parent visiting (25 February 1987), in possession of Judith Young.

26 Anonymous oral interview by author, participant #9, 26 February 2014.

27 Likewise, visiting at Thistletown was permitted from 2 to 4 p.m. on Sundays. Parents could visit seriously and critically ill children "daily as they please," and accident cases "the day following admission for a few minutes." Hospital for Sick Children, Standing Orders (September 1948), 6–7. HSC Archives.

28 Johanne W. Bentzon, "Polio, The Hospital for Sick Children/Thistletown," (c. 1950s), 10, Polio Subject File, HSC Archives.

29 Official name. Trustees Minutes, 21 February 1928.

30 AR 1882, 15.

31 Mary Adelaide Snider, "'T.B.' Amongst the Children The Work of The Heather Club," (January 1913), 10 Miscellaneous Pamphlets, HSC Archives. The Heather Club became a chapter of the Toronto Branch of The Imperial Order of the Daughters of the Empire (IODE) in 1912. A year-round preventorium was established through the IODE in 1913. "The Imperial Order of the Daughters of the Empire Preventorium" (Toronto: University of Toronto Press, 1919), 5, 19.

32 AR 1921, 5, 14.

33 Geoffrey Reaume, *Lyndhurst: Canada's First Rehabilitation Centre for People with Spinal Cord Injuries, 1945–1998* (Montreal: McGill-Queen's Press, 2007), 11.

34 Roy Hanes, "Linking Mental Defect to Physical Deformity: The Case of Crippled Children in Ontario: 1890–1940," *Journal on Developmental Disabilities* 4, no. 1 (1995): 37. See H.J. Prueter, "Facing the Future: The Care and Education of Crippled Children in Ontario" (Toronto: OSCC [published PhD Thesis, U of T], 1937), 63–5; "Survey Completed to Aid in Problem of Disabled Child," *The Globe*, 1 January 1924, 16; "Classes for Cripples to Open at Easter," *Toronto Daily Star*, 9 March 1926, 7.

35 Trustees Minutes, Executive Committee and MAB 21 December 1921. For Gallie's call, see AR 1921, 14; AR 1923, 30. See also Katherine McCuaig, *The Weariness, the Fever and the Fret: The Campaign against Tuberculosis in Canada, 1900–1950* (Montreal: McGill-Queen's University Press, 1999), 44–5.

36 Trustees Minutes, 9 June 1925. For the prior visits, see Trustees Minutes, 1 August 1923.

37 Quotation Chairman H.H. Williams, "A Letter About Your Children," 1926, Appeals Subject File #1, HSC Archives. See also Trustees and MAB joint meeting, Trustees Minutes, 28 July 1925; J. Stuart Crawford, *A History of the Hospital for Sick Children 1918 to 1958* (Toronto: HSC Archives, 1959), 21; Trustees Minutes, 18 August 1925.

38 Trustees Minutes, 1 February 1926, 9 February 1926, 13 July 1926, 6 August 1929, and 29 January 1951; Chairman H.H. Williams, "A Letter About Your Children" (1926) and Letter, H.H. Williams to all Clergymen in the three Toronto Presbyteries of the United Church of Canada (4 March 1926), Appeals Subject File #1; Crawford, *A History of the Hospital for Sick Children*, 22. For the promised provincial grant of $100,000, see Trustees Minutes, 1 September 1925, 8 September 1925, and 10 November 1925.

39 Trustees Minutes, 27 April 1926 and 5 June 1928; "Hospital Campaign Exceeds Objective with Huge Surplus," *The Globe*, 13 March 1926, 27; "Cry of Little Children Touches Human Hearts," *The Globe*, 10 March 1926, 11.

40 Trustees Minutes, 6 August 1929.

41 Trustees Minutes, 9 July 1935; AR 1929, 21; Trustees Minutes, 21 May 1931; "Crippled Children get Vote of $25,000," *The Globe*, 28 November 1931, 13. The Shriners regularly brought entertainment to the children at Thistletown. "Shriners Entertain Children at Home," *The Globe*, 9 July 1932, 11; "Clowns to Entertain Children in Hospital," *The Globe*, 15 November 1933, 15.

42 H.H. Williams, president of the hospital board of trustees, quoted in AR 1927, 7.

43 Trustees Minutes, 5 July 1927; "Sick Children's Home Cornerstone Laid," *Toronto Daily Star*, 5 July 1927; "Premier to Attend Hospital Opening," *Toronto Daily Star*, 23 October 1928, 14.

44 Trustees Minutes, 1 November 1927.

45 Trustees Minutes, 9 October 1928.

46 Trustees Minutes, 17 July 1928.

47 Paraphrased in "Hospital for Sick Children at Thistletown Officially Opened," *The Evening Telegram*, 25 October 1928. Thistletown Subject File #1, HSC Archives.

48 As quoted in "Hospital for Sick Children at Thistletown Officially Opened," *Evening Telegram*, 25 October 1928.

49 "It is somewhat difficult to name the generic style of architecture; specifically it has the Romanesque appearance with a suggestion of the French chateau." *The Hospital for Sick Children, College Street, Toronto; The Lakeside Home for Little Children, The Convalescent Branch of the Hospital on Gibraltar Point, Toronto Island: History of These Institutions, Toronto, Canada* (Toronto: 1891), 57–8.

50 Quotation "Children's Hospital Triumph of Science, Dr. Gallie Declares," *The Globe* 25 October 1928, 13. See Trustees Minutes, 4 December 1928; "Spacious Country Hospital For Suffering Little Ones Is Dream to Be Realized," *The Globe*, 5 July 1927, 9; Superintendent Joseph Bower to Dr. J.L. McDonald, Unsigned Memo, 26 October 1932, 5pp, Thistletown Subject File, HSC Archives.

51 Trustees Minutes, 26 October 1926; Trustees Minutes, 5 July 1927.

52 Crawford, *A History of the Hospital for Sick Children*, 23.

53 "Hospital for Sick Children at Thistletown Officially Opened," *Evening Telegram*, 25 October 1928. Thistletown Subject File #1, HSC Archives.

54 Crawford, *A History of the Hospital for Sick Children*, 34.

55 Kathleen S. Syme, R.N. P.H.N., Info Sheet, HSC Country Branch, Thistletown Subject File.

56 The Thistletown supervisor was directly responsible to the HSC General Superintendent. Trustees Minutes, 1 May 1928. Crawford, *A History of the Hospital for Sick Children*, 30.

57 Superintendent Joseph Bower to Dr. J.L. McDonald, Unsigned Memo, 26 October 1932, 1. Thistletown Subject File. Trustees Minutes, 8 January 1929.

58 Trustees Minutes, 31 July 1928.

59 AR 1929, 51.

60 Trustees Minutes, 19 March 1929; Trustees Minutes, 20 November 1928.

61 Trustees Minutes, 13 December 1927

62 Superintendent Joseph Bower to Dr. J.L. McDonald, Unsigned Memo, 26 October 1932, 5; Trustees Minutes, 28 May 1929 and 7 July 1931; Kathleen S. Syme, R.N. P.H.N., Info Sheet, HSC Country Branch, Thistletown Subject File.

63 It was planned to move the patients on Wednesday, 10 October 1928. Trustees Minutes, 9 October 1928. One sufferer of TB of the hip had attended Lakeside Home for the past three summers. "Island Patients in New Home at Thistletown," *Evening Telegram*, 3[?] October 1928.

64 Superintendent Joseph Bower to Dr. J.L. McDonald, Unsigned Memo (26 October 1932), 4. Thistletown Subject File, HSC Archives.

65 Bentzon, "Polio, The Hospital for Sick Children/Thistletown," 10, Polio Subject File, HSC Archives.

66 AR 1930, 12. H. Willenegger, "Troop Activity of the R.L.S. Troop," (c. 1930s) Boy Scouts and Girl Guides Subject File, HSC Archives. A Girl Guides troop was formed soon after. Discharged patients transitioned to new troops in the community. "Getting Well in the Country," *The Canadian Nurse* 31, no. 2 (1935): 57–8.

67 Bentzon, "Polio, The Hospital for Sick Children/Thistletown," 10, Polio Subject File, HSC Archives.

68 AR 1937, 52.

69 AR 1943, 43.

70 Gregory Clark, "Polio Fight: Childhood's Cruellest Enemy is Being Cornered By Canadian Medical Research," *The Standard,* 16 April 1949, 8. Polio Subject File, HSC Archives. See also AR 1930, 12.

71 Harvey Agnew, "The Care of Convalescent Patients," *Canadian Medical Association Journal* 26, no. 5 (1932): 597.

72 Quotation from Agnew, "The Care of Convalescent Patients," 596.

73 "Combine to Build Convalescent Home," *The Globe,* 27 October 1928, 23. The Anglican
Sisters of St. John the Divine undertook to open a convalescent hospital. "Rev. C.J.S. Stuart
Lauds Sisters' Work," *The Globe,* 22 November 1933, 11.

74 Crawford, *A History of the Hospital for Sick Children,* 44.

75 Trustees Minutes, 29 January 1935; Trustees Minutes, 30 June 1936.

76 Miss Doris Muckle, "Preliminary Student Experience, Introduction to Thistletown," 28
October 1948, 2 p, Thistletown Subject File, HSC Archives.

77 AR 1930, 29.

78 Ibid., 49.

79 Superintendent Joseph Bower to Dr. J.L. McDonald, Unsigned Memo (26 October 1932), 4,
Thistletown Subject File, HSC Archives. The 1929 Annual Report stated that the 112 beds had
been "continuously occupied" since the opening day. AR 1929, 10.

80 The Chairman's Address, AR 1933, 11.

81 At that time there were sixty-seven surgical patients. Superintendent Joseph Bower to Dr. J.L.
McDonald, Unsigned Memo (26 October 1932), 4, Thistletown Subject File, HSC Archives.

82 Anne Evans, quoted in Janice Tyrwhitt, "The Hospital Where Parents are Partners," *Reader's
Digest,* March 1975, 139, Parenting Subject File, HSC Archives.

83 Anonymous, interviewed by Judith Young, 21 March 1987, in possession of Judith Young.

84 Ruth McCamus, quoted in Sharon McKay, "From Birth to One. This Issue: Infants in
Hospital," *Today's Parent* (May 1987), 38, Parenting Subject File, HSC Archives.

85 Bentzon, "Polio, The Hospital for Sick Children/Thistletown," 4, Polio Subject File, HSC
Archives.

86 Alice Boxill to Director of Nursing Services, Boston Children's Hospital, re Parents Personal
Service, 15 July 1966. Letter obtained from Barbara Fox. File on the Psychosocial Care of
Children, in possession of Judith Young.

87 See Report of the Superintendent, AR 1931, and AR 1932, 26–7; MAB 30 September 1930.
This was reaffirmed 7 November 1930 after the trustees submitted another protocol that the
MAB deemed "impractical" because "it might forbid adequate treatment, which adequate
treatment would be carried out in the interest of the patient, and that the one so doing
would render himself liable to legal action."

88 MAB 4 December 1930.

89 Tanner, "Too Many Mothers?" 154.

90 W.H.R., "Out of the Iron Lung," (Toronto, 28 May 1952), 5, Polio Subject File, HSC Archives.

91 Details unstated. MAB 30 September 1930.

92 AR 1931, 26.

93 J.H.W. Bower, "General Outline of Duties of Follow-Up Nurse," 11 July 1930, 1, Parents
Personal Service (PPS) Subject File.

94 J.H.W. Bower, Original letter of reference, covering duties of follow up nurse in PPS, 11 July
1930, PPS Subject File Service, Blue Binder, Women's Auxiliary Boxes, Box 1, HSC Archives.

95 Alice Boxill to Director of Nursing Services, Boston Children's Hospital, re Parents Personal
Service, 15 July 1966. Letter obtained from Barbara Fox. File on the Psychosocial Care of
Children, in possession of Judith Young.

96 AR 1931, 27.

97 See, for example, John Bowlby, "Visiting in Children's Wards," letter to the editor, *The Lancet*
235, no. 6076 (1940): 291; H. Edelston, "Visiting in Children's Wards," letter to the editor, *The
Lancet* 235, no. 6078 (1940): 391; R.A. Spitz, "Hospitalism: An Inquiry into the Genesis of
Psychiatric Conditions in Early Childhood," *The Psychoanalytic Study of the Child* 1 (1945): 53–74;
"Children in Hospital," editorial comment, *Canadian Medical Association Journal* 74 (1956):
221; Philip E. Rothman, "A Note on Hospitalism," *Pediatrics* 30, no. 6 (1962): 995–9, http://
pediatrics.aappublications.org/content/30/6/995.full.pdf. Frank C.P. van der Horst and René

van der Veer, "Changing Attitudes towards the Care of Children in Hospital: A New Assessment of the Influence of the Work of Bowlby and Robertson in the UK, 1940–1970," *Attachment & Human Development* 11, no. 2 (2009): 119–42.

98   Young, "Changing Attitudes Towards Families of Hospitalized Children," 1424.

99   The film showed the experience of a two-year-old hospitalized for eight days, and the creators argued that her constant stress and "fretting" should not be accepted as normal, but should be studiously avoided. Lindsay, "'A 2-Year-Old Goes to Hospital,'" 17–26.

100 Young, "A 'Necessary Nuisance,'" 85.

101 Young, "Changing Attitudes Towards Families of Hospitalized Children," 1424.

102 Brown, "Preventive Paediatrics and its Relation to the General Practitioner," 520–1.

103 Lindsay, "'A 2-Year-Old Goes to Hospital,'" 20.

104 Lindsay, "Pariahs or Partners?," 121.

105 "Polio Hospital Empty, Suggest Home for Aged," *Toronto Daily Star,* 19 October 1956, 3; Bethune L. Smith (vice-chairman, board of trustees), Statement Issued re Sale of Thistletown, February 1957, Thistletown Subject File, HSC Archives; AR 1957, 10.

106 Chairman R.A. Laidlaw was approached about the possible sale of the country branch for use as a tuberculosis sanitarium for children. Trustees Minutes, 2 April 1951.

107 Trustees Minutes, 23 August 1951; Trustees Minutes, 12 November 1951.

108 Trustees Minutes, 24 November 1955.

109 Bethune L. Smith (vice-chairman, board of trustees) Statement Issued re Sale of Thistletown, February 1957, Thistletown Subject File, HSC Archives.

110 Florence Schill, "Centre for Disturbed Badly Needed," *Globe and Mail,* 20 February 1957; "Ontario Buys Thistletown Hospital," *Telegram,* 26 February 1957; "New Mental Hospital Planned for Children," *Globe and Mail,* 26 February 1957; all in Thistletown Subject File, HSC Archives.

111 Young, "A 'Necessary Nuisance,'" 96, 98.

112 Trustees Minutes, 31 May 1966; 28 June 1966; 25 September 1967.

113 See AR 1977–8 ("A Salute to Parents – Partners in Care"), 9; See WA Slide Presentation on the Parents' Post-Operative Service, Blue Binder, Women's Auxiliary Boxes, Box 1, HSC Archives.

9   THE RABBIT-WARREN

1   "A Worthy Cause," *Rouyn Noranda Press* PQ, 29 November 1949. In 1949 Scrapbook no. 2, 185, HSC Archives.

2   Brown forwarded this report to the trustees. The trustees merely responded that this was a common complaint in city hospitals at the time. MAB Minutes, 17 December 1937; Trustees Minutes, 4 January 1938.

3   "Amended Report as Proposed by the MAB to Submit to the Board of Trustees," (Report on the Condition of 67 College Street), 10 February 1944, with signatures of MAB, Hospital 5th Subject File, HSC Archives, 1.

4   Ibid., 2–6.

5   J. Stuart Crawford, *A History of The Hospital for Sick Children 1918 to 1958* (Toronto: HSC Archives, 1959), 36.

6   "Conditions in Existing O.P.D. Noted During Visits and comments by Miss Baxter and Others," (July 1946) in Binder, *Construction Plans,* quotations 67 and 69.

7   "Amended Report as Proposed by the MAB to Submit to the Board of Trustees," (Report on the Condition of 67 College Street), 10 February 1944, 2, Hospital 5th Subject File, HSC Archives.

8   Ibid.

9   Lawrence Solomon, *Toronto Sprawls: A History* (Toronto: University of Toronto Press, 2007), 17, 21.

10 Edward J. Chambers, "New Evidence on the Living Standards of Toronto Blue Collar Workers in the Pre-1914 Era," *Social History* 18, no. 36 (1986): 298.

11   Alan Brown, Report of the Physician-in-Chief, Annual Report 1942, 43. See also MAB Minutes, 13 May 1941.

12   "Report on the Condition of 67 College Street, 10 February 1944, Amended Report as proposed by the MAB to Submit to the Board of Trustees," with signatures of MAB (6 pp.), Hospital 5th Subject File, HSC Archives.

13   R.A. Laidlaw, Chairman's Address, AR 1942, 11.

14   Quotation AR 1943, 22. For medical staff shortages see A.B. LeMesurier, for Report of the Surgeon-in-Chief see AR 1943, 49; Crawford, *A History of The Hospital for Sick Children*, 55; AR 1945, 54.

15   AR 1943, 33; AR 1942, 40–1; "Hospital for Sick Children Makes Appeal for Nurses," *Globe and Mail*, 3 July 1945, 10; Jack Hambleton, "Schoolgirls Are Proving Capable Nurses' Aides," *Globe and Mail*, 5 July 1945, 11.

16   Trustees Minutes, Monthly Meeting, 11 May 1926; Crawford, *A History of The Hospital for Sick Children*, 27; Joseph H.W. Bower, "Serving Sick Children," reprint from *The Canadian Hospital* (Jan & Feb 1951): 3. Hospital 6th Subject File #3; James Govan, "The Hospital for Sick Children," reprint from *Royal Architectural Institute of Canada Journal* 28, no. 6 (1951): 5–6. Hospital 6th Subject File #3; Trustees Minutes, 9 June 1930; Superintendent Joseph Bower R. Laidlaw, "The Growth and Expansion of the Hospital for Sick Children," (Report on necessity of providing new city hospital), 12–14, 10 June 1938, Hospital 5th Subject File.

17   Pierre Berton, *The Great Depression: 1929–1939* (Toronto: Anchor Canada, 2001), quotation 31, 42.

18   Charis Cotter, *Toronto Between the Wars: Life in the City, 1919–1939* (Richmond Hill, ON: Firefly Books, 2004), 112.

19   James Struthers, *The Limits of Affluence: Welfare in Ontario, 1920–1970* (Toronto: University of Toronto Press, 1994), 92.

20   Berton, *The Great Depression*, 155.

21   Trustees Minutes, 15 November 1932; Gagan and Gagan, *For Patients of Moderate Means*; Crawford, *A History of The Hospital for Sick Children*, 40.

22   Trustees Minutes, 7 February 1933.

23   Trustees Minutes, 14 March 1932.

24   Bower, "The Growth and Expansion of the Hospital for Sick Children," (Report on necessity of providing new city hospital), 5, 10 June 1938, Hospital 5th Subject File.

25   [crossed out] "The Medical Advisory Board regrets that the Board of Trustees would debate the question of whether a Large City Hospital is necessary. A Large City Hospital is urgently required," MAB, 17 September 1936 (Bower to MAB, Report, Plans for New City Hospital); MAB 26 November 1936.

26   Trustees Minutes, 5 June 1934; J.S. Crawford, "The First Seventy-Five Years," *Bulletin of the HSC* 16, no. 4 (1964): 17 (Hospital 6th Subject File #5); See Trustees Minutes, 6 February 1945, 1 April 1947; Mary E. James, "In Seven Houses, Nurses Hope for Central Residence," *Globe and Mail*, 29 November 1949, 14.

27   Crawford, *A History of The Hospital for Sick Children*, 46.

28   Eva-lis Wuorio, "The Hospital Prayer Built," *Maclean's Magazine,* 1 February 1951, 21, 42.

29   Joseph Bower to R. Laidlaw, "The Growth and Expansion of the Hospital for Sick Children," (Report on necessity of providing new city hospital), 10 June 1938, 6, 10, Hospital 5th Subject File. Waiting lists grew. Between September 1935 and September 1936, there were averages of 14 medical, 66 surgical, and 35 nose and throat patients awaiting admission. Trustees Minutes, 22 September 1936. See also MAB Minutes, 17 December 1937.

30   AR 1937, 28.

31   "Hospital Campaign to Open June 18," *Globe and Mail,* 18 May 1945, 11. By 1949, the figures of 400 and even 800 patients waiting treatment were cited in newspapers, though one wonders whether the higher figure was used to bolster the campaign's impact. Jack Brehl, "'Always 800 Waiting' Sick Children's Needs $4,000,000 for Building," *Toronto Daily Star,* 17

November 1949, 1, 10; "Hospital Needs $4,000,000 as 800 Children Waiting," *Toronto Daily Star,* 18 November 1949, 12.

32 Trustees Minutes, 15 May 1934 and 20 April 1937, inter alia; Joseph Bower, "Report to Board on Site for New Hospital," 12 March 1937 (31 pp.), Hospital 6th Subject File #2.

33 Trustees Minutes, 13 April 1937, 20 April 1937, 25 May 1937, 1 June 1937, 13 September 1938, and 22 November 1938; Joseph Bower, "Report to Board on Site for New Hospital." A transportation study of 474 individuals revealed that 65 per cent of patients walked one block or more to take the streetcar to the hospital, 25 per cent of patients walked the entire way, and 10 per cent drove (34).

34 Quotation from Trustees Minutes, Special Meeting, 29 February 1944; See Trustees Minutes, 13 April 1937, 20 April 1937, 25 May 1937, 29 November 1938, and 29 April 1942.

35 Lesley Marrus Barsky, *From Generation to Generation* (Toronto: McClelland and Stewart, 1998), 49–53, quotation 52–3. The situation was recapitulated, and illustrated by a map, in "Ask City for $300,000 for Hospital," *Toronto Daily Star,* 15 June 1944, 18.

36 Trustees Minutes, 8 February 1944 and Trustees Minutes, Special Meeting, RE: Question of New Hospital Site, 29 February 1944.

37 Alan Brown, "Memorial to the Late Dr. D.E. Robertson," read before the Faculty of Medicine, 6 April 1944, (DE Robertson Subject File) published in AR 1944, HSC Archives.

38 Allison Brown Kingsmill, *Portrait of a Tyrant* (Markham, ON: Fitzhenry & Whiteside for Associated Medical Services and The Hannah Institute for the History of Medice, 1995), 94–5, 204n42 (interview with Dr. J.J. Slavens), 204n40. See also A.I. Willinsky, *A Doctor's Memoirs* (Toronto: Macmillan, 1960), 83–5.

39 Barsky, *From Generation to Generation,* 5; Trustees Minutes, 23 May 1944. To help negotiations with Mount Sinai, in February 1945 HSC purchased the Fasken Property on University Avenue for $34,000. Trustees Minutes, 6 February 1945.

40 Trustees Minutes, 11 January 1938, 27 December 1938, 14 February 1939, 10 March 1939, 24 March 1939, 5 June 1945, 25 June 1945, and 17 July 1945.

41 Quotation *Minute Book, Hospital for Sick Children, New Hospital,* 20 March 1944, 993.011–001. See Minutes of the Sub-Committee of the Board of Trustees, 1 March 1944, and Organization Committee Minutes, 20 March 1944, *Minute Book, Hospital for Sick Children, New Hospital,* 993.011–001; "New Noranda Director," *Toronto Star,* 30 January 1942, 16; "Norman C. Urquhart on Red Cross Board," *Toronto Star,* 21 April 1944, 2; "Market Sidelights," *Toronto Star,* 2 January 1942, 13; Norman C. Urquhart, Chairman, Royal Ontario Mining Commission, *Report of the Royal Ontario Mining Commission* (Toronto, 1944).

42 "Employee Committees Take Hold," editorial, *Globe and Mail,* 20 June 1945, 6; "Magnificent Response by Firms for Hospital," *Globe and Mail,* 20 June 1945, 15; "Firms Assisting Hospital Drive Reach New High," *Globe and Mail,* 22 June 1945, 15.

43 "A Plea to Mining Hearts," *Northern Miner,* 22 December 1949.

44 Quotation "Small Gifts are Needed," editorial, *Globe and Mail,* 28 June 1945, 6. See "Employees Plunge Into Collecting To Help Hospital," *Globe and Mail,* 28 June 1945, 15; "Packers' Staff Donations Mount In Hospital Drive," *Globe and Mail,* 4 July 1945, 7; "General Canvass In Firms Is Best Way to Aid Fund," *Globe and Mail,* 3 July 1945, 13.

45 "Union Support of Hospital Drive Asked by Leader," *Globe and Mail,* 19 June 1945, 4.

46 "Subscriptions Total $2,899,688.91," *Globe and Mail,* 23 June 1945, 15; "Small Gifts are Needed," editorial, *Globe and Mail,* 28 June 1945, 6.

47 "A Magnificent Achievement," *Globe and Mail,* 6 August 1945, 6. In total, the campaign raised $7,452,413.39. J.S. Crawford, "The First Seventy-Five Years," 18.

48 Report of the Property Committee to the Board of Trustees, Trustees Minutes, 15 April 1952.

49 "Remarks by J.G. Glassco at the laying of the cornerstone of the HSC," 22 April 1949 (8 pp.), Hospital 6th Subject File #3.

50 "Fact Sheet for Hospital for Sick Children Building Fund Campaign," (c. 194-?), Campaign Folder, R.A. Laidlaw Fonds, HSC Archives.

51 Interim Report of the Building Committee to the Board of Trustees, appended to Trustees Minutes, 4 February 1947. The children's hospital in Alberta experienced the same challenge when attempting to construct a new building, opened in March 1951. Arty Coppes-Zantinga and Ian Mitchell, *The Child in the Centre: 75 Years at the Alberta Children's Hospital* (Calgary: University of Calgary Press, 1997), 105–7.

52 Report of the Property Committee to the Board of Trustees, Trustees Minutes, 15 April 1952; Bethune L. Smith and J. Grant Glassco, Confidential, Report to the Board of Trustees on the Activities of the Building Committee, Trustees Minutes, 12 December 1947.

53 "Hospital Needs $4,000,000 as 800 Children Waiting," *Toronto Daily Star,* 18 November 1949, 12; MAB Minutes, 10 April 1946.

54 Jack Brehl, "Even Leave Doors off to Cut Hospital Cost Still Short $593,633," *Toronto Daily Star,* 31 December 1949, 1, 2.

55 Trustees Minutes, 19 June 1947.

56 See image in Mike Filey, *A Toronto Album 2: More Glimpses of the City That Was* (Toronto: Dundurn Press, 2002), 84. For context, see Sean Purdy, "'It Was Tough on Everybody': Low-Income Families and Housing Hardship in Post-World War II Toronto," *Journal of Social History* 37, no. 2 (2003): 457–82; Kevin Brushett, "Where will the People Go: Toronto's Emergency Housing Program and the Limits of Canadian Social Housing Policy, 1944–1957," *Journal of Urban History* 33, no. 3 (2007): 375–99; Humphrey Carver, *Houses for Canadians: A Study of Housing Problems in the Toronto Area* (Toronto: University of Toronto Press, 1948).

57 Trustees Minutes, 5 May 1947; "Trailer Colony Action Deferred," *Globe and Mail* 21 November 1945, 4; "Legal Actions Face Trailerites On Hospital Site," *Globe and Mail,* 30 May 1947, 5.

58 Quotation in "Furniture Moved Out While University Ave Folk Plead Case," *Toronto Daily Star,* 8 October 1947, 2. See "100 Trailerites to Fight Downtown Camp Loss," *Globe and Mail,* 24 April 1947, 5; "57 Families Protest Order to Vacate Site of Hospital," *Toronto Daily Star,* 19 May 1947, 3; "Child Death Jury Deplores Play on Streets," *Globe and Mail,* 22 August 1946, 5; "Trailer Families Will be Housed At Long Branch," *Globe and Mail,* 22 May 1947, 5; "Boulevard Before Barracks Home, Says Trailerite," *Globe and Mail,* 2 July 1947, 5; "Trailerites May Set New Site Next Week," *Globe and Mail,* 31 October 1947, 5.

59 Trustees Minutes, 12 December 1947.

60 Trustees Minutes, 5 May 1947, 19 June 1947, 9 August 1949, and 5 December 1949; Bethune L. Smith and J. Grant Glassco, Confidential, Report to the Board of Trustees on the Activities of the Building Committee, included in Trustees Minutes, 12 December 1947; Gordon L. Wallace and Clare D. Carruthers, "Outline of Structure," reprint from *Royal Architectural Institute of Canada Journal* 28, no. 6 (1951): 24–5, Subject File, Hospital 6th, #3.

61 "Laborers Vote For Strike Action In Building Trade," *Globe and Mail,* 29 April 1949, 5; "Laborers Set Deadline, May Halt City Building: Will Picket Every Job In Toronto," *Globe and Mail,* 3 May 1949, 1; "Toronto Building Strike May Be Settled Today: Expect Work Will Resume Next Monday," *Globe and Mail,* 26 May 1949, 1; Trustees Minutes, 15 April 1952.

62 Remarks by J.G. Glassco at the laying of the cornerstone of the HSC, 22 April 1949, 8 pp. Hospital 6th Subject File #3; Trustees Minutes, 2 May 1949; "250 Attend Ceremony Despite Driving Rain," *Globe and Mail* 23 April 1949, 17; "At Hospital Since Opening Helps As New One Started," *Toronto Daily Star,* 20 April 1949, 2.

63 "Chartered Banks Clearing Posts in Hospital Drive," *Toronto Daily Star,* 22 November 1949, 9; "Had Humble Start Need New Building for Sick Children," *Toronto Daily Star,* 12 December 1949, 1. By the third week, three quarters was raised ($3,110,750.85). "Hospital Research Defeats Diseases But Task Unending," *Toronto Daily Star,* 22 December 1949, 1.

64 "Where No Child Knocks in Vain," editorial, *Globe and Mail,* 10 December 1949, 1.

65 Jack Brehl, "Need $320,000 Daily if Hospital to Reach Goal of $4,000,000," *Toronto Daily Star,* 30 December 1949, 1; J.W. Cochrane, "Administration, Resume of Preparation for 1949 Campaign," 2 May 1950, Campaign Folder, R.A. Laidlaw Fonds; "$100,000 Eaton gift

assures hospital fund of its $4,000,000 goal," *Toronto Daily Star,* 6 January 1950, 1, 3; Trustees Minutes, 12 September 1949, 6 February 1950, and 6 March 1950. As of July 1951, after the hospital's opening, there was an overdraft of $200,000 in building fund account (Trustees Minutes, 23 July 1951). As of August 1951, this amount stood at $451,000 (Trustees Minutes, 23 August 1951). J.W. Cochrane, Chairman, "Administration, Resume of Preparation for 1949 Campaign," 2 May 1950, Campaign Folder, Laidlaw Fonds, HSC Archives.

66 Lester Velie, "'The Sick Kids' – A Share and a Prayer," *Colliers,* 22 July 1950, 24–5, 36–7. Hospital 6th Subject File #3; "The New 'Sick Kids,'" *The Star Weekly,* 9 December 1950, 2. Boston Children's Hospital undertook a similar campaign for $11,500,000 in the spring of 1949, but struggled to raise even half of that amount ($6,500,000), forcing the institution to scale back its plans for a new building, from twelve to eight floors. See also, "Children's Hospital Construction Expected to Begin Early in 1950," *Daily Boston Globe,* 12 December 1949, 4. "Legislature Adopts Measure Urging Hospital Fund Aid," *Daily Boston Globe,* 26 May 1949, 10.

67 John Brehl, "Wide Area of Service Typified as Patients Open New Hospital," *Toronto Star,* 13 January 1951, 2.

68 Ken MacTaggart, "Steal the Show: Six Children Open Doors Of Hospital," *Globe and Mail,* 16 January 1951, 13.

69 Ken MacTaggart, "Hospital to Be Opened By Six Small Patients," *Globe and Mail,* 13 January 1951, 15.

70 "Celebrities for a Day," photograph (photo standalone 1, no title), *Globe and Mail,* 16 January 1951, 1.

71 In Minutes, Meeting of tours and organization re opening of new hospital, 14 November 1950, "Opening" Folder, R.A. Laidlaw Fonds.

72 J.W. Cochrane to W.C. Harris, memo, 16 November 1950, Hospital 6th Subject File #3.

73 Quotation in "Successful 'Open House,'" editorial, *Globe and Mail,* 22 January 1951, 6; J.S. Crawford, "The First Seventy-Five Years," 19.

74 "Hospital 'Wishing Well' Yields 800 Lbs. Coins," *Telegram,* February 1951, clipping, Hospital 6th Subject File #3.

75 Report of the HSC Property Committee to the Board of Trustees, Trustees Minutes, 15 April 1952. James Govan, "The Hospital for Sick Children," reprint from *Royal Architectural Institute of Canada Journal* 28, no. 6 (1951): 5–6. 67 College Street could accommodate 190 patients, and, with extensions and Thistletown, came to a total of 320 beds. Bower, "Serving Sick Children," 32.

76 Bower, "Serving Sick Children," 6.

77 Report of the Property Committee to the Board of Trustees, Trustees Minutes, 15 April 1952.

78 Bower, "Serving Sick Children," 4–8.

79 "Special Features in New Hospital," *Canadian Hotel Review and Restaurant,* 15 March 1951, 18, Hospital 6th Subject File #2; Edith B. Toland, "Where No Child Knocks in Vain," *Hydro News* (Toronto), May 1951, 8–12, Hospital 6th Subject File #4.; G.D. Wilson, "The Use of Shielding in Hospital Construction," *Hospital Administration in Canada* 6, no. 10 (1964): 27. Hospital 6th Subject File #2, HSC Archives.

80 J.C. Montgomery, "Color Therapy for the Kids," *Canadian Hotel Review and Restaurant,* 15 March 1951, 16, 28, Hospital 6th, Subject File #2, HSC Archives.

81 H.S. Parish, "Refrigeration in Toronto's Hospital for Sick Children," *Canadian Refrigeration Journal,* May 1951, 17–19.

82 Charles Coady, "Transfer Tiny Patients to $12,500,000 Hospital in Clockwork Manner," *Toronto Daily Star,* 4 February 1951, 23.

83 Anonymous oral interview by author, participant #12, 12 December 2013.

84 75th Anniversary Dinner Program (1961), 10. Nursing School Subject File #10 (Anniversary 1961), HSC Archives.

85 "The Women's Auxiliary," *Hospital for Sick Children News* 1, no. 1 (1960), 3.

86 See, inter alia, Veronica Strong-Boag, "Their Side of the Story: Women's Voices from Ontario Suburbs, 1945–60," in *A Diversity of Women: Ontario, 1945–1980,* ed. Joy Parr (Toronto: University of Toronto Press, 1995), 47.

87 Dr. A.L. Chute quoted in Joanne Strong, "The Informal Dean Chute," *Globe and Mail,* 2 April 1973, 8. See also Kingsmill, *Dr. Alan Brown,* 61; Carlotta Hacker, *The Indomitable Lady Doctors* (Toronto: Clarke, Irwin & Company Limited, 1974), 213–14; MAB Minutes, 8 January 1936, 11 January 1937 (Helen Reid, Dorothy Tebbe), 22 January 1937 (5 total, including Dorothy Tebbe, Frances Mulligan, and Genevieve Delfs).

88 Henry B.M. Best, *Margaret and Charley: The Personal Story of Dr. Charles Best, The Co-Discoverer of Insulin* (Toronto: Dundurn Press, 2003), 163. For Reid's biography, see Rose Sheinin and Alan Bakes, *Women in Medicine in Toronto Since 1883: A Who's Who* (Toronto: University of Toronto Press, 1987), 81.

89 Leone Kirkwood, "Some Thoughts on Passing 40," *Globe and Mail,* 2 February 1967, W1.

90 Quotation Leone Kirkwood, "Some Thoughts on Passing 40," W1; Joan Hollobon, "Doctor Helps Scientists Say What They Think," *Globe and Mail,* 25 April 1968, W3.

91 Women's Auxiliary (hereafter WA) Minute Book, 8 March 1950-May 1955, Minutes of 8 March 1950, WA Box 1, HSC Archives.

92 As quoted in Max Braithwaite, *Sick Kids: The Story of the Hospital for Sick Children in Toronto* (Toronto: McClelland and Stewart, 1974), 1121. The official auxiliary minutes state only that Glassco "suggested that one of [the] primary objects might be the organization of toys and materials for recreation for the children in the new hospital." WA Minutes, 19 April 1950. Minute Book, Box 1, HSC Archives. See also Anne MacInnis "50 Years of Caring" (History of the WA, 2000, 2 pp); WA Minutes, 28 April 1950, Box 118, HSC Archives.

93 Quotation Trustees Minutes, 23 October 1950. See WA Minutes, 19 April 1950 and 28 April 1950, Box 118, HSC Archives.

94 WA Minutes, 19 April 1950. Minute Book, Box 1, HSC Archives; "HSC Women's Auxiliary Reports Successful Year," *Globe and Mail,* 22 May 1953, 15; Anne MacInnis, "50 Years of Caring" (History of the WA, 2000, 2 pp); "Hold Open House: HSC Volunteer Tasks Increase," *Globe and Mail,* 25 October 1957, 12; Jean Baker, "New Fields for Hospital WA," *Globe and Mail,* 23 March 1962, 10.

95 "Doctors, Nurses, Guides, To Greet Hospital Visitors," *Globe and Mail,* 5 January 1951, 12.

96 Braithwaite, *Sick Kids,* 121; Mona Purser, "The Homemaker," *Globe and Mail,* 13 November 1950, 15; WA Minutes, 8 January 1951 and 21 February 1951.

97 Quotation WA Minutes, 23 November 1951, Box 118, HSC Archives; Trustees Minutes, 12 November 1951.

98 Trustees Minutes, 26 November 1951 and 27 October 1958; Anne MacInnis, "50 Years of Caring" (History of the WA, 2000, 2 pp).

99 Quotation "HSC Women's Auxiliary Reports Successful Year," *Globe and Mail,* 22 May 1953, 15. See WA Minutes, 21 February 1951, Box 1, HSC Archives; "HSC Auxiliary Fills Sewing Needs," *Globe and Mail,* 27 October 1954, 15; "HSC Auxiliary Reviews Projects," *Globe and Mail,* 28 May 1954, 17.

100 Anonymous oral interview by author, participant #8, 29 January 2014.

101 Trustees Minutes, 19 May 1952. See also "HSC Women's Auxiliary Reports Successful Year," *Globe and Mail,* 22 May 1953, 15; "WA Presents $9,000 Cheque To Hospital," *Globe and Mail,* 23 May 1957, 14; "Four Nursing Scholarships Offered," *Globe and Mail,* 25 February 1960, 15; "New Shop To Be Opened At Hospital," *Globe and Mail,* 25 February 1965, W2; "Gift of $11,800: WA Helps New Hospital Projects," *Globe and Mail,* 22 May 1958, 18.

102 "$15,000 WA Cheque Benefits Sick Children," *Globe and Mail,* 28 February 1963, 21; John T. Law, "The Director's Corner," *Paediatric Patter* 4, no. 5 (1963): 2; "Women's Auxiliary Grows At Sick Children's Hospital," *Globe and Mail,* 29 May 1952, 12.

103 "Hold Open House: HSC Volunteer Tasks Increase," *Globe and Mail,* 25 October 1957, 12.

104 Mary E. James, "Tender, Loving Care: Nurses at Hospital for Sick Children Have Extra Duties," *Globe and Mail,* 1 December 1955, 21.

105 "Gift of $11,800: WA Helps New Hospital Projects," *Globe and Mail,* 22 May 1958, 18. See also Polly Thompson, "Mary Bailey: 60 Years of Service to Children and Families at the Hospital for Sick Children," *Smock Talk* (WA Newsletter), Fall 2013, 3. Repr. "Two Weeks"; "HSC Auxiliary Reviews Projects," *Globe and Mail,* 28 May 1954, 17.

106 "Hold Open House: HSC Volunteer Tasks Increase," 12; WA Minutes, 10 May 1951.

107 Trustees Minutes, 23 March 1959 [date of project approval]; "Auxiliary Gives Hospital $14,106," *Globe and Mail,* 21 May 1959, 14; "$15,000 WA Cheque Benefits Sick Children," *Globe and Mail,* 28 February 1963, 21; "WA Gives $6,000 to Hospital," *Globe and Mail,* 27 May 1960, 13; "Projects Approved by Women's Auxiliary," *Paediatric Patter* 4, no. 8 (1963): 1; "Volunteer and Recreation Department," *Paediatric Patter* 5, no. 2 (1964): 3; AR 1964, 6.

108 John T. Law, "The Director's Corner," *Paediatric Patter* 4, no. 5 (1963): 2. See also Jane Baker, "New Fields for Hospital WA," *Globe and Mail,* 23 March 1962, 10.

109 Campaign Committee Meeting Minutes, 21 November 1950 in "Opening" Folder, R.A. Laidlaw Fonds, HSC Archives.

110 Dr. Nelles Silverthorne, "My Most Unforgettable Character," *Readers' Digest,* April 1962, 92–100.

111 "Meet the Staff," *Paediatric Patter* 3, no. 5 (1962): 2; Kay Kritzwiser, "The Toronto Clubwoman: Is She a Do-Gooder, a Busybody, or Does She Play a Vital Role in the Community?" *Globe and Mail,* 7 February 1963, 13.

112 "Young Patients Are Opening 'Officials,'" *Telegram,* 16 January 1951. See also C.A. Sage, 2 April 1951, To Board of Trustees, Re February Statement Folder – Finance Committee, R.A. Laidlaw Fonds.

113 "The New Hospital for Sick Children," *Toronto Calling,* January 1951, 10–11. "They all speak wistfully of the great 'family feeling' in the old Hospital, the friendliness of the place. The feeling that you knew everyone and they knew you. 'At first,' one doctor commented wistfully, 'it just seemed you couldn't find anybody or anything'" (Braithwaite, *Sick Kids,* 124).

114 Trustees Minutes, 4 December 1950 and 8 January 1951.

10 BLUE BABIES

1 Anonymous interview by author, participant #12, 26 March 2014. See also the recollection in Hilda Rolstin, *History of the School of Nursing, The Hospital for Sick Children* (Toronto: Alumnae Association, 1972), 30.

2 John E. Lesch, *The First Miracle Drugs: How the Sulfa Drugs Transformed Medicine* (Oxford: Oxford University Press, 2007), 3 and passim.

3 Shorter, *Partnership for Excellence,* 180–1.

4 In particular, streptococcal septicaemia, streptococcal meningitis, and streptococcal peritonitis.

5 Nelles Silverthorne, Alan Brown, and W.J. Auger, "Sulphanilamide and Sulphapyridine in the Treatment of Disease in Children," *Canadian Medical Association Journal* 41, no. 1 (1939): 16–21, http://www.ncbi.nlm.nih.gov/pmc/articles/PMC537305/pdf/canmedaj00206-0025.pdf.

6 D.E. Robertson, "The Medical Treatment of Hematogenous Osteomyelitis," *Annals of Surgery* 118, no. 2 (1943): 322; Mark M. Ravitch, "The American Surgical Association: The Peaks of Excitement," *Annals of Surgery* 192, no. 3 (1980): 282–7.

7 Edward Corrigan, *Tales of a Forgotten Theatre* (Winnipeg: D. Day Publishers, 1969), 45–7; Joanne Strong, "The Informal Dean Chute," *Globe and Mail,* 2 April 1973, 8.

8 Shorter, *Partnership for Excellence,* 464.

9 "Toronto Studies on Penicillin," editorial, *Canadian Medical Association Journal* 49, no. 5 (1943): 422–3.

10 Shorter, *Partnership for Excellence,* 464.

11 Harry M. Marks, *The Progress of Experiment: Science and Therapeutic Reform in the United States, 1900–1990* (Cambridge: Cambridge University Press, 2000), 106.

12 Nelles Silverthorne, "Penicillin in the Treatment of Haemolytic Staphylococcal Septicaemia," *Canadian Medical Association Journal* 49, no. 6 (1943): 516–17, http://www.ncbi.nlm.nih.gov/pmc/articles/PMC1828022/pdf/canmedaj01709-0148.pdf.

13 "Aldershot Girl is Improved by Penicillin," *Globe and Mail*, 17 August 1943, 20.

14 Trustees Minutes, 3 October, 1944. Bower advised an increase to a flat $3.50 per day, with additional charges for blood transfusions and penicillin.

15 MAB Minutes, 8 November 1944, 1 November 1945, and 16 December 1946.

16 Empyema is a collection of pus within a naturally existing anatomical cavity.

17 Bethune L. Smith (vice-chairman, board of trustees), "Statement Issued RE Sale of Thistletown," February 1957, Thistletown Subject File, HSC Archives.

18 AR 1946, 18.

19 The prize, one of which became controversial in terms of scientific credit, was awarded in 1952. See Milton Wainwright, "Streptomycin: Discovery and Resultant Controversy," *History and Philosophy of the Life Sciences* 13, no. 1 (1991): 97–124; William Kingston, "Streptomycin, Schatz v. Waksman, and the Balance of Credit for Discovery," *Journal of the History of Medicine and Allied Sciences* 59, no. 3 (2004): 441–62; Milton Wainwright, "A Response to William Kingston, 'Streptomycin, Schatz v. Waksman, and the Balance of Credit for Discovery,'" *Journal of the History of Medicine and Allied Sciences* 60, no. 2 (2005): 218–20; Albert Schatz, "The True Story of the Discovery of Streptomycin," *Actinomycetes* 4, no. 2 (1993): 27–39.

20 Wainwright, "Streptomycin," 106–9; Albert Schatz, Elizabeth Bugle, and Selman A. Waksman, "Streptomycin, a Substance Exhibiting Antibiotic Activity Against Gram-Positive and Gram-Negative Bacteria," *Experimental Biology and Medicine* 55, no. 1 (1944): 66–9.

21 Katherine McCuaig, *The Weariness, the Fever, and the Fret: The Campaign Against Tuberculosis in Canada, 1900–1950* (Montreal: McGill-Queen's University Press, 1999), 197.

22 Annmarie Adams, Kevin Schwartzman, and David Theodore, "Collapse and Expand: Architecture and Tuberculosis Therapy in Montreal, 1909, 1933, 1954," *Technology and Culture* 49, no. 4 (2008): 908–42, 929.

23 Geoffrey Reaume, *Lyndhurst: Canada's First Rehabilitation Centre for People with Spinal Cord Injuries, 1945–1998* (Montreal: McGill-Queen's University Press, 2007), 42.

24 "Distribution of Streptomycin," editorial comments, *Canadian Medical Association Journal* 55, no. 3 (1946): 298.

25 "Streptomycin," editorial comments, *Canadian Medical Association Journal* 56, no. 2 (1947): 215.

26 McCuaig, *The Weariness, the Fever, and the Fret*, 197, 221.

27 Gladys L. Boyd, "Streptomycin in Childhood Tuberculosis," *Canadian Medical Association Journal* 60, no. 5 (1949): 480.

28 Nelles Silverthorne, "Meningitis in Childhood," *Canadian Medical Association Journal* 58, no. 3 (1948): 256–7.

29 Charlotte Burt, "An Older Nurse Looks Back," *Paediatric Patter* 8, no. 6 (1967): 2, 9.

30 Nelles Silverthorne, "Meningitis in Childhood," *Canadian Medical Association Journal* 58, no. 3 (1948): 257, 255–8.

31 McCuaig, *The Weariness, the Fever, and the Fret*, 221.

32 George Jasper Wherrett, *The Miracle of the Empty Beds: A History of Tuberculosis in Canada* (Toronto: University of Toronto Press, 1977), 46.

33 Christopher J. Rutty, "The Middle-Class Plague: Epidemic Polio and the Canadian State, 1936–37," *Canadian Bulletin of Medical History* 13 no. 2 (1996): 248; Christopher Rutty, "'Do Something! ... Do Anything!,'" 209–12, 291–329.

34 Luis Barreto, Rob Van Exan, and Christopher J. Rutty, "Polio Vaccine Development in Canada: Contributions to Global Polio Eradication," *Biologicals* 34 (2006): 92–4; see also Paul Bator and Andrew James Rhodes, *Within Reach of Everyone: A History of the University of Toronto School of Hygiene and the Connaught Laboratories*, vol. 1 (Ottawa: Canadian Public Health Association, 1990).

35 Heather MacDougall, *Activists and Advocates: Toronto's Health Department, 1883–1983* (Toronto: Dundurn Press, 1990), 152–7.

36 Doug Owram, *Born at the Right Time: A History of the Baby Boom Generation* (Toronto: University of Toronto Press, 1997).

37 AR 1946, Alan Brown, Report of the Physician-in-Chief, 29.

38 William Mustard, interviewed by Valerie Schatzker (AMS Interviews, U of T Faculty of Medicine), 19 August 1981–12 September 1981, HSC Archives, 130.

39 Ibid., 12, 131.

40 A.W. Farmer interviewed by Valerie Schatzker (AMS Interviews, U of T Faculty of Medicine), March–April 1979, HSC Archives, 60–1.

41 William Mustard, interviewed by Valerie Schatzker (AMS Interviews, U of T Faculty of Medicine), 19 August 1981–12 September 1981, HSC Archives, 12.

42 AR 1921, 19.

43 Maude Abbott, *Atlas of Congenital Cardiac Disease* (New York: American Heart Association, 1936).

44 AR 1922, 24–5; AR 1925, 28; AR 1938, 46, inter alia.

45 Hugh O'Brodovich, with the assistance of Elizabeth Uleryk, Susan Belanger, Daune MacGregor, and Michelle O'Brodovich, *Doctors Who Care for the Future: The History of Medical Care at Toronto's Hospital for Sick Children* (December 2008, unpublished manuscript, Hospital for Sick Children Archives), 89.

46 Contemporaries tend to contrast Keith and Mustard: "He [Mustard] had a puckish sense of humour, and was one of the few people prepared to pull John Keith's leg, which was not an easy thing to do when John was in his dour Scottish mood." Peter M. Olley, Arnold L. Johnson, and Robert Beamish, "Lest We Forget: Canadian Contributions to the Care of Children With Congenital Heart Malformations," *Canadian Journal of Cardiology* 17, no. 6 (2001): 705–9.

47 Joan Hollobon, "Gairdner Awards to Canadians: 30 Years of Saving Babies Honored," *Globe and Mail*, 30 October 1975, F10. See J. H. Gardiner and John D. Keith, "Prevalence of Heart Disease in Toronto Children: 1948–1949 Cardiac Registry," *Pediatrics* 7 (1951): 713–21.

48 For recording data he had devised a four-page folded sheet with a striped right edge that became known as his zebra form. There were separate zebra forms for clinical findings, catheterization, and post-op information. These sheets were easily recognizable in the hospital chart and were filed in a separate cardiac records room in the cardiology division. Information from these sheets was coded and punched into cards that could then be sorted and collated. Anonymous interview by author, participant #15, 26 May 2014, Hospital for Sick Children.

49 AR 1947, 24.

50 Joan Hollobon, "Survey Tracks Heart Disease in Children," *Globe and Mail*, 3 August 1964, 4.

51 AR 1946, 35.

52 Shelley McKellar, *Surgical Limits: The Life of Gordon Murray* (Toronto: University of Toronto Press, 2003), 53–6; "Rare, Dangerous Operation Returns Child to Normal Life," *Globe and Mail*, 4 May 1940, 3.

53 McKellar, *Surgical Limits*, 56.

54 "A congenital malformation of the heart characterized by a defect in the ventricular septum, misplacement of the origin of the aorta, narrowing of the pulmonary artery, and enlargement of the right ventricle. Also called Fallot's tetrad, *tetralogy of Fallot*." *The American Heritage Medical Dictionary* (Boston: Houghton Mifflin, 2007), s.v. "Fallot's tetralogy."

55 Tetralogy of Fallot was the most common cyanotic heart malformation, and transposition of the great vessels the second. McKellar, *Surgical Limits*, 57.

56 "Long Branch Blue Baby Sure Of Life-Saving Operation," *Globe and Mail*, 24 December 1945, 4. "Two More 'Blue' Babies Come to Johns Hopkins for Relief," *Washington Post*, 25 January 1946, 14; "Vancouver's Blue Baby 'Janet' en Route to Baltimore Hospital," *Globe and Mail*, 23 April 1946, 4.

57 McKellar, *Surgical Limits,* 58–9. The next survived: "Toronto Doctor Gives Blue Baby 'New Heart,'" *Globe and Mail,* 4 July 1946, 5; "Boy, 18, a Former 'Blue Baby,' Dies as Parents Rush to Side," *Globe and Mail,* 4 November 1946, 4.

58 McKellar, *Surgical Limits,* 61–4. For example: "B.C. Miner's 'Blue Baby' in Toronto for Operation," *Globe and Mail,* 24 January 1947, 5; "Blue Baby Treatments on 'Assembly Line' Basis," *Globe and Mail,* 1 March 1947, 5; "Scottish-Born Blue Baby To Be Operated On Here," *Globe and Mail,* 6 June 1947, 4.

59 William Mustard, interviewed by Valerie Schatzker (AMS Interviews, U of T Faculty of Medicine), 19 August 1981–12 September 1981, HSC Archives, 71–5.

60 Hollobon, "Gairdner Awards to Canadians," F10.

61 Olley, Johnson, and Beamish, "Lest We Forget," 707; Kelly Ivers, "'Incredible' Technique Explores Babies' Hearts: 'Blue Baby' Operations Increase in Toronto," *Globe and Mail,* 17 December 1947, 3.

62 James Y. Nicol, "Study Heart in Action with Cinematic X-Ray," *Globe and Mail,* 25 May 1948, 5.

63 McKellar, *Surgical Limits, 64.*

64 Shafie Fazel, William G. Williams, and Bernard S. Goldman, "Thinned Blood, Monkey Lungs, and the Cold Heart," *Surgical History* 19, no. 3 (2004): 278; Marilyn Dunlop, *Bill Mustard: Surgical Pioneer* (Toronto: Dundurn Press for the Hannah Institute for the History of Medicine, 1989), 56.

65 Shorter, *Partnership for Excellence,* 95–6, 765n104; W.G. Bigelow, W.T. Mustard, and J.G. Evans, "Some Physiologic Concepts of Hypothermia and Their Applications to Cardiac Surgery," *Journal of Thoracic Surgery* 28, no. 5 (1954): 463–80.

66 "Toronto M.D.'s Report Success in Operation on 'Frozen' Hearts," *Toronto Daily Star,* 15 May 1954, 28b, 52.

67 Andreas P. Naef, "The Mid-Century Revolution in Thoracic and Cardiovascular Surgery: Part 4," *Interactive Cardiovascular and Thoracic Surgery* 3, no. 2 (2004): 213.

68 Dunlop, *Bill Mustard,* 53. See Campbell Cowan, "Physiological Perfusion Pump," *Journal of Applied Physiology* 4, no. 8 (1952): 695–7.

69 Ibid.

70 W.T. Mustard and A.L. Chute, "Experimental Intracardial Surgery with Extracorporeal Circulation," *Surgery* 30, no. 4 (1951): 684–8.

71 William Mustard, interviewed by Valerie Schatzker (AMS Interviews, U of T Faculty of Medicine), 19 August 1981–12 September 1981, HSC Archives, 14, 84.

72 Mustard and Chute, "Experimental Intracardial Surgery," 684–8.

73 "Use Monkey Lung to Keep Babies Alive for Surgery – U of T Doctor," *Toronto Daily Star,* 19 April 1952, 1.

74 W.T. Mustard, A.L. Chute, J.D. Keith, A. Sirek, R.D. Rowe, and P. Vlad, "A Surgical Approach to Transposition of the Great Vessels with Extracorporeal Circuit," *Surgery* 36, no. 1 (1954): 39–51.

75 Ibid., 51; William Mustard, interviewed by Valerie Schatzker (AMS Interviews, U of T Faculty of Medicine), 19 August 1981–12 September 1981, HSC Archives, 84.

76 W.T. Mustard, "Mortality in Congenital Cardiovascular Surgery," *Canadian Medical Association Journal* 72, no. 10 (1955): 740.

77 Ibid., 740–4.

78 W.T. Mustard, and J.A. Thomson, "Clinical Experience with the Artificial Heart Lung Preparation," *Canadian Medical Association Journal* 76, no. 4 (1957): 268, 265–9.

79 William Mustard, interviewed by Valerie Schatzker (AMS Interviews, U of T Faculty of Medicine), 19 August 1981–12 September 1981, HSC Archives, 119–20.

80 Ibid.

81 Shafie Fazel, William G. Williams, and Bernard S. Goldman, "Thinned Blood, Monkey Lungs, and the Cold Heart," *Surgical History* 19, no. 3 (2004): 276–7.

82   Dunlop, *Bill Mustard*, 57.

83   HSC Research Institute (hereafter HSC RI), Annual Report 1956, 20.

84   Fazel, Williams, and Goldman, "Thinned Blood, Monkey Lungs, and the Cold Heart," *Surgical History* 19, no. 3 (2004): 275–8.

85   Olley, Johnson, and Beamish, "Lest We Forget," 707.

86   "Meet the Staff, Dr WT Mustard," *Paediatric Patter* 4, no. 10 (1963), 2, HSC Archives.

87   HSC RI Annual Report 1959, 6th AR January–December 1959.

88   HSC RI Annual Report 1958, 61–2.

89   HSC RI Annual Report 1959, 6th AR January–December 1959, 6.

90   HSC RI Annual Report 1962, 77.

91   William Mustard, interviewed by Valerie Schatzker (AMS Interviews, U of T Faculty of Medicine), 19 August 1981–12 September 1981, HSC Archives, 106.

92   See Dunlop, *Bill Mustard*, 66; and Max Braithwaite, *Sick Kids: The Story of the Hospital for Sick Children in Toronto* (Toronto: McClelland and Stewart, 1974), 136–7.

93   Dunlop, *Bill Mustard*, 66–7.

94   William Mustard, interviewed by Valerie Schatzker (AMS Interviews, U of T Faculty of Medicine), 19 August 1981–12 September 1981, HSC Archives, 97.

95   Ibid., 86–7; Marilyn Dunlop, "The Surgeon's Joy in Saving Lives," *Toronto Star*, 1 August 1989, A14.

96   William Mustard, interviewed by Valerie Schatzker (AMS Interviews, U of T Faculty of Medicine), 19 August 1981–12 September 1981, HSC Archives, 86–9; Mustard, "Successful Two-Stage Correction of Transposition of the Great Vessels," *Surgery* 55, no. 3 (1964): 469–72.

97   Dunlop, *Bill Mustard*, p. 68, quoting Dr. George Trusler.

98   See P. Swyer, *Babies: The Fight for Intact Survival at the Hospital for Sick Children, Toronto, Canada, 1875–2000, A Personal View* (Toronto, 2000), 9–10 and table 1; AR 1960, 15; AR 1961, 15.

99   Anonymous interview by author, participant #9, 26 February 2014.

100 G.W. Chance, M.J. O'Brien, and P.R. Swyer, "Transportation of Sick Neonates, 1972: An Unsatisfactory Aspect of Medical Care," *Canadian Medical Association Journal* 109, no. 9 (1973): 847–51.

101 The Sabin vaccine "used small numbers of live viruses in a sweet syrup to take the viruses directly to the alimentary canal, where they multiplied and produced antibodies which circulated in the bloodstream" (MacDougall, *Activists and Advocates*, 156, 152–7).

102 John T. Law, "Director's Corner," *Paediatric Patter* 2, no. 1 (1961): 2.

103 AR 1961, 17.

104 See, for example, Ronald Kotulak, "New Surgery Saving Lives of Blue Babies," *Chicago Tribune*, 23 October 1965, 7.

105 June Callwood, "The Informal Dr. Mustard," *Globe and Mail*, 14 October 1974, 8.

106 Hollobon, "Gairdner Awards to Canadians," F10.

107 Anonymous interview by author, participant #15, 26 May 2014.

108 Olley, Johnson, and Beamish, "Lest We Forget," 707.

109 Shorter, *Partnership for Excellence*, 89.

11 A SISTERHOOD OF NURSING

1   Quoted by Roul Tunley, "Why Not Compulsory Hospital Insurance?" *Saturday Review*, 8 July 1967, 14.

2   This vignette has been told and retold several times in biographies of Douglas. As quoted in Lewis H. Thomas, ed., *The Making of a Socialist: The Recollections of T.C. Douglas* (Edmonton: University of Alberta Press, 1982), 6–7. See also Doris French Shackleton, *Tommy Douglas* (Toronto: McClelland and Stewart, 1975), 17; Thomas H. McLeod and Ian McLeod, *Tommy Douglas: The Road to Jerusalem* (Edmonton: Hurtig Publishers, 1987), 145; Dave Margoshes, *Tommy Douglas: Building the New Society* (Montreal: XYZ Publishing, 1999), 7.

3   Quoted in McLeod and McLeod, *Tommy Douglas*, 145.

4   Quoted in Thomas, ed., *The Making of a Socialist*, 7.

5   Malcolm G. Taylor, *Health Insurance and Canadian Public Policy: The Seven Decisions that Created the Health Insurance System and Their Outcomes* (Montreal: McGill-Queen's University Press, 2009), 102.

6   C. Stuart Houston and Merle Massie, *36 Steps on the Road to Medicare: How Saskatchewan Led the Way* (Montreal: McGill-Queen's University Press, 2013), 100.

7   C. David Naylor, *Private Practice, Public Payment: Canadian Medicine and the Politics of Health Insurance, 1911–1966* (Montreal: McGill-Queen's Press, 1986), 177; Gregory Marchildon, ed., *Making Medicare: New Perspectives on the History of Medicare in Canada* (Toronto: University of Toronto, 2012).

8   See Naylor, *Private Practice, Public Payment* and Charles Webster, *The National Health Service: A Political History*, 2nd ed. (Oxford: Oxford University Press, 2002).

9   Dominique Jean, "Family Allowances and Family Autonomy: Quebec Families Encounter the Welfare State, 1945–1955," in *Canadian Family History: Selected Readings*, ed. Bettina Bradbury (Toronto: Irwin Pub, 2000), 401–37.

10   Outpatient diagnostic services, medical services in the community, and psychiatric care were not included in the plan.

11   Quotation from *Statutes of Ontario* 1957, The Hospital Services Commission, bill no. 165 (Assented to 3 April 1957) ch. 46; R.W.I. Urquhart, "The Ontario Hospital Services Commission" in "The Public Health Significance of Recent Legislation in the Fields of Hospital Insurance and Home Care: A Symposium" *Canadian Journal of Public Health* 50, no. 2 (1959), 47–9. *An Act to Establish the Hospital Services Commission of Ontario* (The Hospital Services Commission Act), bill no. 112, *Statutes of Ontario* (1956) Chapter 31, 2nd Session, 25th Legislature, Ontario, 4–5 Elizabeth II, 1956.

12   Taylor, *Health Insurance and Canadian Public Policy*, 157–8; Ontario Hospital Services Commission, *Questions and Answers about Hospital Care Insurance for Residents of Ontario* (Toronto: Ontario Hospital Services Commission, 1958), 3.

13   Taylor, *Health Insurance and Canadian Public Policy*, 157; Ontario Hospital Association, submission to the *Royal Commission on Health Services* 50 (Hearings, 10 May 1962, Toronto), 9487.

14   Trustees Minutes, 22 December 1960; See Executive Director Douglas E. Snedden to E.H. Shuter, HSC Sec. 1 March 1972, Paediatric Research Foundation of Toronto, Pablum & Nutrition Subject File, HSC Archives.

15   John T. Law, "Director's Corner," *Paediatric Patter* 2, no. 2 (1961): 2, HSC Archives.

16   Although Medicare is often dated from the Medical Care Act of 1966, it did not take effect until 1 July 1968, and even then, provinces were required to pass their own legislation in conformity with the principles of Medicare. As a consequence, different provinces "joined" Medicare at different times. In Ontario, it was 1969. Gregory P. Marchildon, "Canadian Medicare: Why History Matters," in *Making Medicare: New Perspectives on the History of Medicare in Canada*, ed. Gregory P. Marchildon (Toronto: University of Toronto Press, 2012), 8.

17   Trustees and Medical Policy Committee Special Meeting, 10 November 1966, and Appendices (in Trustees Minutes) see Appendix A, "O.M.S.I.P.," November 1966. HSC Archives.

18   Around 80 per cent of RNs were in practice 1951–61. *Report of the Royal Commission on Health Services in Canada,* vol. 1 (Ottawa: Queen's Printer, 1964), 264–6.

19   Canadian Nursing Association, "A Statement on Nursing in Canada," (excerpt of brief submitted to Hall Commission) *Canadian Nurse* 58, no. 6 (1962): 533–5. See recommendation 12, "That the Education of Nurses be under the Jurisdiction of Institutions whose Primary Function is Education," submission of Canadian Nurses' Association to the Royal Commission on Health Services, Hearings, vol. 38, Ottawa, 26 March 1962, 7560–659. The RNAO was more divided about the desired location of training, but did advocate for

the expansion of university nursing schools. See also Submission of Registered Nurses Association of Ontario to the Royal Commission on Health Services, vol. 49, 9 May 1962, 9211–65.

20 John T. Law, "Director's Corner," *Paediatric Patter* 3, no. 9 (1962): 2. See also his later response to "A number of articles ... that foster discontent among the members of the nursing profession." John T. Law, "Director's Corner," *Paediatric Patter* 4, no. 8 (1963): 2. For media criticisms of nursing schools, see for example David Spurgeon, "WANTED: A New System for Training Nurses; Evidence of Exploitation at some Hospital Schools has Revealed that Students Pay for Education with Hard Labor," *Globe and Mail,* 23 May 1963, 13; "Hospital Schools Criticized, Praised," *Globe and Mail,* 30 October 1963, 11; Michele Landsberg, "New Education Program Urged to Replace Nursing Apprenticeship," *Globe and Mail,* 14 December 1963, 16.

21 Hilda Rolstin, *History of the School of Nursing, The Hospital for Sick Children* (Alumnae Association, 1972), 38–9, quotation 38. See also AR 1972, 2; AR 1971, 6.

22 AR 1972, 2; Rolstin, preface to *History of the School of Nursing,* 38; Elsbeth Geiger, "What's Going On in Nursing Education in Ontario Today?" *Alumnae News* (Spring 1966). By 1968, nearly half of Ontario's nursing schools had switched from a three-year program to the 2+1 program. "Dymond Says Not Enough Grade 13 Graduates to Fill Nursing Needs," *Hospital Highlights,* (Spring 1968); OHSC Annual Report 1965 and 1966, 10; Rolstin, *History of the School of Nursing,* 36–9.

23 J. Douglas Snedden, "Director's Corner: HSC Will Support New Training System," *What's New* (August 1973): 2.

24 Quotation in Alumnae Association, *100 Years: A Celebration of the Alumnae Association of the School of Nursing, The Hospital for Sick Children* (Toronto: The Alumnae Association, 2003), 41; J.D. Snedden, "HSC will Support New Training System," *What's New* (August 1973): 2.

25 *Sick Kids Book of Memories, Class of 1960,* 50th Reunion, 15 September 2010, 3. 2010–209–001, HSC Archives.

26 A national study reported that 16.3 per cent of the dropouts of the class of 1950 left for marriage, up from 14 per cent in 1948. Marriage was the third most common reason for withdrawal, after failure in class work and health reasons. Margery Walker, "Student Nurses in Canada," *Canadian Nurse* 48, no. 6 (1952): 472–4. HSC appears to have made exceptions from time to time, such as a Mrs. Marguerite Gray, '46, who appears to have been the first married woman to graduate from the school of nursing. The hospital authorities may well have provided an exception based on the fact that her husband, Gordon, was a prisoner in Hong Kong (Alumnae Association, *100 Years,* 47).

27 Trustees Minutes, 29 December 1958.

28 "37 Graduates of Hospital for Sick Children are Last to Take Entire Course in Present Building," *Toronto Star,* 11 June 1950, 28; *Sick Kids Book of Memories,* 3, 5, 7, 11, 17; Lynda (Fallis) McKean, "(CL'66) Lynda – A Room of My Own," Alumnae Association of the School of Nursing, The Hospital for Sick Children, last modified 2011, http://hscnursingalumnae.org/cl66-lynda-a-room-of-my-own/.

29 *Sick Kids Book of Memories,* 14.

30 Alumnae Association, *100 Years,* 49; Mary E. James, "In Seven Houses: Nurses Hope for Central Residence," *Globe and Mail,* 29 November 1949, 14.

31 Quotation from *Sick Kids Book of Memories,* 8; "Student Nurses Moving Into New Residence," *Globe and Mail,* 21 March 1952, 3; "Residence Addition for 1960," *Globe and Mail,* 14 February 1959, 32; "What's In A Nurses' Residence?" *What's New* (September 1970): 16.

32 Alumnae Association, *100 Years,* 45.

33 Ibid., 39, 44, 49; *Sick Kids Book of Memories;* "What's In A Nurses' Residence?" 16.

34 Kathryn McPherson, *Bedside Matters: The Transformation of Canadian Nursing, 1900–1990* (Toronto: University of Toronto Press, 2003), 238–9. See also *Report of the Royal Commission on Health Services in Canada,* vol. 1 (Ottawa: Queen's Printer, 1964), 276–7.

35 *Sick Kids Book of Memories*, 2.

36 Ibid., 16.

37 Joan (Ford) Raymond, S'57 quoted in Alumnae Association, *100 Years*, 47.

38 *Sick Kids Book of Memories*, 12.

39 The quotation was attributed to Eli (Lainchbury) Dandy (HSC 1941) in "Memories of HSC Nurses Who Served in WWII," *Alumnae News* 69, no. 2 (2009): 5.

40 McPherson, *Bedside Matters*, 32, 40.

41 "Beth (Bailey) Bartlett Tells Us How it Was," *Alumnae News* 68, no. 2 (2008): 12–13.

42 "Professional Etiquette," (typed, given to probationers 1938–1941), Nursing School Subject File 3, HSC Archives.

43 Handwritten notes on Professional Etiquette (some differences from typed version), Nursing School Subject File 3, HSC Archives.

44 Masten quoted by Director John T. Law in "The Director's Corner," *Paediatric Patter* 1, no. 7 (1960): 2; Anonymous oral interview by author, participant #12, 26 March 2014.

45 Anonymous oral interview by author, participant #6, 8 January 2014.

46 Ibid.

47 *Sick Kids Book of Memories*, 5.

48 Ibid., 8.

49 Anonymous oral interview by author, participant #12, 26 March 2014.

50 "HSC '62 Stories, The Hospital for Sick Children School of Nursing Class of 1962 Memoirs," memoirs, Class of 1962, collected for 50th reunion, compiled by Janet (Barker) Saunders (April 2012), 20, HSC Archives.

51 Ibid., 13.

52 Anonymous oral interview by author, participant #5, 12 December 2013.

53 Medical staff member, quoted in Max Braithwaite, *Sick Kids: The Story of the Hospital for Sick Children in Toronto* (Toronto: McClelland and Stewart, 1974), 86.

54 *Sick Kids Book of Memories*, 12

55 Mary E. James, "Jean Masten Retiring As Nursing Director," *Globe and Mail,* 1 February 1961, 11; Alumnae Association, *100 Years*, 38; Rolstin, *History of the School of Nursing*, 31–2; "Trend in Nursing: The School Cap," *Canadian Nurse* 49, no. 3 (1953): 209.

56 Quotation from Alumnae Association, *100 Years*, 53; Rolstin, *History of the School of Nursing,* 31, 38.

57 Quotation in Rolstin, *History of the School of Nursing,* 32.

58 Rolstin, *History of the School of Nursing,* 31, 38; *Sick Kids Book of Memories*; Alumnae Association, *100 Years*, 53. See Christina Bates, *A Cultural History of the Nurse's Uniform* (Gatineau, QB: Canadian Museum of Civilization, 2012).

59 Agnes Calliste, "Women of 'Exceptional Merit': Immigration of Caribbean Nurses to Canada," *Canadian Journal of Women and the Law* 6 (1993): 85–102; Karen Flynn, "Beyond the Glass Wall: Black Canadian Nurses, 1940–1970," *Nursing History Review* 17, no. 1 (2009): 129–52; McPherson, *Bedside Matters*, 211.

60 HSC School of Nursing Graduating Class Photographs, HSC Archives, http://hscnursingalumnae.org/imagegalleries/classes/; "Trying on Cap," *Globe and Mail,* 25 October 1962, 20.

61 Rolstin, *History of the School of Nursing*, 35.

62 Ibid., 32. See excerpts from Registered Nurses' Association of Ontario, *Curriculum and Information for Schools of Nursing in Ontario* (Toronto: The Association, 1953), 50–3.

63 Rolstin, *History of the School of Nursing*, 33; AR 1965, 9; "Nurses From All Ontario Train at Hospital for Sick Children," *Globe and Mail,* 28 June 1945, 15; AR 1960, 18; AR 1965, 9. See recollection of Sioux Lookout in Alumnae Association, *100 Years*, 52.

64 Rolstin, *History of the School of Nursing*, 31.

65 AR 1949, 19; AR 1953, 67; AR 1958, 15; AR 1961, 18; AR 1962, 4; "Affiliates at Hospital Reach Record Number," *Globe and Mail,* 10 September 1964, W2.

66 Quoted by Andrew Webster, "Hospital Manager Likened to Head of Company," *Globe and Mail,* 28 October 1964, B5; Claus A. Wirsig, "John Thomas Law 1917–1977 A Tribute," *Hospital Administration in Canada* 20, no. 2 (1978): 35–6; "John T. Law Child Care Innovator," *Globe and Mail*, 31 December 1977, 4; Braithwaite, *Sick Kids*, 133.

67 Wirsig, "John Thomas Law," 36.

68 "Sick Children's Flies to No. 1 Spot on New Wing," *Globe and Mail,* 7 May 1964, 5; Ron Lowman, "Addition makes Sick Kids Largest on the Continent," *Toronto Daily Star*, 7 May 1964, 35.

69 Quotation from John T. Law, "Director's Corner," *Paediatric Patter* 4, no. 8 (1963): 2; "Meet the Staff, Olive Hargreaves, Personnel Officer," *Paediatric Patter* 5, no. 10 (1964): 2.

70 "Personnel Quiz," *Paediatric Patter* 4, no. 1 (1963): 3–4; Arthur Kruger, "Collective Bargaining in Ontario Public Hospitals," *Relations industrielles/Industrial Relations* 40, no. 1 (1985): 48–67, quotation 52.

71 "Meet the Staff," *Paediatric Patter* 3, no. 5 (1962): 2.

72 Arthur Kruger, "Collective Bargaining in Ontario Public Hospitals," 64n12.

73 Duncan L. Gordon, "The Hospital for Sick Children Board of Trustees," 19 January 1968, appended to Trustees Minutes, 5 February 1968.

74 Duncan L. Gordon, "The Changing Role of The Board of Trustees," 30 November 1967, appended to Trustees Minutes, 5 February 1968, 3.

75 John T. Law, "Impact of the Canadian Federal-Provincial Hospital Program on the Voluntary Hospital," in "Canadian-American Conference on Hospital Programs," supplement, *Medical Care* 7, no. 6 (1969): 36.

76 Quotation from Arthur Brydon, "Hospital's Drive Runs $5,000,000 Short — Fund-Raisers Blame Good Image," *Globe and Mail*, 21 August 1965, 1; HSC Foundation, "Retrospective on the First Decade 1973 to 1983," May 1983, 6, HSC Foundation Subject File #2, HSC Archives; Law, "Impact of the Canadian Federal-Provincial Hospital Program," 37–9.

77 *Hospital for Sick Children News*, March 1960.

78 Clinton A. Stephens, MD, *Annual Report of Admissions and Discharges Committee for 1959*, appended to Medical Advisory Council Minutes, 9 March 1960.

79 Medical Policy Committee Minutes 2 April 1957, memo of discussion by the heads of the four services (Chute, Farmer, Morgan, Whaley).

80 Stephens, *Annual Report of Admissions and Discharges.*

81 Trustees Minutes, 27 August 1956.

82 Anonymous oral interview by author, participant #1, 30 October 2013. See also Francesca Grosso, *The History of Sunnybrook Hospital: Battle to Greatness* (Toronto: Dundurn Press, 2014), 80–1.

83 Dr. J. Harry Ebbs, interviewed by Valerie Schatzker, 20 February, 22 February, 27 February, and 6 March 1979 (Hannah Institute for the History of Medicine / Associated Medical Services, Inc.), 203.

84 Quotation MPC Minutes, HSC Memo of Matters Discussed at a meeting of the MPC held Thursday 21 March 1957.

85 Quoted in Trustees Minutes, 7 August 1957, Special Meeting at the York Club, 7–10:25 p.m., Board and Farmer, to consider report of the MPC on the subject of enlarging the hospital, dated 3 July 1957: Xerox of MPC report, Minutes from special meeting, 7 August 1957 (Xeroxed and appended to Trustee Minutes 27 June 1966).

86 MPC Minutes 2 April 1957, Memo of discussion by the heads of the four services.

87 J. Grant Glassco to ON Hospital Services Commission 23 October 1957, Appendix to Trustees Minutes 31 October 1966.

88 HSC Memo of Matters Discussed at a meeting of the MPC held Thursday 21 March 1957.

89 AR 1964, 16; AR 1966, 9.

90 Italics added. Quoted in Trustees Minutes, 7 August 1957.

91 MPC Minutes, 3 July 1957.

92 Quoted in Trustees Minutes, 7 August 1957; MPC Minutes, 2 April 1957 Memo of discussion by the heads of the four services (Chute, Farmer, Morgan, Whaley).

93 Trustees Minutes, 10 September 1957.

94 "Research Affected: Too Many Minor Cases Tax Hospital for Sick Children," *Toronto Daily Star*, 9 March 1961, 1. See also "Hospital Beds For Children Running Short," *Globe and Mail*, 9 March 1961, 5.

95 Committee for Survey of Hospital Needs in Metropolitan Toronto, *Hospital Accommodation and Facilities for Children in Metropolitan Toronto: Part Six of a Study by the Committee for Survey of Hospital Needs in Metropolitan Toronto* (Toronto: The Committee, 1962), quotation 2–3, 17.

96 Ibid., 33.

97 Ibid., 42, 65–6, 69.

98 John T. Law, "The Director's Corner," *Paediatric Patter* 5, no. 6 (1964): 2.

99 Report of the Budget & Finance Committee, Trustees Minutes, 27 April 1967. See John T. Law to Mr. Stanley W. Martin (OHSC Chairman), (8 December 1966, copy) appendix B to Trustees Minutes, 3 January 1967.

100 "IODE," North York General Hospital, last modified 2016, http://www.nygh.on.ca/Default.aspx?cid=1403&lang=1.

101 Law, "Impact of the Canadian Federal-Provincial Hospital Program," 35.

102 Taylor, *Health Insurance and Canadian Public Policy*, 158.

103 Law, "Impact of the Canadian Federal-Provincial Hospital Program," 38.

104 Anonymous oral interview by author, participant #1, 30 October 2013; Martin L. Friedland, *The University of Toronto: A History*, 2nd ed. (Toronto: University of Toronto Press, 2013), 508–10.

105 Anonymous oral interview by author, participant #1, 30 October 2013.

12 TRAGEDY AND TRANSFORMATION

1 Roy McMurtry, *Memoirs and Reflections* (Toronto: University of Toronto Press, 2013), 281–2.

2 Quotation in Mr. Justice Charles L. Dubin (Chairman), Joan Gilchrist, Hugh McDonald, and Henry Nadler Report (Committee Members), *Report of The Hospital for Sick Children Review Committee* (Toronto: January 1983), 164; "4 MDs Disagree on X-rays of Boy, 8, Inquest Hears," *Globe and Mail*, 30 April 1980, 4; Arthur Johnson and Ian Mulgrew, "Deaths Blacken Hospital's Record," *Globe and Mail*, 5 May 1980, 5.

3 Quotation David Logan, "Cardiac Arrest Suffered by Boy on Release Day," *Globe and Mail*, 2 May 1980, 1, 2; "Death of Boy Due to Faulty Treatment, Jury Finds," *Globe and Mail*, 3 May 1980, 1. On the recommendation of the coroner's jury, HSC's Board initiated an external review in May 1980, which was chaired by McGill Medical Professor Dr. Maurice McGregor and made public upon its completion. See Dubin et al., *Report of The Hospital for Sick Children Review Committee*, 164–9.

4 David Logan, "Hospital Records Ripped Out and Stolen, Inquest Told," *Globe and Mail*, 1 May 1980, 1; "Remedy Sick Kids' Ills," editorial, *Toronto Star*, 16 August 1980, B2; David Logan, "Cardiac Arrest Suffered by Boy on Release Day," 1, 2.

5 "Eight MDs Face a Fight for Licences," *Globe and Mail*, 18 May 1982, 3; Rick Haliechuk, "Court Defers Ruling in Hospital Death of Boy, 8," *Toronto Star*, 8 April 1987, A27; Rick Haliechuck, "Court Rejects Bid for Secret Hearing into MDs' Treatment of Boy who Died," *Toronto Star*, 4 June 1987, A2; Michael Bociurkiw, "Supreme Court Upholds Public Medical Hearing," *Globe and Mail*, 8 June 1987, A2; Paul Taylor, "Hearing Faults 2 MDs in Death Boy Misdiagnosed at Sick Kids' Hospital," *Globe and Mail*, 18 May 1991, A1; Paul Taylor, "Two Doctors Reprimanded 11 Years After Death of Child: 'It's a Joke,' Mother of Steven Yuz Says of Penalty Dealt Out after Her Long Struggle to Bring Case to Judgment," *Globe and Mail*, 2 November 1991, A7.

6 Dubin et al., *Report of The Hospital for Sick Children Review Committee*, quotation 164, 169–72.

7 "Remedy Sick Kids' Ills," B2; See Dubin et al., *Report of The Hospital for Sick Children Review Committee*, 164–5.

8 J.D. Snedden, "Outside Experts Will Review Jury Recommendations," *What's New* 13, no. 1 (1980): 1.

9 Dubin et al., *Report of The Hospital for Sick Children Review Committee*. When complete, the report was initially given only to the Medical Officer of Health, HSC trustees, legislature, and attorney general for review, although it was leaked to the press. See "When an Inquiry Needs an Audience," editorial, *Globe and Mail*, 3 June 1982, 6; Ontario Legislature, Debates (Hansard transcripts), Official Records Session 32:2, 5 January 1983, http://hansardindex.ontla.on.ca/hansardeissue/32-2/l191.htm and Session 32:2, 9 February 1983, http://hansardindex.ontla.on.ca/hansardeissue/32-2/l206.htm; H.W. Bain, "Report of the Assessment of 44 Deaths on Wards 4A and 4B of the Hospital for Sick Children, Toronto," (24 June 1982 and clarifications 23 November 1982), HSC Archives; James W. Buehler, Lesbia F. Smith, Evelyn M. Wallace, Clark W. Heath Jr., Robert Kusiak, and Joy L. Herndon, "Unexplained Deaths in a Children's Hospital: An Epidemiologic Assessment," *New England Journal of Medicine* 313, no. 4 (1985): 211.

10 Sarah Jane Growe, *Who Cares? The Crisis in Canadian Nursing* (Toronto: McClelland and Stewart, 1991), 38.

11 S.G.M. Grange, *Report of the Royal Commission of Inquiry into Certain Deaths at the Hospital for Sick Children and Related Matters* (Toronto: Ontario Ministry of the Attorney General, 1984), 7, 9–10, 12.

12 Grange, *Report of the Royal Commission of Inquiry*, 175–7, quotation 175.

13 She was originally only charged with one count of first-degree murder; three counts were added days later. Harold Levy, "Nelles Deserves a Break from Court," *Toronto Star*, 17 August 1989, A22.

14 Steven L. Solomon, Evelyn M. Wallace, E.L. Ford-Jones, W. Mark Baker, William J. Martone, Irwin J. Kopin, Ann D. Critz, and James R. Allen, "Medication Errors with Inhalant Epinephrine Mimicking an Epidemic of Neonatal Sepsis," *New England Journal of Medicine* 310, no. 3 (1984): 166–70, quotation 166. See also *Her Majesty the Queen v. Susan Nelles: Submissions of Counsel before His Honour Judge D. Vanek*, vol. 21 (Toronto: Ministry of the Attorney General, 1982), 56–66.

15 Dubin et al., *Report of The Hospital for Sick Children Review Committee*, 177–8. See Leslie Scrivener, "Nurse Believed Drug was Vitamin, Baby Inquest Told," *Toronto Star*, 20 May 1982, A8.

16 *Her Majesty the Queen v. Susan Nelles*, 64. See also HSC Memo, J. Douglas Snedden to all staff and trustees, 4 May 1983, Susan Nelles Subject File, HSC Archives.

17 Dubin et al., *Report of The Hospital for Sick Children Review Committee*, 173.

18 The Dubin committee commented that "[n]urses inexperienced in tracheotomy care were often assigned together" (Dubin et al., *Report of The Hospital for Sick Children Review Committee*, 175).

19 Dubin et al., *Report of The Hospital for Sick Children Review Committee*, 175.

20 McMurtry, *Memoirs and Reflections*, 279; R. Roy McMurtry, Press Release Statement, *The Grange Report, Ontario, Royal Commission of Inquiry into Certain Deaths at the Hospital for Sick Children and Related Matters* (Toronto, 3 January 1985), 17.

21 Rodney Singleton Fowler, Testimony during Preliminary Hearing, *Her Majesty the Queen v. Susan Nelles*, vol. 19 (Toronto: Ministry of the Attorney General, 1982), 46–7. See also *Her Majesty the Queen v. Susan Nelles: Reasons for Judgment on Preliminary Inquiry before His Honour D. Vanek, Provincial Judge* (Toronto: Ministry of the Attorney General, 1982), 53; *Her Majesty the Queen v. Susan Nelles: Preliminary Inquiry Hearings*, vols. 1–34 (Toronto: Ministry of the Attorney General, 1983). For a critique, see *Registered Nurses' Association of Ontario, RNAO Responds: A Nursing Perspective on Events at The Hospital for Sick Children and the Grange Inquiry* (Toronto: RNAO, 1986/1987?), 6–7.

22 Fowler, Testimony during Preliminary Hearing, *Her Majesty the Queen v. Susan Nelles*, vol. 19, 66–7.

23 During the hearing, it became known that Lombardo's exhumed tissues had tested positive for digoxin. Grange, *Report of the Royal Commission of Inquiry*, 204–5.

24 *Her Majesty the Queen v. Susan Nelles*, 81–2.

25 Trish Wood, "A Cloud of Suspicion," *The Fifth Estate* (Toronto: Canadian Broadcasting Corporation, 10 October 1995). See also Growe, *Who Cares?*, 30.

26 David Vanek, *Fulfilment: Memoirs of a Criminal Court Judge* (Toronto: Dundurn Press, 1999), 298.

27 Ibid.

28 Elaine Buckley Day, "A 20th Century Witch Hunt: A Feminist Critique of the Grange Royal Commission into Deaths at the Hospital for Sick Children," *Studies in Political Economy* 24, no. 1 (1987): 20–1; Grange, *Report of the Royal Commission of Inquiry*, 37.

29 Day, "A 20th Century Witch Hunt," 20.

30 Buehler et al., "Unexplained Deaths in a Children's Hospital," 212.

31 Ibid., 213–14, quotation 214.

32 Ibid., 215.

33 Hon. Mr. McMurtry, Ontario Legislature, Debates (Hansard transcripts), Official Records for Session 32:2, 21 February 1983, http://hansardindex.ontla.on.ca/hansardeissue/32-2/l218.htm; Kevin Cox, "Hospital Demands Release of Report into Infant Deaths," *Globe and Mail*, 24 February 1983, 5; "Air the Sick Kids' Report," editorial, *Toronto Star* 23 February 1983, A24.

34 Grange, *Report of the Royal Commission of Inquiry*, 36–7.

35 Italics added. Day, "A 20th Century Witch Hunt," 21.

36 Mr. Peterson, Oral Questions, Ontario Legislature, Debates (Hansard transcripts), Official Records Session 32:2, 25 May 1982, http://hansardindex.ontla.on.ca/hansardeissue/32-2/l056.htm

37 Hon. Mr. McMurtry: Ontario Legislature, Debates (Hansardtranscripts), Official Records Session 32:3, 22 April 1983, http://hansardindex.ontla.on.ca/hansardeissue/32-3/l004.htm; McMurtry, *Memoirs and Reflections, 282–3.*

38 Quotation in J.D. Snedden, "Director's Message," *Telescope* (April 1983), Box 63, Anne Evans Fonds, HSC Archives; Ontario Legislature, Debates (Hansard transcripts), Official Records Session: 32:3, 22 April 1983, http://hansardindex.ontla.on.ca/hansardeissue/32-3/l004.htm; Rosemary Speirs and Sylvia Stead, "Appeal Court Judge will Inquire into 28 Baby Deaths at Hospital," *Globe and Mail*, 22 April 1983, 1, 2; Kevin Cox, "Judge Promises a Full Airing of Hospital Deaths," *Globe and Mail*, 23 April 1983, 1, 2; "Statement on Inquiry into Baby Deaths," *Globe and Mail*, 23 April 1983, 5.

39 Grange, *Report of the Royal Commission of Inquiry*, 223, quotation 2; Day, "A 20th Century Witch Hunt," 21.

40 Grange, *Report of the Royal Commission of Inquiry*, 2.

41 Quotation in Grange, *Report of the Royal Commission of Inquiry*, appendix two: Amendment to Order-in-Council 24 May 1984, 231, 246–51; Paul S.A. Lamek in Royal Commission of Inquiry into Certain Deaths, *Hearings*, vol. 132, 18 April 1984, 426–9; "Court Says Grange Can't Name Names," *Toronto Star*, 13 April 1984, A1, A13.

42 Royal Commission of Inquiry into Certain Deaths, *Hearings*, vol. 118, 19 March 1984, 6753.

43 Grange, *Report of the Royal Commission of Inquiry*, xii–xvi. See Royal Commission of Inquiry into Certain Deaths, *Hearings* (Transcripts of Evidence).

44 Grange, *Report of the Royal Commission of Inquiry*, 160.

45 Kathryn McPherson, *Bedside Matters: The Transformation of Canadian Nursing, 1900–1990* (Toronto: University of Toronto Press, 2003), 256.

46 Ms. E. McIntyre, RNAO Counsel, *Hearings of the Royal Commission of Inquiry into Certain Deaths at the Hospital for Sick Children and Related Matters Ontario*, vol. 144 (Transcript of Evidence for 10 May 1984), 3228, 3230, 3246 and vol. 145 (14 May 1984), 3271.

47   Growe, *Who Cares?*, 32.

48   Grange, *Report of the Royal Commission of Inquiry*, 37; Day, "A 20th Century Witch Hunt,"
      32; *Royal Commission of Inquiry into Certain Deaths at the Hospital for Sick Children and Related
      Matters Ontario*, Transcript of Evidence for 15 May 1984, vol. 146, 3529–663.

49   Marian McGee, quoted in Léo Charbonneau, "The Grange Report: Nurses Criticize
      Commission's Report for Lack of Answers," *Canadian Nurse* 81, no. 3 (1985): 17.

50   Baumgart in M. Allen, "Women, Nursing and Feminism: An Interview with Alice J.
      Baumgart, RN, PhD," *Canadian Nurse 81*, no. 1 (1985): 21. See also Judith Banning, "Feeling
      Numb," editorial, *Canadian Nurse* 81, no. 3 (1985): 7.

51   Lorraine Rosenal, "Letter to the Editor," *Canadian Nurse* 81, no. 5 (1985): 10.

52   Growe, *Who Cares?*, 35, quotation 33–4.

53   Quotation Lynn Kelly, "The Grange Ordeal: One Hundred and Ninety-One Days of Personal
      and Professional Dilemmas," *Ryerson Review of Journalism* (9 April 1985) http://rrj.ca/the-
      grange-ordeal/; T. Bissland, *Death Shift: The Digoxin Murders at "Sick Kids"* (Toronto: Methuen,
      1984).

54   Mary E. Thomas, "Letter to the Editor," *Canadian Nurse* 81, no. 5 (1985): 10.

55   Jane C. Haliburton, "Letter to the Editor," *Canadian Nurse* 80, no. 10 (1984): 9. See also
      "(Grange Commission) Baby Probe Blasted as Witch-Hunt," *Vancouver Sun*, 2 March 1984,
      A9; "Grange Inquiry called 'Witch Hunt,'" *Toronto Star*, 19 April 1984, A4; Sandra Walton,
      "Inquiry Recalls Witch Trials," letter to the editor, *Globe and Mail*, 12 May 1984, 7; John
      Munch, "Not on a Witch-Hunt Grange Lawyer Says," *Toronto Star*, 5 June 1984, A2; "Grange
      Commission Inquiry," Ontario Legislature, Debates (Hansard transcripts), Official Records
      Session 32:4, 18 April 1984, http://hansardindex.ontla.on.ca/hansardeissue/32-4/l015.htm.

56   Day, "A 20th Century Witch Hunt," 13; Kathleen Connors, "Plight of Nurses," *Ottawa Citizen*,
      25 March 1989, B2; Kathleen Connors, "No More Witch Hunts Among Nurses," *Toronto Star*,
      26 March 1989, B2.

57   Quoted in *Royal Commission of Inquiry into Certain Deaths at the Hospital for Sick Children and
      Related Matters Ontario*. Transcript of Evidence for 22 February 1984, vol. 108, 4500 and Kevin
      Cox, "Threatened by Police over Stress Meetings, Nurse Says at Inquiry," *Globe and Mail*, 14
      February 1984, 1.

58   Quoted in *Royal Commission of Inquiry into Certain Deaths at the Hospital for Sick Children and
      Related Matters Ontario*. Transcript of Evidence for 22 February 1984, vol. 108, 4497–9.

59   Kevin Cox, "Liberties Group Loses Appeal Bid on Nurses' Behalf," *Globe and Mail*, 27 March
      1984, M1.

60   Grange, *Report of the Royal Commission of Inquiry*, 162–9, quotation 40–1.

61   Day, "A 20th Century Witch Hunt," 36.

62   J. Douglas Snedden, "Director's Corner: Budget May Put Constraints on Service," *What's
      New* 5, no. 1 (1972): 2.

63   "Budget Cut Reduces HSC Beds by 6," *What's New* 5, no. 12 (1972): 1.

64   J. Douglas Snedden, "Would Hold Nursing Graduation in Spring," *What's New* 6, no. 8
      (1973): 2.

65   J. Douglas Snedden, "Director's Corner: All Staff Must Cut Costs to Save Jobs," *What's New* 8,
      no. 1 (1975): 2.

66   Sharon Richardson, "Unionization of Canadian Nursing" in *On All Frontiers: Four Centuries
      of Canadian Nursing*, ed. Christina Bates, Dianne Dodd, and Nicole Rousseau (Ottawa:
      University of Ottawa Press, 2005), 220.

67   J. Douglas Snedden, "Director's Corner: Neonatal Ward Must Have Staffing Priority," *What's
      New* 8, no. 7 (1975): 2.

68   J. Douglas Snedden, "Would Hold Nursing Graduation in Spring," 2.

69   "Irresponsible Charges: 'Useless' Description Angers Ontario Nurses," *Toronto Star*, 16 March
      1976, 1.

70 Edward J. Elliot, "'Experts' Say Nurses to Blame," letter to the editor, *Toronto Star*, 23 March 1976, B3.

71 D. Hunter, M. Sellenkowitsch, J. Hasler, R. Whitehead, "Nurses Forced into Program," letter to the editor, *Toronto Star*, 23 March 1976, B3.

72 Pat Farmer, "Nurses are Not Uneducated, Over-Paid," letter to the editor, *Toronto Star*, 23 March 1976, B3.

73 Craig Heron, *The Canadian Labour Movement: A Short History*, 3rd ed. (Toronto: James Lorimer and Co., 2012), xi.

74 Richardson, "Unionization of Canadian Nursing," 223.

75 This conclusion has been alluded to in several retrospectives, and given force by the book by Gavin Hamilton, *The Nurses are Innocent: The Digoxin Poisoning Fallacy* (Toronto: Dundurn Press, 2011). See also "A Cloud of Suspicion," *The Fifth Estate* (Toronto: Canadian Broadcasting Corporation, 10 October 1995); Warren Kinsella, "Research Clouds Case of Sick Kids' Murders," *Ottawa Citizen*, 14 March 1989, A1; Kathleen Kenna, "Bodies Make Copy-Cat Drug like Digoxin Doctor Says," *Toronto Star*, 24 February 1989; Lawrence Surtees, "Former Grange Inquiry Lawyers Disputes Claim of New Evidence," *Globe and Mail*, 24 February 1989, A15; Anne Dawson, "Hospital Deaths: Father Wants New Probe," *Toronto Sun*, 25 February 1989, 3; Dale Brazao and Marilyn Dunlop, "Lawyers See No Reason to Alter Baby Verdict," *Toronto Star*, 25 February 1989, A1, A4; Linda Barnard, "Grange Insists It Was Murder," *Toronto Sun*, 24 February 1989, 3; William Walker, "No New Inquiry into Baby Deaths," *Toronto Star*, 24 February 1989, A1; "Doubt Cast that Babies Murdered at Sick Kids," *Toronto Star*, 23 February 1989, A1, A7.

76 Grange, *Report of the Royal Commission of Inquiry*, 4, 254–62. See also Richard W. Pound, *History of Stikeman Elliott* (Montreal: McGill-Queen's University Press, 2002), 347–50.

77 "'My Life has Changed,' Says Nurse Cleared in Baby Deaths," *Toronto Star*, 23 March 1991, A8.

78 "Nurse Describes Her Futile Job Hunt," *Globe and Mail*, 3 April 1984, M1; "Nelles to Now: Evolution of Criminal Legal Support," CNPS Annual Report 2013, 7; Janet Beed to Claudia Anderson, "Your Request RE: Grange," HSC Memorandum, 10 December 1984, Susan Nelles Subject Files.

79 Michael Tenszen, "Dr. David Nelles Was Pediatrician," *Toronto Star*, 1 December 1988, A9.

80 See Don Stuart, "Prosecutorial Accountability in Canada," in *Accountability for Criminal Justice: Selected Essays*, ed. Philip C. Stenning (Toronto: University of Toronto Press, 1995), 341; Judy Mungovan, *Report of the Joint Criminal/Civil Section Working Group On Malicious Prosecution* (Charlottetown, PEI: Uniform Law Conference of Canada, 2007).

81 "Hospital Integration Project," Memo, 30 September 1983, Box 63, Anne Evans Fonds, HSC Archives.

82 Peter Larson, "Hospital Revamp Born Out of Baby Deaths Probe," *Edmonton Journal*, 18 August 1990, G6.

83 Eva Innes and Lesley Southwick-Trask, *Turning It Around: How Ten Canadian Organizations Changed Their Fortunes* (Toronto: Random House, 1989), 35–7. See also "Meet the New Boss: David Martin to be HSC's New President," *This Week* 3, no. 1 (1986): 1.

13 THE ATRIUM

1 Quoted in "A Miracle Renewed," *Globe and Mail*, 25 January 1993, special advertising supplement, C1.

2 Christian Kugler and Franz Stanzel, "Tracheomalacia," *Thoracic Surgery Clinics* 24, no. 1 (2014): 51.

3 Nicolaas van Rijn "'Help-Herbie' Drive to Aid Baby," *Toronto Sunday Star*, 18 February 1979, A4.

4 "N.Y. Infant with Choking Ailment Has Successful Corrective Surgery," *Los Angeles Times*, 27 February 1979, A14. See also G.K. Blair, R. Cohen, and R.M. Filler, "Treatment of Tracheomalacia: Eight Years' Experience," *Journal of Pediatric Surgery* 21, no. 9 (1986): 781–5.

5 "Toronto Operation for 'Baby Herbie,'" *Newsday* (NY), 23 February 1979, 30Q.

6   Quotation Dale Brazao, "Red Tape Stalls Tiny Herbie's Fight for Life," *Toronto Star*, 22 February 1979, A12; "N.Y. Infant with Choking Ailment Has Successful Corrective Surgery," *Los Angeles Times*, 27 February 1979, A14; Dick Beddoes, "A Tug at the Heart," *Globe and Mail*, 26 February 1979, 8.

7   van Rijn, "'Help-Herbie' Drive," A4.

8   Peter Goodspeed, "Baby Herbie Is Counting on Toronto MD to Save His Life," *Toronto Saturday Star*, 17 February 1979, A1.

9   Alex Nino Gheciu, "Herbie Day Brings Smile to Children's New Faces," *National Post*, 9 June 2012, http://news.nationalpost.com/posted-toronto/herbie-day-brings-smile-to-childrens-new-faces; Stefan Morrone, "Retiring Herbie Fund Founder Gina Godfrey on the Charity that Has Provided Medical Care for 765 Children," *National Post*, 29 November 2014, http://news.nationalpost.com/posted-toronto/retiring-herbie-fund-founder-gina-godfrey-on-the-charity-that-has-provided-medical-care-for-765-children.

10   Quotation Nicolaas van Rijn, "Metro Opens Its Heart to Herbie," *Toronto Star*, 19 February 1979, A1; Beddoes, "A Tug at the Heart," 8; van Rijn, "'Help-Herbie' Drive," A4; Gillian Cosgrove, "Raising a Glass to Herbie: First Recipient of Herbie Fund Now 24 and Happy to Be Here," *National Post* (Toronto Edition), 14 December 2002, TO1/front.

11   Hospital for Sick Children, "$50,000 Launches Permanent 'Herbie Fund,'" news release, 12 June 1979, Herbie Fund Subject File, HSC Archives.

12   Beddoes, "A Tug at the Heart," 8.

13   "A Little Man with Many Fans," *What's New* 12, no. 1 (1979): 16.

14   "U.S. Pays Herbie's $5,000 Tab," *Toronto Star*, 3 March 1979, A3; Dale Brazao, "Healthy and Happy Herbie goes home," *Toronto Star*, 21 March 1979, A9; "NAMES... FACES," *Boston Globe*, 28 February 1979, 4; "Infant Said Doing Well after Throat Operation," *The Hartford Courant*, 28 February 1979, 43; Photo, *Newsday* (NY), 15 March 1979, 9; Photo, *Chicago Tribune*, 15 March 1979, 2; Clyde Haberman and Albin Krebs, "Notes on People: Quinones Infant Goes Home From Toronto Hospital," *New York Times*, 21 March 1979, C16; "Has Throat Ailment: Canadians Come to Aid of New York Baby," *Los Angeles Times*, 21 February 1979, B4.

15   Carola Vyhnak, "Most U.S. Herbie Tales Have Unhappy Endings," *Toronto Star*, 28 February 1979, A13.

16   "Health: Donations by Toronto Citizens for the Treatment of Herbie Quinones – Motion Under S.O. 43," Canada House of Commons Debates, 30th Parliament, 4th Session, 27 February 1979, http://parl.canadiana.ca/view/oop.debates_HOC3004_04/227?r=0&s=1.

17   "Gift to Herbie Fund Reflects Confidence in HSC" (internal HSC document), 15 July 1982, 5–6, Herbie Fund Subject File 2, HSC Archives; SickKids Herbie Fund, "About Us: The Herbie Fund at SickKids: Our Past, Present and Future," http://www.herbiefund.com/aboutus.asp. See also "The Story of the Herbie," SickKids International Patient Program Website, http://www.sickkids.ca/IPP/The%20Herbie%20Fund/The%20Herbie%20Fund.html; "$50,000 to 'Herbie Fund' on Friday," *Toronto Sun*, 12 June 1979; HSC, "$50,000 Launches Permanent 'Herbie Fund'"; "Metro Endorses Herbie Fund," *Toronto Star*, 11 April 1979, A3; Michael McAteer, "Metro, Province Match Cheques and Herbie Fund Gets $100,000," *Toronto Star*, 16 June 1979, A3; Ontario Ministry of Health, "Health Minister Announces $50,000 Grant to Hospital for Sick Children's Herbie Fund," news release, 15 July 1982, Herbie Fund Subject File #2, HSC Archives.

18   Dr. Filler, quoted in Arlene Waite, "The Gift of Giving," *Country Estate*, November 1990, 5, The Herbie Fund Subject File 2, HSC Archives. See also Information Sheet, "The Herbie Fund," August 1979, The Herbie Fund Subject File 1, HSC Archives.

19   Bill Houston, "Girl Dies Despite Herbie-Fund Help," *Sunday Sun*, 1 April 1979, Herbie Fund Subject File 1; "Family Mourns Lost Child," *Toronto Star*, 2 April 1979, A3.

20   Jackie Smith, "Man Offers $2,000 to Aid Sick Boy," *Toronto Star*, 2 December 1980, Herbie Fund Subject File #1, HSC Archives. See Kathy English, "Bid to Save a Little Boy," *Toronto Sun*, 2 December 1981, Herbie Fund Subject File #1, HSC Archives; Waite, "The Gift of Giving," 5,

The Herbie Fund Subject File 2. Although she was funded by the community and was not a Herbie fund patient: "Girl here for gift of life," *Toronto Sun*, 24 July 1979, Herbie Fund Subject File, HSC Archives; John Munch, "Metro Arabs Rally Round Girl," *Toronto Star* 25 July 1979, A4.

21 *Our Day, Our Decade: Ten Years of the Herbie Fund at the HSC*, The Herbie Fund Subject File 1. See Claudia Anderson, Director of Public Affairs, letter to the editor, *Canadian Medical Association Journal* 140, no. 1 (1989): 11–12. http://www.ncbi.nlm.nih.gov/pmc/articles/PMC1268512/pdf/cmaj00182-0013b.pdf.

22 Marina Jimenez, "The Great Divide," *Toronto Life*, February 2006, 46–53; The Herbie Fund, "Success Stories: Who is Herbie Helping?," http://www.herbiefund.com/childrenTinashe.asp; Jan Wong, "Twin Peaks (10 Things Canada Does Best: A Series Exploring How This Land Leads the World)," *Globe and Mail*, 25 June 2005, F1.

23 Herbie Hoedown invitation card, Herbie Fund Subject File #2, HSC Archives.

24 Brianne Hogan, "More than 30 Years of Life-Changing Surgeries," *Post City Magazine*, 29 September 2011, http://www.postcity.com/Post-City-Magazines/October-2011/More-than-30-years-of-life-changing-surgeries/. See booklet and program, the Cartier Mistletoe Ball 1991, The Herbie Fund Subject File 2; Sheila Sotton, "Herbie Fund Gets Big Boost," *Toronto Star*, 29 December 1988, B2.

25 Quotation in Rosemary Sexton, "Ball Raises $175,000 to Save Children's Lives," *Globe and Mail*, 12 December 1989, A19; Rosemary Sexton, "Holt Renfrew Fashion Show Helps the Herbie Fund," *Globe and Mail*, 25 November 1989, A14.

26 Rosemary Sexton, "Cartier Mistletoe Ball Attracts the Cream," *Globe and Mail*, 8 December 1990, C6.

27 Ian Harvey, "Herbie Fund: Cash Means Lease on Life," *Toronto Sun*, 18 February 1988, 26, Herbie Fund Subject File #2, HSC Archives; Rosemary Sexton, "Flashy Times are Over," *Globe and Mail*, 10 October 1992, A1, A10; Nomi Morris, "Herbie's So Devoted to Metro He'll Even Cheer Jays over Mets," *Toronto Star*, 31 March 1989, A10.

28 Ludia Zajc, "Mexican Girl's 4 Operations Eat up Money in Herbie Fund," *Toronto Star*, 22 August 1988, A7; Lillian Newbery, "Herbie Fund Aids World's Children," *Toronto Star* 29 May 1997, G19.

29 L. Cohen and P.P. Morgan, "Medical Dramas and the Press: Who Benefits from the Coverage?" *Canadian Medical Association Journal* 139, no. 7 (1988): 659, http://www.ncbi.nlm.nih.gov/pmc/articles/PMC1268260/pdf/cmaj00176-0059.pdf.

30 Cohen and Morgan, "Medical Dramas and the Press," 657–61.

31 Polly Thomson, "Re 'Medical Dramas and the Press: Who Benefits from the Coverage?,'" letter to the editor, *Canadian Medical Association Journal* 140, no. 1 (1989): 11, http://www.ncbi.nlm.nih.gov/pmc/articles/PMC1268510/pdf/cmaj00182-0012c.pdf.

32 Claudia Anderson, "The Director of Public Affairs at The Hospital for Sick Children responds," letter to the editor, *Canadian Medical Association Journal* 140, no.1 (1989): 11. http://www.ncbi.nlm.nih.gov/pmc/articles/PMC1268511/pdf/cmaj00182-0013a.pdf

33 AR poster 1987–8.

34 "Because of the nursing shortage, we seldom had been able to open more than half our intensive care beds. Surgery often was cancelled; children were referred to other centres." Allan L. Beattie and David H. Martin, "A Servant to the Public," in AR 1990–1, 1; Richard Mackie, "Children's Hospital to Bar All but Essential Surgery," *Globe and Mail*, 15 June 1990, A1; Christie McLaren, "No Inquest Called in Case of Child Who Died Waiting," *Globe and Mail*, 13 February 1990, A15.

35 Children's Miracle Network, "SickKids Foundation," http://childrensmiraclenetwork.ca/Hospital/SickKidsFoundation; William Olcott, "Helping Sick Kids – Children's Miracle Network," *Fund Raising Management* 19, no. 10 (1988): 30–1; Roger H. Cook, "Miracles in the Making: The Story behind the Success of Children's Miracle Network," *Fund Raising Management* 31, no. 7 (2000): 10.

36 Mike Shannon, president of the Osmond Foundation, quoted in Olcott, "Helping Sick Kids," quotation 31, 30–2.

37 "A Chronology of the Marathon of Hope," *Globe and Mail*, 29 June 1981, 11; Salem Alaton, "Charity Knows No Bounds," *Globe and Mail*, 4 December 1982, F3; Jane Gadd, "Smaller Groups Feel the Pinch: Charities Compete for Funds," *Globe and Mail*, 9 April 1983, C16; Joanne Strong, "Charity Is TV Host's Specialty," *Globe and Mail*, 26 January 1984, L8; David Tatt, "The Diary," *Globe and Mail*, 22 March 1986, A18.

38 "HSC Foundation and CFTO-TV to Join June Telethon," *This Week* 2, no. 4 (985): 4; "Four Other Canadian Children's Hospitals Join the Miracle Network," *This Week* 2, no. 21 (1985): 2; Children's Miracle Network Television, *This Week* 2, no 11. (14 March 1985): 1; "That 1.13 Million Dollar Feeling!" *This Week* 2, no. 23 (1985): 1; *This Week* 3, no. 25 (1986): 1.

39 Karen Pallarito, "Children's Miracle Network Continues Raising Money, Public's Consciousness," *Modern Healthcare* 22, no. 25 (1992): 96.

40 Crouzon syndrome is an autosomal genetic disorder (chromosome 10) that affects craniofacial structure and development whereby bones prematurely "fuse," thus impeding normal bone growth.

41 HSC Telethon 1987, edited footage (2005–028–031–004); 1985 HSC Telethon Highlight Package 2005–028–031–001, HSC Archives; "Telethon Film Crew May Visit Your Area," *This Week* 3, no. 8 (1986): 1.

42 1985 HSC Telethon Highlight Package 2005–028–031–001, HSC Archives.

43 "Multicultural Efforts Here," *Toronto Star*, 1 June 1989, M9; CHIN Radio, "Johnny Lombardi," www.chinradio.com/about/johnny-lombardi.

44 *This Week* 3, no. 25 (1986): 1; "Volunteer Leaders Ready to Roll for June Telethon," *What's New* 3, no. 10 (1986): 1; David Taft, "The Diary," *Globe and Mail*, 18 May 1985, M2; Jack Lakey, "Zoo Raises Funds for Sick Kids," *Toronto Star*, 10 June 1986, 9; Lilana Novakovich, "Lilana's Diary," *Toronto Star*, 4 April 1987, 68; Bill Taylor, "Stars Coming Out for Kids' Hospital: Telethon Aims to Raise $1 million," *Toronto Star*, 12 June 1986, H1.

45 David Martin, "Swallowing the Bitter Pill," *The Empire Club of Canada Addresses* (Toronto, 16 November 1989), 109–18, http://speeches.empireclub.org/61220/data?n=33.

46 Paul Taylor, "New Medical Wing a Family Affair," *Globe and Mail*, 12 January 1993, A10. See AR 1985–6, 11.

47 "A Miracle Renewed," *Globe and Mail*, 25 January 1993, special advertising supplement, C1.

48 "Becoming Partners in a Consumer-Oriented World," *Kaleidoscope*, Winter 1993–4, 5, HSC Archives.

49 Madeleine Grey, "Brightening Up Sick Kids!" *DownWrite Special*, April–May 1993. Hospital 6th Subject File, HSC Archives.

50 Haslam quoted in "Changes Reflect New Needs," *Globe and Mail*, 25 January 1993, special advertising supplement, C5.

51 Mary Lou Lobsinger, Review, "Animation for Sick Kids (Toronto's New Hospital for Sick Children)," *Canadian Architect* 38, no. 4 (1993): 20; *Insider Report on the Capital Campaign for the HSC* (accompaniment to *This Week*) no. 1 (April 1985): 1; AR 1992–3, 1–2.

52 Quotation in "Annual Report of the Chairman of the Board of Trustees and the President and Chief Executive Officer," AR 1984–5, 10. See "Building a Strong Foundation: The Capital Campaign Gets Started," *This Week* 3, no. 9 (1985): 1; Duncan L. Gordon, "Report of the Chairman of the Board of Trustees and the Executive Director," AR 1982, 3; Leslie Fruman, "Remarkable Reva," *Toronto Star*, 8 July 1986, B1.

53 Louise Brown, "11 hospitals' Special Campaign Fundraising Goals," *Toronto Star*, 18 January 1987, H4. See "Insider Report on the Capital Campaign for the HSC," *This Week*, no. 1 (1985).

54 Quotation Walter Stefaniuk, "'Eat Dust, Guys,' Says Media Racer: Star Reporter Places Second via Rolls and Priority Post," *Toronto Star*, 9 May 1986, final edition, A11; "Famous Faces Will Show at the Capital Campaign Launch," *This Week* 3, no. 17 (1986): 2.

55 Louise Brown, "Why Metro Hospitals are Pleading for Money," *Toronto Star*, 18 January 1987, H1. See "Ontario Gives $60 million to Sick Kids Hospital" *Toronto Star*, 9 May 1986, A1.

56 Rona Maynard, "Tightwads, Ltd.: Corporate Canada is Drowning in Requests for Money for Worthy Causes – and It's Doling Out Less than Ever Before," *Report on Business Magazine*, April 1987, 30–2, quotation 34.

57 AR 1986–7, n.p.; "What's Going On at the Atrium on Bay?: An Update on Capital Campaign Activities," *This Week* 3, no. 42 (1986): 1; AR 1989–90, n.p.; *This Week* 3, no. 25 (1986): 1.

58 Tom Spears, "Inquest Jury Says Wrecking Firm 'Somewhat deficient' in Safety," *Toronto Star*, 20 April 1988, A6; Anonymous oral interview by author, participant #7, 15 January 2014; Don Dutton, "Falling Slab Kills Woman at Sick Kids," *Toronto Star*, 19 November 1987, A2.

59 Phinjo Gombu, "Demolition Firm Cleared in Death," *Toronto Star*, 6 January 1990, A17; "Worker's Death Draws $600,000 Fine," *Toronto Star*, 13 February 1993, A6; AR 1990–1, 1; AR 1991–2, 1.

60 "Nurse Shortage Restricts Work at Sick Kids," *Ottawa Citizen*, 15 June 1990, final edition, A13; Craig McInnes, "Living with Death: The Strains of Daily Tragedy Feed Chronic Shortage of Nurses," *Globe and Mail*, 4 August 1987, A1; Joseph Hall, "Nurses Wage Daily War on Death at Sick Kids Intensive Care Unit," *Toronto Star*, 18 March 1990: A1. This issue became a point of intense political debate. See, for example, Hansard Debates of the Ontario Legislature 1989–91 inter alia session: 34:2, date: 1989–06–15, http://hansardindex.ontla.on.ca/ hansardeissue/34-2/l026.htm; session: 35:1, date: 1991–11–06, http://hansardindex.ontla. on.ca/hansardeissue/35-1/l081.htm; and session: 34:2, date: 1990-06-14, http://hansardindex. ontla.on.ca/hansardeissue/34-2/l047_90.htm.

61 Lisa Priest, "Sick Children's Addition Full of High-Tech Wonder," *Toronto Star*, 12 January 1993, A7.

62 AR 1992–3, 5; Frank Calleja, "It's a Moving Time at Revamped Sick Kids," *Toronto Star*, 15 March 1993, A7.

63 "*Congratulations!!* The Hospital for Sick Children Opens Its New Doors," *Alumnae News* (Spring 1993), 1, HSC Archives.

64 Annmarie Adams and David Theodore, "Designing for "the Little Convalescents": Children's Hospitals in Toronto and Montreal, 1875–2006," *Canadian Bulletin of Medical History* 19, no. 1 (2002): 229–33.

65 Madeleine Grey, "Brightening Up Sick Kids!" *DownWrite Special*, April–May 1993, in Hospital 6th Subject File #13, HSC Archives.

66 "Pediatric Care Finds Its Jerusalem. The Perfect Setting," *Globe and Mail*, 25 January, 1993, special advertising supplement, C3. Quoted also by Edward Shorter, *Partnership for Excellence: Medicine at the University of Toronto and Academic Hospitals* (Toronto: University of Toronto, 2013), 257.

67 HSC Spokesperson Claudia Anderson, quoted in "A Great Big Thanks," *Globe and Mail*, 25 January 1993, C4.

68 Quoted in "A Miracle Renewed," *Globe and Mail*, 25 January 1993, C4.

69 Quotation from anonymous oral interview by author, participant #15, 24 May 2014; AR 1983–4, titled "Sicker Children, Greater Care."

70 "*Congratulations!!* The Hospital for Sick Children Opens Its New Doors in 1993," *Alumnae News*, Spring 1993, 1; AR 1994–5, 31.

71 Peter Larson, "Hospital Revamp Born Out of Baby Deaths Probe," *Edmonton Journal*, 18 August 1990, G6.

72 Eva Innes and Lesley Southwick-Trask, *Turning It Around: How Ten Canadian Organizations Changed Their Fortunes* (Toronto: Random House, 1989), 34–5; David Martin, "A Letter from the President," *This Week* 3, no. 49 (1986): 2–3. See also AR 1986–7.

73 Innes and Southwick-Trask, *Turning It Around*, 36.

74 Martin, "A Letter from the President," 2.

75 Miriam Shuchman, *The Drug Trial: Nancy Olivieri and the Science Scandal that Rocked the Hospital for Sick Children* (Toronto: Random House Canada, 2005), 228.

76 Anonymous interview by author, participant #14, 16 April 2014.

77 Anonymous interview by author, participant #1, 30 October 2013.

78 See Innes and Southwick-Trask, *Turning It Around*, 31–50; Martin "Swallowing the Bitter Pill."

79 Quotation Gillian Cosgrove, "Raising a Glass to Herbie: First Recipient of Herbie Fund Now 24 and Happy to be Here," *National Post*, 14 December 2002, T01/front; "Herbie Gets a Kick," *The Medical Post* (Toronto), 1 December 1981, The Herbie Fund Subject File 1; Gus Carlson, "It's Not 'Baby Herbie' Any More," *Toronto Sun*, 25 November 1981, 30, The Herbie Fund Subject File 1, HSC Archives.

80 Dale Brazao, "Star Finds Herbie Quinones Jr. Healthy at 30," *The Star*, 18 April 2009 http://www.thestar.com/life/health_wellness/2009/04/18/star_finds_herbie_quinones_jr_healthy_at_30.html

81 "Campaign Was Big Winner," *Globe and Mail*, 25 January 1993, C4 (Special Advertising Supplement).

82 Annmarie Adams, David Theodore, Ellie Goldenberg, Coralee McLaren, and Patricia McKeever, "Kids in the Atrium: Comparing Architectural Intentions and Children's Experiences in a Pediatric Hospital Lobby," *Social Science & Medicine* 70, no. 5 (2010): 658–67.

83 Smoking had been banned in corridors, elevators, stairwells, patient areas, labs, and anywhere with flammable liquids or medical gases since the 1970s. Jim Finlay, "Don't Strike Your Match on that Oxygen Tank!" *What's New* 8, no. 6 (1975): 3, 5. At the end of 1986, the policy banned smoking in children's areas of the building. It was permitted only in designated areas and single-occupant offices. At that time, it was decided to remove the cigarette machine. "HSC Adopts Healthier Policy on Smoking," *This Week* 3, no. 51 (1986): 1. The (old) cafeteria had had a smoking section, which was eliminated with the new cafeteria adjacent to the Atrium.

14 A GENETIC WILDERNESS

1 Helen Pearson, "One Gene, Twenty Years," *Nature* 460 (2009): 166.

2 Quotation Pat Ohlendorf, "The Taming of a Once-Certain Killer," *Maclean's*, 7 October 1985, 50; Wendy Herman, "Passion for Life: Susan Has No Time to Waste in Self-Pity over Fatal Disease," *Toronto Star*, 15 October 1980, A10; "Victim of Cystic Fibrosis Cheats Death Every Day," *Montreal Gazette*, 16 October 1980, 88; "The Wish," mini-doc in Telethon Highlight Package VHS (1985) 2005–028–031–001, HSC Archives.

3 "Victim of Cystic Fibrosis Cheats Death Every Day," 88.

4 Sherwin Huth, quoted by The Canadian Press, "Susan McKellar Dead at 42," *Calgary Herald*, final edition, 4 September 1997, A12; "Victim of Cystic Fibrosis Cheats Death Every Day," 88; Ohlendorf, "The Taming of a Once-Certain Killer," 50; Mary Hynes, "CF Victims Defy Fatal Disease," *Globe and Mail*, 28 May 1982, 11; Lillian Newberry, "CF Victims Celebrate 'Old Age,'" *Toronto Star*, 29 July 1984, D4.

5 Hynes, "CF Victims Defy Fatal Disease," 11; Newberry, "CF Victims Celebrate 'Old Age,'" D4; Passages from *Maclean's*, 15 September 1997, 11.

6 Quoted in Donna Jean MacKinnon, "Susan McKellar, 42, Fought to Help Cystic Fibrosis Patients," *Toronto Star*, final edition, 4 September 1997, A8; "Victim of Cystic Fibrosis Cheats Death Every Day," 88.

7 Passages from *Maclean's*, 15 September 1997, 11; "The Wish," mini-doc; MacKinnon, "Susan McKellar, 42," A8.

8 Peter S. Harper, ed., *Landmarks in Medical Genetics: Classic Papers with Commentaries* (Oxford: Oxford University Press, 2004), 67ff. See Joe Hin Tjio and Albert Levan, "The Chromosome Number of Man," *Hereditas* 42, no. 1–2 (1956): 1–6.

9   Fritz Fuchs and Povl Riis, "Antenatal Sex Determination," *Nature* 177, no. 4503 (1956): 330; Harper, ed., *Landmarks in Medical* Genetics, 67ff; Ruth Schwartz Cowan, "Medicine, Technology, and Gender in the History of Prenatal Diagnosis," in *Feminism in Twentieth-Century Science, Technology, and Medicine*, ed. Angela N.H. Creager, Elizabeth Lunbeck, and Londa L. Schiebinger (Chicago: University of Chicago Press, 2001), 186–96; Ruth Schwartz Cowan, "Women's Roles in the History of Amniocentesis and Chorionic villi Sampling," in *Women and Prenatal Testing: Facing the Challenges of Genetic Technology*, ed. Karen H. Rothenberg and Elizabeth J. Thomson (Columbus: Ohio State University Press, 1994): 35–48.

10 Joan Hollobon, "Fluid Test Gives Warning of Retardation," *Globe and Mail*, 11 November 1968, 13; Lydia Dotto, "The Search for the Disabling Gene," *Globe and Mail*, 20 July 1972, W1; Hospital for Sick Children, Annual Report 1974, 19–20.

11 William Leeming, "The Early History of Medical Genetics in Canada," *Social History of Medicine* 17, no. 3 (2004): 492–3; Fiona Miller, "A Blueprint for Defining Health: Making Medical Genetics in Canada" (PhD diss., York University, 2000).

12 Manuel Buchwald, interview with Susan Belanger (21 December 2006), History of the Department of Paediatrics Fonds, Folder 2007-230-031 in Box 44, HSC Archives; Minutes of the Service, Education and Research Committee, 18 October 1979 and 13 September 1979; Hugh O'Brodovich with Elizabeth Uleryk, Susan Belanger, Daune MacGregor, and Michelle O'Brodovich, (unpublished manuscript, December 2008, HSC Archives), 109; Robert Cook Deegan, (New York: W.W. Norton and Company, 1994), 62.

13 Pearson, "One Gene, Twenty Years," 166; Margaret W. Thompson, Roderick R. McInnes, Huntington F. Willard, eds., *Thompson & Thompson Genetics in Medicine*, 5th ed. (Toronto: W.B. Saunders Company, 1991), 2–3; "Human Molecular Genetics," in *A Short History of Medical Genetics*, ed. Peter Harper (New York: Oxford University Press, 2008), 363–71; Elise Hancock, "The Short Course That's Long on Influence," *Johns Hopkins Magazine*, November 1996, 10. See also Victor McElheny, *Drawing the Map of Life: Inside the Human Genome Project* (New York: Basic Books, 2010), 30ff; Deegan, *Gene Wars*, 64.

14 Marilyn Dunlop, "'Curtain of Silence' Hid Hunt for Deadly Cystic Fibrosis Gene," *Toronto Star*, 8 September 1989, A20.

15 Quotation in Steven Scherer, Steacie Prize Award Address, 26 February 2004, Current HSC News (archived and printed webpage), History of the Department of Paediatrics Fonds, Box 45, Folder 2007–230-031, HSC Archives; Victor A. McKusick, "History of Medical Genetics," in *Emery and Rimoin's Essential Medical Genetics*, ed. David L. Rimoin, Reed E. Pyeritz, and Bruce R. Korf (Waltham, MA: Elsevier, 2013), 7; Ronald G. Worton and Margaret W. Thompson. "Genetics of Duchenne Muscular Dystrophy," *Annual Review of Genetics* 22 (1988): 602; Dunlop, "'Curtain of Silence,'" A20.

16 Pearson, "One Gene, Twenty Years," 166.

17 Lawrence Surtees, "Hospital for Sick Children Scientists Identify Cystic Fibrosis Gene Defect," *Globe and Mail*, 24 August 1989, A14; Pearson, "One Gene, Twenty Years," 166.

18 Jean L. Marx, "The Cystic Fibrosis Gene Is Found," *Science* 245, no. 4921 (1989): 923–5.

19 Marx, "The CF Gene Hits the News," *Science* 245, no. 4921 (1989), 924; Marx, "The Cystic Fibrosis Gene Is Found," 923; John R. Riordan, Johanna M. Rommens, Bat-sheva Kerem, Noa Alon, Richard Rozmahel, Zbyszko Grzelczak, and others, "Identification of the Cystic Fibrosis Gene: Cloning and Characterization of Complementary DNA," *Science* 245, no. 4922 (1989): 1066–73.

20 Buchwald, interview with Susan Belanger, 7; Marx, "The CF Gene Hits the News," 924; Marx, "The Cystic Fibrosis Gene Is Found," 923–5; "Telling the World about the CF gene," *This Week* 6, no. 35 (1989): 1.

21 Anonymous oral interview by author, participant #13, 14 January 2015.

22 André Picard, *The Gift of Death: Confronting Canada's Tainted-Blood Tragedy* (Toronto: HarperCollins, 1995). For a father's account of a child infected by tainted blood, see Vic

Parsons, *Bad Blood: The Tragedy of the Canadian Tainted Blood Scandal* (Toronto: Lester Publishing, 1995).

23 Claudia Anderson, quoted in Mary Williams Walsh, "AIDS Crisis Hits Home in Canada," *Los Angeles Times*, 17 April 1993, A21; André Picard, "Surveys Show 1985 a Bad Year for Blood," *Globe and Mail*, 26 March 1994, A9.

24 "AIDS ALERT: Sick Kids Hospital Warns of '79–'86 Blood Risk," *Toronto Sun*, 16 April 1993, 1. See "Hospital Launches HIV Information Project," *This Week* 10, no. 15 (1993): 1. See also Picard, *The Gift of Death*, 152–3; "Parents Call HSC for Details on HIV Information Project," *This Week* 10, no. 16 (1993): 1.

25 Debra Black, "Living with a Killer," *Toronto Star*, 26 April 2002, F01.

26 Walsh, "AIDS Crisis Hits Home in Canada," A21.

27 Ciaran Ganely and Linda Barnard, "Hotline Swamped," *Toronto Sun*, 17 April 1993, 4.

28 Picard, *The Gift of Death*, 153. Of the seventeen, eleven had previously been diagnosed, and six were new diagnoses resulting from the notification project. Susan King, Trudy Murphy, Mary Corey, Alice M. Newman, Carol Major, Brian W. McCrindle, Judry Irwin, Marion Stevens, Margaret Fearon, and Annette O. Poon, "The HIV Information Project for Transfusion Recipients a Decade After Transfusion," *Archives of Pediatrics and Adolescent Medicine* 149 (1995): 680–5; "HIV Information Project Nears End of Phase Three," *This Week* 11, no. 40 (1994): 1.

29 "HSC Sends Letters to Blood Product Recipients," *This Week* 11, no. 14 (1994): 1.

30 Picard, *The Gift of Death*, 153, 154; André Picard, "Find Tainted-Blood Victims, Ottawa Told," *Globe and Mail*, 18 May 1993, A1, A2.

31 "HSC Scientists Involved in AIDS Research," *This Week* 2, no. 35 (1985): 1; Janet Bagnall, "When a Child Gets AIDS, Anguish Is Hard to Take," *Montreal Gazette*, 17 August 1987, A1; Sarah Jane Growe, "Born without Hope," *Toronto Star*, 12 September 1987, F1; Heather Mallick, "'Children Had to Take Chance,' MD Says," *Globe and Mail*, 29 May 1987, A12.

32 Anne Mullens, "Living in Fear: Clotting Breakthrough for Hemophiliacs Carried a Terrible Price," *Vancouver Sun*, 10 June 1987, A12; Herbert H. Denton, "AIDS Reported at Canadian Clinic: Young Hemophilia Patients Exposed Through Blood Transfusions," *Washington Post*, 31 May 1987, A19.

33 "Why I'm Not Worried about [Catching] AIDS, by an HSC Physician," *This Week* 2, no. 39 (1985): 2.

34 Lillian Newberry, "Fear of Getting AIDS from Hemophiliacs Needless, Doctors Say," *Toronto Star*, 29 May 1987, A13.

35 "Infectious Disease Program for Children with HIV, AIDS," *This Week* 6, no. 2 (1989): 1; Marilyn Dunlop, "3 AIDS Babies Doing Well on New Drug, Doctor Says," *Toronto Star*, 6 May 1989, A3.

36 Rod Mickleburgh, "Anger, Tears as Victims Tell of Blood Horror," *Globe and Mail*, 22 February 1994, A1. See also Picard, *The Gift of Death*, 151.

37 Georgina MacDougall (HIV clinic coordinator), "Staff Perspectives" (2013), http://www.sickkids.ca/AboutSickKids/Newsroom/Past-News/2013/HIV-staff-perspectives.html.

38 Leonarda Szewczyk, quoted in "CHAS Advocates, Supports and Educates Parents," *This Week* 8, no. 35 (1991): 2; "Daylong Program Explores Ethics in AIDS," *This Week* 6, no. 15 (1989): 2; "Parents Split on Tests," *Sunday Sun*, 7 May 1989, 26; Dick Chapman, "Kids' AIDS Tests Secret," *Saturday Sun*, 6 May 1989, 16.

39 International Monetary Fund, "Historical Public Debt Database," http://www.imf.org/external/datamapper/index.php?db=DEBT.

40 Cemile Sancak, Lucy Qian Liu, and Taisuke Nakata, "Canada: A Success Story," in *Chipping Away at Public Debt: Sources of Failure and Keys to Success in Fiscal Adjustment*, ed. Paolo Mauro (Hoboken, NJ: John Wiley and Sons, 2011), 5.

41 Aleck Ostry estimates that federal transfers to provincial governments for health-care expenditures dropped from 42.3 per cent of provincial health-care expenditures in 1977

to 32.1 per cent in 1995. Aleck Ostry, *Changes and Continuity in Canada's Health Care System* (Ottawa: CHA Press, 2006), 81–2.

42 Quotation in Duncan Gordon Sinclair, Mark Rochon, and Peggy Leatt, *Riding the Third Rail: The Story of Ontario's Health Services Restructuring Commission, 1996–2000* (Montreal: IRPP, 2005), 1; Raisa Deber, "Rethinking and Re-balancing: The Changing Role of Hospitals in the Canadian Health Care System," in *Survival Strategies: the Life, Death and Renaissance of a Canadian Teaching Hospital*, ed. David Goyette, Dennis William Magill, and Jeff Denis (Toronto: Canadian Scholars' Press, 2006), 23–9.

43 Sinclair, Rochon, and Leatt, *Riding the Third Rail*, 1.

44 Kate Bezanson, *Gender, the State, and Social Reproduction: Household Insecurity in Neo-Liberal Times* (Toronto: University of Toronto Press, 2006), 55.

45 Michael Bliss, *Beyond the Granting Agency: The Medical Research Council in the 1990s* (Ottawa: Medical Research Council of Canada, 2000), 15.

46 Medical Research Council (Canada), *A Legacy of Excellence, 1960–2000, 40 Years* (Ottawa: Medical Research Council of Canada, 2000), 18.

47 Dr. Henry Friesen, *Report of the President 1993–1994* (Ottawa: Medical Research Council, 1994), 8.

48 Bliss, *Beyond the Granting Agency*, 11, 13.

49 Ibid., 13.

50 Health Services Restructuring Commission, "Important Information About Building a Better Health System in Metropolitan Toronto," *Toronto Star*, 24 July 1997, advertisement, A21. See also "HSC Confirms Support of Hospital Restructuring and Accepts Child Health Network Leadership Role," *This Week* 14, no. 14 (1997): 1; Jon Thompson, Patricia Baird, and Jocelyn Downie, *The Olivieri Report: The Complete Text of the Report of the Independent Inquiry Commissioned by the Canadian Association of University Teachers*, A CAUT Series Title (Toronto: James Lorimer and Company, 2001), 228.

51 Arnold Naimark, reviewer, and Bertha Maria Knoppers and Frederick H. Lowy, associate reviewers, *Clinical Trials of L1 (Deferiprone) at The Hospital for Sick Children in Toronto: A Review of Facts and Circumstances* (1998), HSC Archives Version (deposited January 1999), 59–67, 136–7, 146.

52 Miriam Shuchman, *The Drug Trial: Nancy Olivieri and the Science Scandal that Rocked the Hospital for Sick Children* (Toronto: Random House Canada, 2005), 86–7; Thompson, Baird, and Downie, *The Olivieri Report*, 225.

53 Naimark, Knoppers, and Lowy, *Clinical Trials of L1*, 57–9; Thompson, Baird, and Downie, *The Olivieri Report*, 226.

54 Naimark, Knoppers, and Lowy, *Clinical Trials of L1*, 64.

55 Michael Valpy, "Science Friction," *Elm Street*, December 1998, 35.

56 Naimark, Knoppers, and Lowy, *Clinical Trials of L1*, 114; Thompson, Baird, and Downie, *The Olivieri Report*, 230.

57 Thompson, Baird, and Downie, *The Olivieri Report*, 64.

58 Quotation ibid., 4; Shuchman, *The Drug Trial*, 14, 17, 388.

59 Shuchman, *The Drug Trial*, quotation 94–5, 57, 387; Thompson, Baird, and Downie, *The Olivieri Report*, 24, 103–8; Naimark, Knoppers, and Lowy, *Clinical Trials of L1*, 134.

60 Reflecting on the Olivieri-Apotex dispute, David Nathan and David Weatherall would later assert that Ciba-Geigy "abandoned" Deferiprone "in 1993 because of its low therapeutic index in animals without iron overload, its poor stoichiometry ... and its rapid removal from the circulation." David G. Nathan, and David J Weatherall, "Academic Freedom in Clinical Research," *New England Journal of Medicine* 347, no. 17 (2002): 1368.

61 Thompson, Baird, and Downie, *The Olivieri Report*, 120. "The LA-01 protocol and all subsequent modifications were formally approved by the REB, but the contract was formally approved neither by the HSC administration nor the University" (112). See also 111–12 and

115-16; Nancy F. Olivieri et al., "Iron-Chelation Therapy with Oral Deferiprone in Patients with Thalassemia Major," *New England Journal of Medicine* 332, no. 14 (1995): 918–22.

62 Thompson, Baird, and Downie, *The Olivieri Report*, quotation 5, 111, 115. See Miriam Shuchman, "Legal Issues Surrounding Privately Funded Research Cause Furore in Toronto," *Canadian Medical Association Journal* 159, no. 8 (1998): 983, http://www.cmaj.ca/content/159/8/983.full.pdf.

63 Thompson, Baird, and Downie, *The Olivieri Report*, quotation 5, 143ff; HSC Hospital Executive, "Information on The Dr Nancy Olivieri/Apotex Controversy," 1, HSC Archives, Unprocessed Olivieri Material.

64 Thompson, Baird, and Downie, *The Olivieri Report*, 151.

65 Ibid., 115–16.

66 Quotation ibid., 6; HSC, Hospital Executive, "Information on The Dr Nancy Olivieri/Apotex Controversy."

67 Thompson, Baird, and Downie, *The Olivieri Report*, 187–9.

68 Ibid., 6–7.

69 Naimark, Knoppers, and Lowy, *Clinical Trials of L1*, 41–2.

70 Ibid., 43.

71 HSC, Hospital Executive, "Information on the Dr Nancy Olivieri/Apotex Controversy"; Nancy F. Olivieri et al., "Long-Term Safety and Effectiveness of Iron-Chelation Therapy with Deferiprone for Thalassemia Major," *New England Journal of Medicine* 339, no. 7 (1998): 417–23; Kris V. Kowdley, and Marshall M. Kaplan, Editorial "Iron-Chelation Therapy with Oral Deferiprone – Toxicity or Lack of Efficacy?," *New England Journal of Medicine* 339, no. 7 (1998): 468; Michael Strofolino, "To All Staff, Scientists and Clinicians," *This Week* 15, no. 33 (1998): 1; "L1 Clinical Trials Report released," *This Week* 15, no. 49 (1998), 1.

72 Medical Advisory Committee minutes, 1 March 2000, HSC Archives; A.M. Viens and Julian Savulescu, "Introduction to the Olivieri Symposium," *Journal of Medical Ethics* 30, no. 1 (2004): 5.

73 Shuchman, *The Drug Trial*, 292–4; Prof. Rhonda Love (VP Grievances), UFTA news release, 7 January 1999.

74 Shuchman, *The Drug Trial*, quotation 363, 391; Thompson, Baird, and Downie, *The Olivieri Report*, 179.

75 Shuchman, *The Drug Trial*, 391.

76 Thompson, Baird, and Downie, *The Olivieri Report*, 10, 12, 397–402; Laura Bonetta, "Hate-Mail Author Trapped by DNA," *Nature Medicine* 6, no. 4 (2000): 364, http://www.nature.com/nm/journal/v6/n4/pdf/nm0400_364a.pdf; Krista Foss and Andrew Mitrovica, "Sick Kids Battle Turns Bizarre," *Globe and Mail*, 21 December 1999, A1; Scott Simmie, "Hate Mail Scandal Explodes at Sick Kids," *Toronto Star*, 21 December 1999, A1, A8; Krista Foss, "Leading Doctor Steps Down from 3 Posts at Sick Kids, U of T," *Globe and Mail*, 31 December 1999, A2.

77 Harold Levy, "Sick Kids MD Hearing Delayed over New Claims," *Toronto Star*, 5 January 2000, A20.

78 Nicolaas van Rijn and Scott Simmie, "Widen Poison Pen Probe, Lawyers Demand," *Toronto Star*, 4 January 2000, A2.

79 Shuchman, *The Drug Trial*, 340, 341.

80 Ibid., 347.

81 Karen Birmingham, "No Dismissal for Hate-Mail Author," *Nature Medicine* 6, no. 6 (2000): 609.

82 Anne Kingston, "Explosive Judicial Review puts lens on Gideon Koren and SickKids," , 4 January 2016; http://www.macleans.ca/society/health/explosive-judicial-review-puts-lens-on-gideon-koren-and-sickkids/.

83 Karen Birmingham, "Second HSC Researcher Sends Anonymous 'Olivieri' Note," *Nature Medicine* 6, no. 5 (2000): 485.

84 Viens and Savulescu, "Introduction to the Olivieri Symposium," 5.

85 Michael Higgins, "Olivieri, Hospital Settle Dispute," *National Post*, 13 November 2002, A19, front.

86 Anne McIlroy, "Olivieri, Supporters Awarded Settlement," *Globe and Mail*, 13 November 2002, A4.

87 Dalhousie University, "Nancy F. Olivieri: May 2012 Honorary Degree Recipient," http://www.dal.ca/academics/convocation/ceremonies/honorary_degree_recipients/hon_degree_2012/nancy_olivieri.html; "Nancy F. Olivieri, MD, MA, FRCPC," *Research at UHN*, http://www.uhnresearch.ca/researcher/nancy-f-olivieri.

88 Rose M. Morgan, preface to *The Genetics Revolution: History, Fears, and Future of a Life-Altering Science* (Westport Connecticut: Greenwood Press, 2006), viii.

89 Ronald G. Worton and Margaret Thompson, "Genetics of Duchenne Muscular Dystrophy," *Annual Review of Genetics* 22 (1988): 601–29, 623.

90 Jennifer Couzin-Frankel, "The Promise of a Cure: 20 Years and Counting," *Science* 324, no. 5934 (2009): 1504.

91 Pearson, "One Gene, Twenty Years," 167–8.

92 Anonymous oral interview by author, participant #13, 14 January 2015.

93 Quoted in Pearson, "One Gene, Twenty Years," 165; Harper, *A Short History of Medical Genetics*, 373.

94 Shuchman, *The Drug Trial*, 359. Medical Research Council (Canada), Natural Sciences and Engineering Research Council of Canada, and Social Sciences and Humanities Research Council of Canada, *Tri-Council Policy Statement: Ethical Conduct for Research Involving Humans* (Ottawa: Medical Research Council of Canada, 1998).

95 Quotation Vincent di Norcia, "A Compelling Study of the Growing Tensions in Clinical Research," review of *The Olivieri Report* by Thompson, Baird, and Downie, *Science and Engineering Ethics* 9, no. 1 (2003): 130; Tanya Talaga, "Olivieri Case Sparks Research Rules," *Toronto Star*, 28 January 1999, A1; "Sick Kids Investigation Prompts Policy Review," *University of Toronto Bulletin*, 4 December 1998, 3; "Summary of the University of Toronto's Position with Respect to Dr. Olivieri and the Hospital for Sick Children," 3 December 1998, appended to memo from J.R. Prichard to Governing Council. Unprocessed Olivieri Affair Material, HSC Archives.

96 Viens and Savulescu, "Introduction to the Olivieri Symposium," 5. See also Faculty of Medicine, *Harmonization of Research Policies, Schedule 3H* (Toronto: University of Toronto Faculty of Medicine, 2001), 36; D. Naylor, "Early Toronto Experience with New Standards for Industry-Sponsored Clinical Research: A Progress Report," *Canadian Medical Association Journal* 166 (2002): 453–5; L.E. Ferris, P.A. Singer, and C.D. Naylor, "The Olivieri Symposium: Better Governance in Academic Health Sciences Centres: Moving beyond the Olivieri/Apotex Affair in Toronto," *Journal of Medical Ethics* 30, no.1 (2004): 25–9.

97 Quotation in Arthur Schafer, "Biomedical Conflicts of Interest: A Defence of the Sequestration Thesis – Learning from the Cases of Nancy Olivieri and David Healy," *Journal of Medical Ethics* 30, no. 1 (2004): 8. See Anne McIlroy, "Prozac Critic Sees U of T Job Revoked," *Globe and Mail*, 14 April 2001, A1; Anne McIlroy, "Snub to Prozac Critic Upsets Teachers," *Globe and Mail*, 16 April 2001, A12; Tanya Talaga, "U of T Sued over Revoked Job," *Toronto Star*, 25 September 2001, B2; Sarah Boseley, "Bitter Pill," *The Guardian*, 7 May 2001, B2; Anjana Ahuja, "'Incompatible' Views That Could Scupper a Career," *The Times* (London), 7 May 2001, 10; Jenny Manzer, "CAMH Appointment Rejection Remains under Cloud," *Medical Post* 37, no.19 (2001): 5; Ann Silversides, "Hospital Denies that Withdrawal of MD's Job Offer Was Related to Drug-Company Funding," *Canadian Medical Association Journal* 164, no. 13 (2001): 1879.

98 Naimark, Knoppers, and Lowy, *Clinical Trials of L1*, 118.

99 Ferris, Singer, and Naylor, "The Olivieri Symposium."

100 Quotation in Dr. Stanley Read, "Staff Perspectives," http://www.sickkids.ca/AboutSickKids/Newsroom/Past-News/2013/HIV-staff-perspectives.html; Bruce Demara, "Lawsuit Fears Didn't Halt HIV Survey, Probe Told," *Toronto Star*, 11 March 1994, A5; Black, "Living with a Killer."

15 A HOSPITAL WITHOUT WALLS

1   Roger Cromarty, former Sioux Lookout residential school student, *The Survivors Speak: A Report of the Truth and Reconciliation Commission of Canada* (The Truth and Reconciliation Committee of Canada, 2015), 177.

2   Anglican Church of Canada, "Pelican Lake School – Sioux Lookout, ON," General Synod Archives, 23 September 2008, www.anglican.ca/tr/histories/pelican-lake/; Harry W. Bain and Gary Goldthorpe, "The University of Toronto 'Sioux Lookout Project' – A Model of Health Care Delivery," *Canadian Medical Association Journal* 107, no. 6 (1972): 524.

3   Maureen Lux, "Care for the 'Racially Careless': Indian Hospitals in the Canadian West, 1920–1950s," *Canadian Historical Review* 91, no. 3 (2010): 407–34.

4   Sioux Lookout Meno Ya Win Health Centre, "History: A Commitment to Health and Well-Being," www.slmhc.on.ca/history; T. Kue Young, *Health Care and Cultural Change: The Indian Experience in the Central Subarctic* (Toronto: University Toronto Press, 1988), 110.

5   T.K. Young, "Mortality Pattern of Isolated Indians in Northwestern Ontario: A 10-Year Review," *Public Health Reports* 98, no. 5 (1983): 470.

6   Evelyne Michaels, "The Sioux Lookout Program: So Many Problems, So Few Physicians," *Canadian Medical Association Journal* 141, no. 8 (1989): 812; AR 1968, 3–4.

7   Charlotte Gray, "Profile: Harry Bain," *Canadian Medical Association Journal* 129, no. 6 (1983): 614, www.ncbi.nlm.nih.gov/pmc/articles/PMC1875550/pdf/canmedajo1399-0092.pdf.

8   Quotation from John H. Read and F. L. Strick, "Medical Education and the Native Canadian: An Example of Mutual Symbiosis," *Canadian Medical Association Journal* 100, no. 11 (1969): 516; James Burgess Waldram, Ann Herring, and T. Kue Young, *Aboriginal Health in Canada: Historical, Cultural, and Epidemiological Perspectives*, 2nd ed. (Toronto: University of Toronto Press, 2006), 223–4; Harry W. Bain, "Canada's Native Children," *Canadian Medical Association Journal* 123, no. 12 (1980): 1237–8.

9   W.G. Goldthorpe, "Infant Health in an Outpost Area," *Canadian Family Physician* 21, no. 5 (1975): 76 (table 1).

10   Bain and Goldthorpe, "The University of Toronto 'Sioux Lookout Project.'"

11   Gray, "Profile: Harry Bain," 14; Scott-McKay-Bain Health Panel, *From Here to There: Steps along the Way* (Toronto: Scott-McKay-Bain Health Panel, 1989), 8; AR 1968, 3; T. Kue Young, "Primary Health Care for Isolated Indians in Northwestern Ontario," *Public Health Reports* 96, no. 5 (1981): 393–4.

12   Earl Dunn et al., "Telemedicine Links Patients in Sioux Lookout with Doctors in Toronto," *Canadian Medical Association Journal* 122, no. 4 (1980): 484.

13   AR 1968, 3; "Student Nurses at Sioux," *What's New* 2, no. 5 (1970). See also Keith C. Titley and Dennis H. Bedard, "An Evaluation of a Dental Care Program for Indian Children in the Community of Sandy Lake, Sioux Lookout Zone, 1973–1983," *Journal of the Canadian Dental Association,* 11 (1986): 923–8; University of Toronto Department of Psychiatry, "Providing Psychiatric Care and Consultation in Remote Indian Villages," *Hospital & Community Psychiatry,* 29, no. 10 (1978): 678–80.

14   Bain and Goldthorpe, "The University of Toronto 'Sioux Lookout Project,'" 523; Harry W. Bain to Dean R.B. Holmes (U of T Faculty of Medicine), 11 December 1978, Sioux Lookout Subject File, HSC Archives; Scott-McKay-Bain Health Panel, *From Here to There,* 21.

15   Bain, "Sioux Lookout Project," 9 March 1970, Sioux Lookout Subject File, HSC Archives.

16   Quotation in AR 1973, 15. See "First Hospital Heliport Emergency: Nip and Tuck Battle for a Baby's Life," *Globe and Mail,* 23 August 1972, 1; "Baby Girl 6 Hours Old First Emergency Case for Hospital Heliport," *Toronto Star,* 23 August 1972, 3.

17   AR 1972, 15. Joan Hollobon, "Sick Children's Issues Procedure Pamphlet: Helicopter Mercy Flights to Downtown Toronto Saved Three Lives," *Globe and Mail,* 4 October 1972, 12; "Hospital's Heliport Open," *Hospital Highlights* (Winter 1971–2), 2, Heliport and Helicopter Subject File, HSC Archives; David Beaumont, "Bandage 1 Covers Distance between Patients,

Hospital," *The Medical Post*, 15 July 1980, 20; figures in Kue Young, "Primary Health Care for Isolated Indians," 393–4.

18 AR, May 1972, 1–2; "Hospital's Heliport Open," 2; AR 1974, 3; "This Isn't Pie in the Sky!" *What's New* 13, no. 2 (1980): 12. It was later joined by Bandage Two and Bandage Three.

19 "This Isn't Pie in the Sky!"; Marilyn Dunlop, "Heliport 'Quickest' Lifesaver," *Toronto Star*, 19 August 1995, L7; Robert MacLeod, "Sick Kids Facing Crisis over Air Routes," *Globe and Mail*, 28 June 1991, A1.

20 AR 1973.

21 Janice Mawhinney, "High Drama: Neonatal Transport Team Rides to Rescue of Babies in Urgent Need of Treatment," *Toronto Star*, 29 May 1997, G4.

22 Ibid.

23 Chris Higgins, Earl Dunn, and David Conrath, "Telemedicine: An Historical Perspective," *Telecommunications Policy* 8, no. 4 (1984): 311.

24 A.M. House and J.M. Roberts, "Telemedicine in Canada," *Canadian Medical Association Journal* 117, no. 4 (1977): 387.

25 Scott-McKay-Bain Health Panel, *From Here to There*, 30–1; Dunn et al., "Telemedicine Links Patients in Sioux Lookout with Doctors in Toronto," 484.

26 Hospital for Sick Children, Public Affairs, "SickKids Establishes Telehealth Partnership with Trinidad and Tobago," news release, 2005, www.sickkids.ca/AboutSickKids/Newsroom/Past-News/2005/SickKids-establishes-telehealth-partnership-with-Trinidad-and-Tobago-2005-release.html.

27 Lisa Priest, "Reach Out and Treat Someone," *Toronto Star*, 8 February 1996, C6.

28 Andy Shaw, "Telehealth Moves Out of the Incubators, as Provinces and Hospitals Expand Projects," *Canadian Healthcare Technology*, October 1999, 18–19.

29 Priest, "Reach Out and Treat Someone."

30 Christine Wolfl, "SickKids Ophthalmologist Uses Telemedicine to Screen for Serious Eye Disease," SickKids Newsroom, 29 October 2014, www.sickkids.ca/AboutSickKids/Newsroom/Past-News/2014/SickKids-ophthalmologist-uses-telemedicine-to-screen-for-serious-eye-disease.html.

31 IBM later changed the name to Health Network Services or HNS.

32 "eCHN celebrates 10 years of Electronic Health Records for Children," *Canada NewsWire* [Ottawa], 2 March 2009.

33 Andrew Szende, "A Lifeline eHealth Record: The Electronic Child Health Network's State-of-the-Art Connectivity Solution is Revolutionizing the Sharing of Health Information in Ontario," *Canadian Healthcare Manager,* 8, no. 5 (2001): 55, 57.

34 Pat Stephens, "NBGH joins eCHN," *North Bay Nugget*, 14 August 2004, B7; Carol Goar, "Electronic Revolution in Health Care," *Toronto Star*, 11 March 2009, A19.

35 Amanda L. Mayo, "Evaluation of The Hospital for Sick Children's Electronic Patient Chart System," (MHSc thesis, University of Toronto, 2004), 3–6, 54, 65–6, 70–1.

36 Dr. Mark Feldman, quoted by André Picard, "Children's Health Network: Today the Children, Tomorrow ...," *Globe and Mail*, 6 March 2009, B8.

37 "Protect Health Privacy," *Toronto Star*, 12 March 2007, A14.

38 Megan Ogilvie, "Sick Kids Doctor Loses Data on 3,300 Patients," *Toronto Star*, 31 August 2007, A2.

39 Rob Ferguson, "Taxpayers Get $26.9M Bill for Axed eHealth Contract," *Toronto Star*, 19 June 2015, A1; "EHealth Scandal a $1B Waste: Auditor," *CBC News*, 7 October 2009.

40 Sioux Lookout Meno Ya Win Health Centre, "History," http://www.slmhc.on.ca/history.

41 Scott-McKay-Bain Health Panel, *From Here to There*, 21, 46–7, and passim.

42 See David Stymeist, "Indian Health in the North," in *Les Facettes de l'identite amérindienne* [The patterns of "Amerindian" identity], ed. Marc-Adélard Tremblay (Québec: Presses de l'Université Laval, 1976), 282–357 (237–78 de l'édition papier).

43 T. Kue Young, "Part Two: Changing Patterns of Health and Sickness among the Cree-Ojibwa of Northwestern Ontario," *Medical Anthropology* 3, no. 2 (1979): 218–19.

44 Sioux Lookout Meno Ya Win Health Centre, "History," www.slmhc.on.ca/history.

45 Geoffrey Tesson, Geoffrey Hudson, Roger Strasser, and Dan Hunt, eds., *Making of the Northern Ontario School of Medicine: A Case Study in the History of Medical Education* (Montreal: McGill-Queen's University Press, 2009), 197.

46 Commission on the Future of Health Care in Canada, and Roy J. Romanow, *Building on Values: The Future of Health Care in Canada: Final Report* (Saskatoon, SK: Commission on the Future of Health Care in Canada, 2002), xix, 77–80.

47 "Bring Medical Records into the Wired World," *Toronto Star*, 14 January 2007, A14.

16 SICKKIDS INTERNATIONAL

1 "Improving the Health of Children Worldwide: International Fellowship Program Trains Physicians from across the Globe," *Globe and Mail,* 29 November 2006, A21.

2 Andy Shaw, "Telehealth moves out of the incubators, as provinces and hospitals expand projects," *Canadian Healthcare Technology* (October 1999): 18–19; "Telehealth Helps HSC Spread the Word around the World," *This Week* 14, no. 35 (1997).

3 AR 2005–6, 1.

4 Anonymous interview by author, participant #1, 30 October 2013.

5 Anne Snowdon, Alexander Smith, and Heidi Cramm, "SickKids in Qatar – Responding to a Request for Proposal," Richard Ivey School of Business Case Collection, suppl. 9B14M025, 4 April 2014.

6 "SickKids Wins Gold for Innovative Business Model," *Canadian Healthcare Manager* 18, no. 3 (2011): 9.

7 Bernard Marr and James Creelman, *Doing More with Less: Measuring, Analyzing and Improving Performance in the Not-For-Profit and Government Sectors*, 2nd ed. (London: Palgrave Macmillan, 2014), 153–4.

8 "The Hospital for Sick Children: Collaborating with Partners around the World to Advance the Health of Children," *Middle East Health,* (July–August 2013): 54. www.middleeasthealthmag.com/jul2013/feature6.htm.

9 Donovan Vincent, "Sick Kids Helps Cancer in Caribbean: Hospital Wants Improved Care, Better Outcomes for Young Patients," *Toronto Star*, 21 January 2013, GT1.

10 "Toronto Attachments For Local Nursing Students," *Bernews*, 25 September 2013; Lara Pietrolungo, "A Balancing Act: The International Learner Program at The Hospital for Sick Children," presented to the 42nd Biennial Convention of the Sigma Theta Tau International Honor Society of Nursing, 16 November 2013; Lydia Aziato and Adzo Kwashie, eds., *Footprints of the Nursing Profession: Current Trends and Emerging Issues in Ghana* (Accra, Ghana: Sub-Saharan Publishers, 2014), 9.

11 Paul Dalby, "Hands across the Ocean: A Generation at Risk. Joint Nursing Program between SickKids and Ghana Aims to Reduce that Country's High Child-Mortality rate," *Toronto Star*, 6 May 2010, 17; SickKids International, "SickKids Focuses International Strategy," news release, 18 November 2011, www.sickkids.ca/AboutSickKids/Newsroom/Past-News/2011/SickKids-focuses-international-strategy.html.

12 Aziato and Kwashie, eds., *Footprints of the Nursing Profession*, 10–11.

13 Quotation in SickKids Foundation Annual Report (hereafter HSCF AR), 2009–10, 15; "India to Have Year-Long Festival in Canada," *The Hindustan Times* (New Delhi), 7 June 2009.

14 HSCF AR 2009–10, 14–15.

15 "Stanley Zlotkin," SickKids Directory, www.sickkids.ca/AboutSickKids/Directory/People/Z/Stanley-Zlotkin.html.

16 Ann Silversides, "Long Road to Sprinkles," *Canadian Medical Association Journal* 180, no. 11 (2009): 1098; Kylie Taggart, "Anemia May be Sprinkled Away," *Medical Post* 41, no. 11 (2005):

29; Andre Picard, "Sick Kids Pushes Nutrition Frontier," *Globe and Mail*, 25 January 2005, A15. For a discussion of the difficulties of engaging the trust of affected populations, see Sam Loewenberg, "Easier than Taking Vitamins," *New York Times*, 5 September 2012, http://opinionator.blogs.nytimes.com/2012/09/05/easier-than-taking-vitamins/.

17   Stanley Zlotkin, "A New Approach to Control of Anemia in 'At Risk' Infants and Children around the World," 2004 Ryley-Jeffs Memorial Lecture, *Canadian Journal of Dietetic Practice and Research* 65, no. 3 (2004): 138.

18   Zlotkin, quoted in Sheryl Ubelacker, "Just a Sprinkle Has Big Impact: Kids Worldwide Helped by Canadian MD's Invention," *The Canadian Press*, 9 March 2015.

19   Quotation in "The Hospital for Sick Children: Collaborating with Partners around the World to Advance the Health of Children," *Middle East Health* (July–August 2013): 54; SickKids International, "Qatar Update: Project Overview and Staff Experience," 7 November 2011, www.sickkidsinternational.ca/2011/qatar-update-project-overview-and-staff-experience/; Khalid Bin Abdulrahman, Ronald Harden, and Madalena Patricio, "Medical Education in Saudi Arabia: An Exciting Journey," *Medical Teacher* 34, no. s1 (2012): S4–S5. See also "SickKids Signs Historic Partnership to Develop State-of-the-Art Children's Hospital in Qatar," *Marketwire*, 7 February 2010.

20   SickKids International, "SickKids and U of T Accredit 706 Paediatric Nurses from Qatar," 20 June 2013, www.sickkidsinternational.ca/2013/sickkids-and-u-of-t-accredit-706-paediatric-nurses-from-qatar/; SickKids International, "Qatar Update: Department of Paediatrics," 19 December 2011; www.sickkidsinternational.ca/2011/qatar-update-department-of-paediatrics/.

21   HSCF AR 2014–15, 6–7.

22   Quotation in SickKids, "A Commitment to Healthier Children and a Better World," news release, 4 May 2010; "Ontario Promises to Kick in $75 Million for Toronto Sick Kids' Research Tower," *The Canadian Press* (Toronto), 15 August 2011; SickKids, "SickKids Receives over $91 Million in CFI Funding to Support Research Infrastructure," news release, 20 August 2008; HSCF AR 2009–10, 1; "Taking a Chance on the Market," *National Post*, 12 December 2009, FP2; "SickKids Closes $200 Million Offering to Fund Construction of Research Tower," *Marketwire*, 17 December 2009.

23   Hockey, quoted in Joseph Hall, "Tower of Discovery: New $400-million Highrise Will Gather 2,000 Far-Flung SickKids Researchers in One Place. Now the Fundraising Begins," *Toronto Star*, 6 May 2010, 23.

24   "A $400M Shot in the Arm, Peter Gilgan Centre for Research and Learning," *National Post*, 12 October 2013, FP13; "Research & Learning Tower Campaign Wins Strong, Early Support from Toronto," *Canada NewsWire*, 28 September 2010; SickKids Foundation, news release, "Peter Gilgan, Founder, Mattamy Homes Helps Build Future Home of SickKids Researchers with Historic $40 Million Gift," 7 March 2012.

25   Tom Blackwell, "Building Chemistry: To Encourage More Mingling, New Research Facility Has Been Divided into 'Neighbourhoods' of Two to Three Storeys," *National Post*, 27 August 2013, A8.

26   Hall, "Tower of Discovery."

27   Anna Mehler Paperny, "Vertical City: Sick Kids Tower to Make Research More Visible," *Globe and Mail*, 4 May 2010, A12.

28   Quotation in "Projects," *The Canadian Architect* 58, no. 10 (2013): 11; Anonymous, "SickKids Starts Construction of Research Tower," *Canadian Healthcare Manager* 17, no. 3 (2010): L6; Alex Bozikovic, "One Giant Leap for Building Design: The Staircase has Become Central to a Building's Form and Function – Providing both Beauty and a Venue for Social Interaction," *Globe and Mail*, 26 March 2015, L4; Hall, "Tower of Discovery"; Anna Mehler Paperny, "Vertical City: Sick Kids Tower to Make Research More Visible," *Globe and Mail*, 4 May 2010, A12.

29   Conversation with Wayne Walker, 29 October 2012.

30   HSCF AR 2005–2006, 12.

31 Sandra Martin, "Harold Joseph Hoffman 1932–2004," *Globe and Mail*, 20 November 2004, S11.

32 "Improving the Health of Children Worldwide: International Fellowship Program Trains Physicians from across the Globe," *Globe and Mail*, 29 November 2006, A21.

EPILOGUE

1 Letter printed in Hospital for Sick Children Annual Report 1876, 16.

2 Cyndy DeGiusti quoted in Paul Waldie, "Black Giving Sick Kids $5-miIlion Just after Launching New Paper," *Globe and Mail*, 20 October 1998, A10.

3 Lillian Newberry, "Donors Sought for Endowed Chairs," *Toronto Star*, 30 May 1996, G10.

4 SickKids Foundation Annual Report (hereafter HSCF AR) 1997–8; HSCF AR 1994–5.

5 SickKids, "SickKids Launches $82 Million Campaign and Garth Drabinsky Gift," news release, 15 September 1997; James Rusk, "Sick Kids Gets Millions in Donation from Labatts," *Globe and Mail*, 8 February 2007, A11; Paul Northcott, "Hospitals Receive Gifts of $5-Million Apiece" *Globe and Mail*, 22 December 2000, A18; Tanya Fanagan, "Largest-Yet Donation Bestowed on Sick Kids: Same Family Gives Twice," *National Post*, 7 February 2007, A10; "SickKids Foundation Receives $3.5 Million Gift from FirstPro Shopping Centres," 14 July 2005; Waldie, "Black Giving Sick Kids $5-MiIlion"; Paul Waldie and Richard Blackwell, "Black's Woes Stir Concern about Hospital Pledge," *Globe and Mail*, 5 April 2004, B4.

6 University Health Network (UNH), "UHN Honours Peter and Melanie Munk," news release, 1 October 2013, www.uhn.ca/corporate/News/Pages/UHN_honours_Peter_Munk.aspx.

7 Quotation in SickKids,"Robert Harding, Chair of SickKids Board, named to Order of Canada," news release, 31 December 2013, www.sickkids.ca/AboutSickKids/Newsroom/Past-News/2013/Robert-Harding-named-to-Order-of-Canada-web-story.html; Michael Valpy, "Jewish Tradition of "Tzedakah" a Boon for Toronto Institutions," *Globe and Mail*, 28 October2006, A2; Tanya Fanagan "Largest-Yet Donation Bestowed on Sick Kids: Same Family Gives Twice," *National Post*, 7 February 2007, A10.

8 HSCF AR 2014–15, 31.

Illustration Credits

City of Toronto Archives: 2.4 (Goad's Atlas, 1890, Plate 15); 5.2 (Fonds 200, series 372-1)

Creative Services Studio, The Hospital for Sick Children: back endpaper (photograph by Rob Teteruck and Diogenes Baena)

Getty Images: 12.1 (#5022236871, Michael Styuparyk for the *Toronto Star*); 12.2 (#499322247, Mike Slaughter for the *Toronto Star*); 12.3 (#502512351, Ron Bull for the *Toronto Star*); 13.1 (#499815590, Dale Brazao for the *Toronto Star*); 14.1 (#499798042, Doug Griffin for the *Toronto Star*, 15 October 1981); 14.3 (#515086845, Jim Rankin for the *Toronto Star*); 15.1 (#502832487, Bob Olsen for the *Toronto Star*, 31 October 1971)

The Globe and Mail archives: 11.2 (26 July 1958, p. 3)

Hamad Medical Corporation Marketing Department: 16.2

Hospital Archives, The Hospital for Sick Children, Toronto: front endpaper (0971-001-228); I.1 (0981-028-004-35); 2.1 (*The Hospital for Sick Children*, 1891, p. 6); 2.2 (0971-010-001); 2.3 (*The Hospital for Sick Children*, 1891, p. 21); 3.1 (0973-043-002); 3.2 (0972-080-001); 3.3 (0972-042-001-31); 3.4 (0977-045-014); 4.1 (0971-001-006); 4.2 (0972-078-005); 4.3 (0980-063-001); 4.4 (0971-001-146); 5.1 (0971-001-026); 5.3 (0971-001-034); 5.4 (0971-001-148); 6.1 (0977-036-001); 6.3 (0987-015-002; photo by Rob Teteruck); 6.4 (0972-072-001); 7.1 (0973-061-001); 7.2 (0971-001-049); 7.3 (0973-035-001); 7.4 (0973-036-001b); 8.1 (0971-001-059); 8.2 (0973-040-001); 8.3 (Thistletown subject file); 8.4 (Thistletown subject file); 9.1 (0971-001-076); 9.2 (978-008-004; John E. Milne, 29 May 1947); 9.3 (2006-400-007); 9.4 (Negative 1968 P63430); 10.1 (2004-038-002); 10.2 (0988-009-001; photo by Rob Teteruck); 10.3 (2009-145-002); 11.1 (0980-038-005); 11.4 (Negative 1974 P50263); 13.2 (2008-225-226-27c); 13.3 (2006-412-005); 14.2 (2008-025-084-004b, 1989); 15.3 (scan from Kaleidoscope, Fall 1997); 16.1 (2016-011-001); 16.3 (2016-007-009-4, photo by Rob Teteruck); E.1 (0971-001-282); F.1 (HSC Annual Report, 1970)

Nursing Alumnae Association of The Hospital for Sick Children: 11.3 (with the kind permission of Judy [Cole] Nesbitt)

Toronto Star archives: 6.2 (21 March 1931, p. 10)

Victorian Web: 1.1 (wood engraving by Sol Eytinge, from Charles Dickens, *A Christmas Carol*, Boston: Ticknor and Fields, 1869 [Diamond Edition]; scanned image by Philip V. Allingham)

Wellcome Library, London: 1.2 (49 Great Ormond Street, London, in course of demolition, watercolour by J.P. Emslie, 1882); 1.3 (Underwood, *A Treatise on the Diseases of Children*, vol. 1, new edition, published by J. Mathews, London, 1789); 1.4 ("The Dance of Death" coloured aquatint, by T. Rowlandson, published by R. Ackermann, London [101 Strand], 1 July 1815)

T. Kue Young: 15.2 (with the author's kind permission, "Mortality Pattern of Isolated Indians in Northwestern Ontario: A 10-Year Review," *Public Health Reports* 98, no. 5 [1983], p. 468)

Index

exclusions: contagious diseases and, 13; of developmental disability from HSC, 65; from East London Orphan Asylum, 15; of immigrants with physical/mental impairments, 154; of infants from Great Ormond Street Hospital, 11; from provincial infirmaries, 14. *See also* parent-child separation

"Facts Illustrative of the Need of a Children's Hospital," 42

families of patients: involvement in medical encounters, 299; psychological justification for separation of patient from, 172; telemedicine and, 344; University Avenue hospital and, 299. *See also* mothers; parent-child separation; parents of patients

Family Allowance Act (1944), 245

Farex, 130

Farmer, Alfred W., 226, 233

federal government: funding of Aboriginal care, 154–5; and health care, 338; and Indian affairs, 338

Federal Health Grants program, 222–3

federal-provincial cost-sharing: 1990s recession and cuts to, 321; and hospital insurance, 246; and Medical Care Act, 247

Féré, Dr. (surgeon), 83–4

Ferguson, G. Howard, 179

The Fifth Estate, 275

Filler, Robert, 289–90, 291, 292, 345–6

finances/financing: 1970s fiscal crisis and budget reductions, 283–4; 1990s public funding reductions and budgets, 321–2; block operating grants, 149; budget rebalancing, 307; and budgeting in decision-making, 307; Charity Aid Act and, 62–7, 149; and curative/acute patient care vs. welfare for destitute, 62; deficit, 155; Great Depression and, 150, 155, 195; of Great Ormond Street Hospital, 11; of hospital systems, 164; Ministry of Health global budgets and salaries/wages, 248; non-solicitation of private funds and, 64; of patient care, 149–55; precariousness of voluntary, 14; Robertson and, 3, 62, 68, 365; University of Toronto student fees and, 148. *See also* payment for services

First Nations. *See* Aboriginal populations

First Nations Hospital (earlier Indian Hospital), Sioux Lookout, 350

5Fifty5 (gift shop), 213

Flavelle, Joseph, 114

Fleming, Alexander, 220

Flexner, Simon, 158, 160

Florey, Howard, 220

Food and Drug Act, 126

food(s): bacteriology and preparation of, 136; cereals, 127–30, 134; enriched, 123–4, 125–6, 137; infant, 118–19, 128; iron as additive to, 126; irradiated, 122–30, 134, 137; women and preparation of, 136. *See also* milk; nutrition

Forster, John Cooper, *The Surgical Diseases of Children*, 80

foundling hospitals, 11, 14–15

Fowler, Rodney Singleton, 273–4

Fox, Terry, 295

Franklin, Rosalind, 313

Freedom, Robert, 279

Freemasons, 52–3

Friesen, Henry, *Investing in Canada's Health: A Strategic Plan for the Medical Research Council of Canada*, 322

Fry, Charles P., 205

funding/fundraising: for construction/renovation, 260; health insurance and, 260; media exposure for life-threatening illnesses and, 307–8; Mistletoe Ball, 293, 307–8; for Patient Care Centre, 300–2; for research tower (Gilgan Centre), 358–60, 366; scientific breakthroughs and, 3–4; SickKids International and, 355; subsidization of outside funds raised, 62; telethons, 295–9; for Thistletown convalescent home, 178–9; for University Avenue building/hospital, 199–202, 205–6; Women's Auxiliary and, 211, 212, 213–14. *See also* donations; payment for services

Gagan, David, 150

Gallie, Brenda, 328, 329

Gallie, W.E.: and country convalescent hospital, 174, 175, 178; "Gallie Course" in postgraduate surgical training, 147–8; on hospital expansion as medical vs. treatment centre, 262; and surgical clinics throughout province, 146; on Thistletown, 179

Garron Family Cancer Centre, 366

gastrointestinal ailments, 101–2

general infirmaries/hospitals: children's hospitals vs., 17; expansion of provincial

259–60; Rowell-Sirois Commission and, 244; state and, 164; universal, 164, 315

health records, electronic, 346–9, 350–1

Health Services Restructuring Commission (HSRC), 321–3, 346–7

Healthier Children: A Better World Initiative, 354

HealthyKids International (HKI), 356–7

Healy, David, 334

Heather Club, 174

heliotherapy, 55, 122, 175, 182, 223

heliport, 342, 343

Help Make Sick Kids Better, 365–6

heparin, 210, 229, 240

Hepburn, Mitchell, 113

Herbert, Ruth, 120

Herbie Fund, 290–3

Hess, Alfred, 122

Hillcrest Convalescent Home (Toronto), 182

Hines, Jordan, 276

hip-joint disease, 82–3, 84

HIV/AIDS: AIDS epidemic, 318; anti-retroviral drugs, 320, 335; and blood supply, 318–21; care for paediatric AIDS patients, 319–20, 335; CHAS (children's HIV/AIDS support group), 320–1; Comprehensive Care Clinic, 335; HIV Information Project, 318

Hockey, Tim, 359

Hodder, Edward Mulberry, 38, 45

Hoffman, Harold J., 361

Holland, Jean, 107

Holt, Emmett, 120

homeopathy, 18, 40

Horses to Helicopters (film), 342

hospital care insurance, 150; federal-provincial cost-sharing and, 246; Hospital Insurance and Diagnostic Services Act (HIDS), 246, 248, 262, 266, 321; Hospital Insurance Plan (Ontario), 246; in Saskatchewan, 244

Hospital for Incurables, 65

Hospital for Ruptured and Crippled Children (New York), 82

Hospital for Sick Children Foundation (HSCF): and Atrium, 304, 308; capital funding by, 300; and Children's Miracle Network, 298, 299; establishment of, 259; and HealthyKids International, 356; and Help Make Sick Kids Better, 365; numbers of donors, 367; numbers of volunteers/events, 367; and Peter Gilgan Centre, 358, 359; and research, 358; and staffing levels in

neonatal ward, 284; and telethons, 298

Hospital for Sick Children's Aid, 211

Hospital Services Commission Act, 246

hospitals: 1970s fiscal crisis and, 283; 1970s fiscal crisis and closures of, 284; amalgamations, 321–2; budget reductions, 321–2; care as provincial jurisdiction, 164; closures, 321–2; dispensary services, 37; evolution of, 2; First Nations, 350; free care within, 165; as "gateways to death," 16; Great Depression and, 195; HIDS and emphasis on care, 248; hiring out student nurses, 90, 92; histories, in academic scholarship, 2–3; Indian, 155, 338; information/electronic health records sharing, 350–1; inspections, 63; intersection of multiple parties within, 5; limitation on lengths of patient stays to active treatment, 63–4; nationalization of, 245; operating deficits, 155, 195; place/role in society, 2; post-war boom vs. 1970s fiscal crisis and, 285; public opinion of, 16; racial separation within, 338–9; restructuring, 321–2, 346; specialist, 14, 18–19; standards, 63; in Toronto vs. other parts of province, 343–4

House of Industry (Toronto), 37, 98

House of Refuge (Toronto), 37

Howland, Mrs., 31–2

Hudson, Alan, 348

Hughes, Patricia, 186–7

immigrants: attitudes toward hospitalization, 185; and epidemics, 35; exclusion for physical/mental impairments, 154; health conditions for entry, 154; and payment for hospital services, 154; in The Ward, 114–15

Immigration Act (1952), 256

Immigration Act (1876), 154–5

Indian and Eskimo Child Health Committee (Canadian Paediatric Society), 339

Indian hospitals, 338

indigence. *See* poverty

Indigenous populations. *See* Aboriginal populations

infant deaths at HSC (1980–81): about, 271, 285–6; alleged cover-ups of, 270; causes of, 271–2, 282, 285–6; inquiries into, 272, 273–7, 282; as medication errors, 272; mortality rates at HSC vs., 271–2, 286; from natural causes, 276; as possible murders, 272, 276, 286; of Yuz, 269–70. *See also* Nelles, Susan

infant mortality: breastfeeding and, 102–3; causes, 9–10; decline in, 239; decline of rate in Toronto, 112–13; in early industrial society, 8; in foundling hospitals, 11; gastrointestinal ailments and, 101–2; Indigenous children, 339; and isolation of hospital, 171; Jewish children and, 102; milk quality and, 102–3; nutritional causes, 107; in post-Second World War period, 225; poverty and, 101; premature babies, 236–7; public health and decline in, 239; rates, 95, 101; rates at HSC, 117–18, 271–2, 286; surgical interventions and, 240; and visiting hours, 173; and ward of glass cubicles, 171–2; weaning and, 102–3. *See also* infant deaths at HSC (1980–81)

infantile paralysis, 81, 156. *See also* poliomyelitis

infants: life expectancy, 112; research experimentation with, 134; surgery in, 228; well-baby clinics, 141, 142, 143, 193

infectious diseases: Aboriginal families and, 225; antibiotics and, 224–6; in central Toronto, 100; and child mortality, 9; children's hospitals and, 16; congenital conditions vs., 317–18; evolution of infectious ward, 171–2; exclusion/non-admission of cases, 65, 83; and quarantine, 172, 173; and sterile hospital environment, 171; vaccination and, 239

influenza, 157–8

inpatients: accommodation units in Patient Care Centre (Atrium), 304; average stays, 239; capacity in Avenue Street building, 27; care of infants/children with AIDS, 320; in Great Ormond Street Hospital, 11, 15; medical treatment in 1870s, 37; proportion of outpatients to, 41; public attitudes toward care, 41–2; rise in numbers, 196

insulin, 3, 119, 129

International Nickel Company (INCO), 201–2

Internet. *See* health records, electronic; internationalization; telemedicine/ Telehealth

interns: female, 210; Jewish, 199; nurses and, 254; at Thistletown, 180; wartime shortage, 194

Irish, Howard, 114

iron lungs, 159–61, 163–4, 165, 167, 238

iron-chelation therapy, 324

irradiated food, 122–30, 134, 137

Isolation Hospital, 60

Ivey School of Business, 355

Jackson, Elaine, 206

Jackson, Mrs. (physician's wife), 212

Jarvis, Mrs. Edgar, 33–4

Jenner, Edward, 20

Jewish children: breastfeeding and, 102; Hospital for Sick Children and, 100–1; infant mortality, 102; as outpatients, 101; unpaid fees, 151

Jewish hospitals, 114, 115, 198–9, 245

Johns Hopkins, 121, 228–9, 240

Johnson, Arnold, 229

Johnson, Athol A., 80

Johnston, Marion, 120

Kaake, Mildred, 120

Karlsberger Hospital Consultants, 300

Kauffman, Dr., 280

Keefer, Charles, 221

Keith, John, 227–8, 229, 235, 236, 238

Kemp, Sir Edward and Lady, 178

Kennedy, Ted, 291, 295

Kinder, Annie, 89

King, Susan, 318–19, 320

Kitely, Frances, 282

knock-knees, 81

Koch, Robert, 103

Koren, Gideon, 324, 325, 326–7, 329–30

Kottmeir, Peter, 289

Krever Commission, 320, 335

L1 drug trials, 324–31

Labatt Family Heart Centre, 366

laboratories: children's hospitals as, 72; development in HSC, 119–20; in Europe, 73; patenting/commercialization of products, 132; in Peter Gilgan Centre for Research and Learning, 360; technicians, 136; Tisdall as director, 136. *See also* Nutritional Research Laboratory (NRL); research

Ladies Committee: board of trustees vs., 60; and Cody as superintendent, 58; composition of, 31–2; and convalescent home, 51, 174; and cot sponsorship, 32–3; donations by, 32–3; establishment of, 26; and financing of hospital, 32; functions of, 32, 34–5; fundraising, 33–4; McMaster and, 31; and physical/moral condition of patients, 34–5; reliance on donations vs.

direct appeals, 43–4; rental on 31 Avenue Street, 26–7; Robertson and, 50; and salaries, 58; training of nurses for outside work, 60; and "visiting ladies'" tours of hospital, 34

Laidlaw, Robert A., 178, 194, 205, 207, 209, 211

Lakeside Home: bed capacity/numbers of patients, 52; climatological benefits, 54–5; country branch hospital vs., 174, 175; expenditure on, 52; first nurse graduation ceremony at, 61; gymnasium, 54–5; institutional events held at, 56; McMaster's legal title to, 51, 61; numbers of patients, vs. in College Street, 57; as parallel hospital and summer retreat, 56–7; patients transferred to Thistletown, 179; as "playhouse," 54; rebuilding, 174; Robertson and, 50–4, 55–6, 68; second wing, 52; transfer of patients to, 55–7; visitors to, 56

Lamek, Paul, 280

The Lancet, 18

Langmuir, John Woodburn, 63–5

Law, John T., 1, 5; on admissions policy, 263; and board of trustees, 259–60; encouragement of other paediatric facilities, 265; as first professional administrator, 258–60; on hospital insurance, 246–7; and staff-hospital relations, 259; on Women's Auxiliary, 216

Lebovic, Joseph and Wolf, 366

lecture theatres, 147

Lee, Mrs. Walter, 32

Lehmann, Allie, 282

LeMesurier, Dr., 226, 229

Levan, Albert, 313

Lewis, Jerry, 295

Lister, Joseph, 79

Lombardi, Johnny, 298

Lombardo, Stephanie, 274, 275

lunatic asylums, 36

Lunenfeld, Samuel, 198

lying-in hospitals, 14, 18, 37–8

Lynch, Abbyann, 249

MacBeth, Mrs. George, 90

MacDonald, Lady Agnes, 31, 32

Macklem, Peter, 285–6

MacMurchy, Helen, 102, 107, 122, 156, 157

Malthus, Thomas, *Essay on the Principle of Population*, 15–16

Manley, Margaret, 354

marasmus, 83

Marathon of Hope, 295

Martin, David, 287, 299, 305, 306–7

Martin, Frank, 86–7

Martin, Paul Jr., 322

Martin, Paul Sr., 223

Massachusetts General Hospital and hospital for sick children, 17

Masten, Jean, 169, 194, 211, 214, 255–6

McCormick Manufacturing Company, 124

McCrindle, Brian, 318

McDonald, John L., 113

McGee, Marion, 280–1

McGill University, and children's hospital in Montreal, 44

McGregor Committee, 270

McKellar, Susan, 310f, 311–12

McKenzie, B.E., 72, 86

McMaster, Elizabeth: board of trustees vs., 60–1; early life, 30–1; and Elizabeth McMaster Building, 300; and Elizabeth McMaster Nursing Residence, 251–2; on homeopathy vs. allopathy, 40; on hospital as religious mission, 45; and Ladies Committee, 31, 34, 45; and Lakeside Home, 51, 61; and nurse training school at hospital, 60–1, 88; own nurse training, 60; and professionalization of nursing care, 58; and quiet room for mothers and critically ill children, 173; replacement of Cody, 60; resignation, 61; Robertson and, 30, 45, 50, 57, 59–61, 69

McMaster, Samuel Fenton, 30

McMaster, William, 30

McMurtry, Roy, 269, 277–8, 285, 287

McPherson, Kathryn, 92, 252–3

Mead's Cereal, 127–30, 134

measles, 9, 10, 20, 156

Medicaid, 290, 291

Medical Advisory Board (MAB)/Committee: on conditions at College Street hospital, 193; establishment of, 115; and female interns, 210; and lack of parents' consent to surgical operations, 185; and Olivieri, 327–8; and parental visitation, 186; and penicillin, 222; and repurposing of Thistletown as principal institution, 196; and residencies, 148; and vitamin D research, 134; and women doctors, 120

Medical Care Act, 247, 321

189; Second World War and, 194; at Thistletown, 186–7

Pasteur, Louis, 79, 103, 105

pasteurization: about, 105; as compulsory in Ontario, 113; as mandatory in Toronto, 110; municipal, 104, 106–7, 113; and near-disappearance of bovine tuberculosis, 112; scientific vs. commercial, 105

pasteurization plant/department, 68, 107–10, 117, 118

pathological labs, 178

Patient Care Centre (Atrium): architecture, 304–5, 308; clinical care changes reflected in, 305–6; construction of, 300, 302, 304; and family-centred care, 299–300; funding/financing, 300–2; inpatient units in, 304, 308; numbers of beds, 305–6; social trends/relations reflected in, 308–9

Patterson, Christopher Salmon, 68

payment for services: and ability to pay, 65–6; dwindling numbers of paying patients, 164; free hospital care vs., 165, 245; free paediatric care vs., 164; free/normative immunization/vaccination programs vs., 164, 245; HSC ceasing to give free medicine, 44; HSC hospital charges/fees, and poor, 32; immigrants and, 154; and non-residents as patients, 154; patient liability for fees, 153–4; for private care, 142, 164; public ward patient charges, 149, 150; quarantine and refusal to pay, 173; in semi-private wards, 149, 173; unpaid fees, 150–4

Pearson, Lester B., 247

Pelican Lake residential school, 337–8

penicillin, 220–2

Pernick, Martin, 79

Peter Gilgan Centre for Research and Learning, 343, 358–60, 366

Peters, Dr. (surgeon), 83

Peterson, David, 277, 301

Pharmaceutical Manufacturers Association of Canada, 322

philanthropy. See charity/charities; donations

Phillips, Eric, 122

physical disability: changing attitudes toward, 85–6; and exclusion of immigrants, 154; and prosthetics, 175; as public health concern, 175

physicians: appointments with University of Toronto, 147; attendance at early HSC, 26, 38–44, 45; costs transferred to province,

248; and new management structure, 306–7; private practices, 143; relations with nurses, 92, 253–5, 308, 309; as researchers, 333; and Second World War, 194; in Sioux Lookout Zone, 341; strike, 299; as unsalaried, 143, 147

Picard, André, 321; *The Gift of Death,* 318

Piva, Michael, 101

play spaces, 215

poliomyelitis: about, 156; bulbar, 160; epidemics, 156–60, 163, 165, 238; First World War and, 157; immunization programs, 224; and iron lungs, 159–61, 163–4; mortality from, 156, 159; orthopaedic supplies, 162; paralytic, 156; and parent-child separation, 174; patients at Thistletown, 182; poliovirus, 224; public health reform and, 156; public subsidies for treatment, 161–2, 164; Roosevelt and, 162; scientific medicine and, 157–8; serum for, 158, 162; Underwood's *Treatise* and, 19; vaccine, 158, 164, 188, 224; zinc sulphate nasal spray against, 160

Poliomyelitis Sufferers Act (Alberta), 162

poor, the: blaming of families for children's disabilities/infirmities, 16; city orders (C.O.s) for, 153–4; countryside/nature vs. urban life and, 50–1; education of parents, 142; Great Depression and, 195; habits/conduct blamed for children's disabilities/infirmities, 16; home visiting, 29; hospital expansion/construction and expulsion from The Ward, 115; municipal funding/grants, 149, 153–4; and paediatric research, 134–5; and patient charges/fees, 32; and poor laws, 7, 27; preventive paediatrics and reform of environments of, 142; public monies and acceptance of all needy, 149; respectable, 149; well-baby clinics and, 142

Porter, Roy, 14, 364

Pott's disease, 41, 82

poverty: and children, 8, 25–6; fostering of, 65–6; and infant/childhood mortality, 101; and milk, 106; promotion of, vs. provincial institutional support, 63; and rickets, 121

premature babies, 236–8, 239, 346

Prichard, Robert, 328

Primrose, Alexander, 84, 123–4

Princess Margaret Hospital, 115, 322

Prison and Asylum Inspection Act, 63–4

Program for Global Pediatric Research, 354

Protestantism, 28–9

provincial government (Ontario): 1990s spending cuts, 321; Board of Health, 107; and financing of HSC, 62–7; Milk Act, 107; milk commission, 106; operating costs transfer to, 248; physicians' costs transferred to, 248; and poliomyelitis epidemic, 159–60; and research tower, 359; and Smart Systems for Health, 348. *See also* Ministry of Health (Ontario)

provincial governments: 1990s spending cuts, 321; health care as jurisdiction, 321, 338; hospital care as jurisdiction of, 164; legislation as response to social/epidemiological crises, 27–8; responsibility over medical/charitable institutions, 27

provincial grants/funding: for active medical care, 183; and convalescence, 183; Great Depression and, 195; and indigent, 149; and inspections, 63, 64–5; and rehabilitation, 183; for Thistletown, 178; through Charity Aid Act, 44

psychology: benefits of institutionalization at Thistletown, 182; and care of the whole child, 214–15; and family/parent-child separation, 172, 187; and impact of hospitalization of children, 165, 168–9; mental hygiene as term, 169; psychological services for children, 36–7

public funding. *See* municipal funding/grants; provincial grants/funding

public health: advent of departments in urban areas, 141; and immunity, 156; improvements in, 113; and infant/childhood mortality, 239; institutional medicine vs., 141; and interventions for children as normative/widely accepted, 245; and milk, 104, 113; nurses, 111; in nursing education, 258; physical disability as concern of, 175; and poliomyelitis, 156; and preventive paediatrics, 142; and respectable poor, 149; and St. John's Ward, 98, 100; Toronto City initiatives, 113

quarantine: infectious diseases and, 172; internal hospital, 173

Quinones family, 288f, 289–92, 307–8

racial separation, of hospital services, 338–9

Rae, Bob, 277

Read, Stanley, 319, 320, 335

Reaume, Geoffrey, 175

Recreation and Volunteer Services, Department of, 215

Red Cross, 146, 318, 335

Registered Nurses' Association of Ontario (RNAO), 278, 280

rehabilitation: convalescent branch hospital and, 174–5, 178; provincial grants and, 183

religion: backgrounds of outpatients, 100–1; Jews in St. John's Ward, 98, 99, 114–15; and opening of Hospital for Sick Children, 26, 45; and relief in urban centres, 28; and sectarianism in welfare services, 28–9; traditions of charity, 22, 25, 26, 29. *See also* Catholic Church; Protestantism

Rementeria, Jose Luis, 289

research: 1990s spending cuts and, 322; and academic freedom, 328, 333–4; "cathedral," 358–60; and children in developing countries, 354; clinical care vs., 137; and confidentiality clauses, 324–5, 326; ethical issues (*see* ethical issues); experimentation, 133–5; funding/financing of department, 131–2; HSC's international reputation in, 361; with infants, 134; and international activities, 361; with mothers, 134; royalties, 129–30, 131, 132, 135, 137; trustee management of funds, 131. *See also* laboratories; Peter Gilgan Centre for Research and Learning

research endowment fund, 131, 132, 135

Research Ethics Board, 324–5, 327–8, 330, 333

Research Institute, 135, 234, 237, 241, 314, 358

research tower. *See* Peter Gilgan Centre for Research and Learning

residents/residencies: Medical Advisory Board and broadening of, 148; nurses and, 254; at Sioux Lookout Hospital, 341

respiratory ailments, 12, 237–8, 239

restraint jackets, 213–14

rheumatic heart disease, 227–8

Rhodes, Andrew J., 224

rickets, 81, 83, 121, 122, 134, 136

Riordan, Jack, 332

Robert Harding Chair in Global Child Health and Policy, 356

Robertson, D.E.: anti-Semitic views, 199; attitudes toward, 255; and iron lungs, 113; and Ontario Orthopaedic Hosital, 162; and sulphonamides, 220

Robertson, Elizabeth Chant, 120, 134, 136

Robertson, Helen, 50
Robertson, James, *A Two-Year-Old Goes to Hospital*, 187, 215
Robertson, John Ross: as benefactor of HSC, 3, 62, 68, 365; and board of trustees, 57, 68–9; Brown and, 117–18; and children of Freemasons, 52–3; and *Daily Telegraph,* 47, 48; death, 69, 115; and district/social service nursing, 139–40; early life and education, 48; Endowment Fund, 68; European tours, 72–3; and *Evening Telegram,* 48–9, 68; family losses, 50; as historian, 68; and infant ward mortality, 117–18; and Ladies Committee, 50; and Lakeside Home, 50–4, 55–6, 68; legacy of, 197, 365; and McKenzie's outpatient orthopaedic clinic, 86; McMaster and, 30, 45, 50, 57, 59–61, 69; and new children's hospital at College Street, 72–3; and nurse training, 62, 88; and nurses' residence, 68, 90; as Paper Tyrant, 49; and pasteurization plant, 68, 107, 115; as philanthropist, 68; phrenological profile of, 47–8, 69; political views/life, 49; portraits, 46f, 50; "Round the World Hospitals," 73; temperament, 49–50; and urban reform, 107; wealth/influence of, 67–8
Robertson, Lloyd, 296, 298, 301
Robertson, Maria Louisa, 50, 90
Robertson, Mrs. D.E., 212
Robinson, Elroy, 202
Robinson, J.T., 86–7
Rockefeller Foundation, and University of Toronto, 147
Rockefeller Institute for Medical Research (New York), 158
Roosevelt, Franklin, 162
Rose, Abraham L., 135
Rosebrugh, Abner Mulholland, 37
Ross, Allan, 263
Ross, J.R., 194
Rotary Clubs, 146, 206
Rothstein, Aser, 314
"Round the World Hospitals" (J.R. Robertson), 73
Routley, T.C., 123
Rowe, Richard Desmond, 279
Roy C. Hill Wing, 366
Royal College of Dental Surgeons, 26–7
Royal College of Physicians, 17–18
Royal College of Physicians and Surgeons, 163
Royal Commission of Inquiry into Certain

Deaths at The Hospital for Sick Children. *See* Grange Commission
Royal Commission on Dominion-Provincial Relations (Rowell-Sirois Commission), 244
Royal Commission on Health Care (Romanow Commission), 350–1
Royal Commission on Health Services (Hall Commission), 248–9
Royal Waterloo Hospital for Children and Women, 15
Rusescu, Tudor, 293
Rutty, Christopher, 159, 163–4
Ryerson Polytechnic Institute, 250

Sadowski, Ben, 198, 199
Sainte-Justine hospital (Montreal), 313
salaries/wages: of Cody as matron/superintendent, 58; freezes, 306; Great Depression and, 155; Ministry of Health and, 248; of nurses, 58, 90, 92; of physicians at HSC, 143, 147; unionization and increases in, 284–5; University of Toronto Faculty of Medicine instructor reimbursement, 148
Salk, Jonas, 224
Sandy Lake, 349
SARS outbreak, 355
scarlet fever (scarlatina), 9, 50
Scherer, Stephen, 316
Scheuer, Edmund, 100
Schlich, Thomas, 80
schools: doctors in, 143, 164; medical officers in, 150; nurses in, 143, 150, 164
scientific medicine: advances in, 21; and decline in Thistletown occupancy rates, 188; middle class and, 149; and orthopaedic surgery, 72; and poliomyelitis, 157–8; and professionalization of nursing, 87; University Avenue hospital and, 299
Scott, Isobel, 221
Scott-McKay-Bain Health Panel/report, 349
scurvy, 121, 136
Sea Breeze Hospital (Coney Island), 56
Second World War: and College Street hospital, 194; demobilization, 202; and penicillin, 220; and post-war economy, 203, 282–3; and projected new building, 155, 199–200; and women's role, 209–10
Seidler, Eduard, 51
Sellars, John, 73
Sexton, Rosemary, 293

tenotomy, 72

Tepperman, Paul, 272

tertiary care, 239, 283, 305, 342

tetralogy of Fallot, 228–9, 232–3, 234–5, 240

thalassemia program, 323, 324–31

The Hospital for Sick Children. *See* Hospital for Sick Children (HSC)

Theodore, David, 76

Thistletown convalescent home: additions to, 183–4; architecture, 179; closure of, 189; construction, 179; cot endowment at, 178–9; as country branch hospital, 176–7f; dental clinic, 214; drug revolution and, 188; emotionally disturbed children and, 189; entertainment at, 181, 182; facilities, 179; fundraising campaign for, 178–9; Great Depression and, 183; and heliotherapy, 188; Lakeside Home patients transferred to, 179; location/surrounding environment, 179–81; mandate of, 183; Mustard and, 226; nurses at, 180, 181–2; occupancy rate, 183, 188, 196; parents of patients and, 184–7; patient care, 181–2; and psychological benefits of institutionalization, 182; repurposing as principal institution, 196; sale of, 189; staff, 180–1; streptomycin and, 223–4; tubercular disease patients at, 181–2; University Avenue hospital opening and, 189; visitors to, 181f, 184–5

Thomas Modified Hip Splint, 84

Thompson, Margaret, 331

Thomson, Juanita, 120

Tiny Tim Guild, 22

Tisdall, Frederick, 120, 123–4, 128, 129–30, 131, 135, 136

Tjio, Joe Hin, 313

Toronto: Board of Health, 104; British medical charity in, 22–3; City Dairy, 105; Department of Public Health, 227; East General Hospital, 287; Eye and Ear Infirmary, 37; Free Dispensary, 37; Grace (Homeopathic) Hospital, 88; Great Depression and, 195; Health Department, 108–9, 110–11, 140, 193; infant mortality in, 95; Islands, 50, 51; Lunatic Asylum, 36; medical services for sick children in Victorian era, 35–8; orphan homes/hospices in, 37; pasteurization in, 104, 110, 113; poliomyelitis in, 158–60; population explosion, 193; poverty and living conditions in, 22, 25–6; Psychiatric Hospital, 258; Pure Milk League, 106; religion and relief in, 28; Western Hospital, 261, 322; Women's Christian Association, 29. *See also* municipal funding/grants

Toronto Academy of Medicine, 179; milk commission, 106; and milk pasteurization, 107

Toronto General Hospital: and air ambulance service, 343; blue baby cases at, 229; Burnside Lying-in Hosital and, 38; Confederation and, 35–6; Dispensary, 37; expansion of College Street building, 115; Jewish hospital and, 198, 199; and medical philanthropy, 35; new College Street building, 114; nurse training program at, 57; nursing school, 88, 249, 250; Patterson and, 68; and penicillin, 220; and possible sites for University Avenue building/hospital, 197; private patients' pavilion, 114; proximity to HSC, 45, 146; sick immigrants in, 35; transfers from, 41; and University Health Network, 322

tracheomalacia, 289

trade unions. *See* unionization

Trayner, Phyllis, 274, 278

trisomies, 313

Tröhler, Ulrich, 87

Trudeau, Pierre Elliott, 285

Trusler, George, 234

trustees, board of. *See* board of trustees

Tsui, Lap-Chee, 316, 317

tubercular conditions: Great Ormond Street Hospital and, 12; heliotherapy and, 55, 182; and pasteurization legislation, 113; and preventorium, 174; streptomycin and, 223–4; and Thistletown patients, 181–2

tuberculosis: in Aboriginal populations, 223, 338–9; bacilli, 103–4, 105; bovine, 103, 112; as consumption, in industrial Britain, 9; environmental conditions and, 82; identification of bacteria, 80; incidence among HSC patients, 104; milk and, 103–4; mortality from, 103, 223; pulmonary, 222

typhoid: 9, 83, 101, 102, 106

typhus: 35

Underhill, Kesiah, 58, 61

Underwood, Michael, *A Treatise on the Diseases of Children,* 19

unionization: 1970s as height of, 284–5; and
donations from unionized employees,
202; HSC as non-union hospital, 259; of
nurses, 283, 285; nurses non-unionized at
HSC, 283
United Biscuit Company of America, 124
United States: bone marrow transplant
patients sent to, 304; concentration of
paediatrics in general hospitals in, 265;
Cystic Fibrosis Foundation, 317; health-
care system compared to Canada's, 291;
Medicaid, 290, 291; National Institutes
of Health, 317; numbers of children's
hospitals vs. general hospitals, 21
Universal Dispensary for Children, 15
University Avenue building: architecture, 197;
Bower and, 195; Campaign Executive
Committee, 200–1; College Street hospital
compared to, 217; construction, 203, 205;
conversion of wings for Patient Care
Centre, 300; cornerstone laying, 205;
daily capacity, 261; decorating scheme,
208–9; demobilization and, 202; facilities,
208; funding for, 199–202; and future
of Thistletown, 189; Great Depression
and, 155; Mount Sinai Hospital and,
198–9; move from College Street to,
209; occupancy rates, 261; opening of,
206–7, 212, 216; overcrowding at, 261,
299; preliminary plans for, 195, 197; as
replacement for College Street hospital, 4;
second fundraising campaign, 203, 205–6;
Second World War and, 155, 199–200;
sites for, 197–9, 200–1f, 203–4, 205; size,
208, 217; soil testing for, 202; space in,
203; specifications, 197; as state-of-art at
time of building, 299; technologies in,
208, 299; Toronto General Hospital and
sites for, 197; trade unions and, 202, 205;
and University of Toronto, 197; women
workers/volunteers in, 216–17
University Health Network, 322
University of Toronto: and academic freedom
of researchers, 333–4; affiliation with
HSC, 4, 45, 146; Department of Surgery,
82; discovery of insulin, 119; Faculty
Association, 328, 329; Faculty of Medicine,
37, 146–8; Grievance Review Panel, 329;
and Healy-CAMH affair, 334; household
science students in HSC pasteurization
unit, 112; and insulin, 129; Mount Sinai

and, 198, 199; medical school, 261; and
Olivieri/Apotex dispute, 328–9, 333–4;
and orthopaedic surgery, 82; orthopaedics
at, 93; and penicillin, 220; and research
ethics, 333–4; Rockefeller Foundation and,
147; and telemedicine, 344; University
Avenue building/hospital near, 197
university-industry partnerships: 1990s
research spending cuts and, 322; ethics of,
321; MRC and, 324
Upper Canada College volunteers, 215
urban environment: and living conditions for
poor in Toronto, 22, 25–6; removal of sick
children from, 178; Robertson and reform
of, 107; socio-economic conditions and
return to countryside/nature, 50–1. See
also poverty; socio-demographics; socio-
economic conditions
Urquhart, Norman C., 200–1

vaccination(s): early inoculation, 20;
immunization programs, 164, 224;
normativity of, 245; smallpox, 9, 20
vaccines: and decline in infectious diseases,
239; for poliomyelitis, 158, 164, 188, 224
Vanek, David, 274–6
Victoria Hospital for Sick Children, 75f;
appellation on College Street building,
217; city government loans for expansion,
94; colour of, 74–5; deaths at, 95; debt,
78; Dispensary, 95; domesticity of, 76;
growing importance for surgical care,
87; gymnasium, 78; internal structure,
76; medical casebooks, 82; medical
technology at, 76–8, 97; number of
surgical operations, 85; nurses' training
school, 87, 88; opening, 74; patient socio-
demographics, 82; physical environment,
76; reliance on probationary/pupil nurse
labour, 89; renaming of Hospital for Sick
Children as, 73; style/scale of building,
74–5; surgery at, 78, 82–7, 93, 94, 97;
verandahs, 76, 90; X-ray services, 77, 78,
94. See also College Street building
videoconferencing, 350, 353
visiting, home: by district/social service nurses,
140; and emergence of HSC, 45; to poor
and sick, 25, 29, 31
visitors, hospital: Brown's retirement and, 189;
closure of hospital to all, 173; general
public as, 173; history of, 171; Ladies

Committee and supervision of hospital operations, 34; lifting of restrictions on, 299; restrictions on, 172–4; social class and, 172; to Thistletown, 181f, 184–5; visiting hours, 172–4, 187–8. *See also* parent-child separation

vitamins: A, 121; B, 126; D, 121–3, 125, 130, 134, 137; enrichment of foods, 135, 137; invisibility of, 126–7

volunteerism, 169; health insurance and end of, 245; history of, 217; post-war formalization of, 217; and telethons, 296. *See also* Ladies Committee; Women's Auxiliary

waiting lists, 196, 302, 304
Waksman, Selman, 222
Wansbrough, Jean, 211, 212
Wansbrough, R.M., 194, 255
Ward, The. *See* St. John's Ward (Toronto)
water: chlorination, 113; clean, 104; quality of, 103
Watson, James, 313
Weatherall, Sir David, 328
welfare services/institutions: inspections, 63; municipal governments and, 28; sectarianism in, 28–9; size, compared to hospitals, 37. *See also* charity/charities
well-baby clinics, 141, 142, 143, 193
Wellcome Institute for the History of Medicine, 364
Wellcome Trust, 363–4
Wellesley Hospital, 196, 229, 250
West, Charles, 11–12
Westlake, Robert, 206
Whaley, J.B., 194
White, Michael, 302
Willard, De Forest, *The Surgery of Childhood*, 81
Willenegger, H., 182
Williams, H.H., 178
Williamson, Robert, 316–17
Wirsig, Claus, 259
Wisconsin Alumni Research Foundation (WARF), 123, 125, 126
women: attitudes toward breastfeeding, 118, 119; entering professional middle class, 209; and food preparation, 136; higher education, 209–10; Hillcrest Convalescent Home for, 182; as laboratory technicians,

136; as percentage of HSC staff, 259, 263f; as pioneers of children's hospitals, 23, 45, 57; post-Second World War domestic role, 209; as volunteers, 210; as workers/volunteers in University Avenue hospital, 216–17. *See also* Ladies Committee; mothers; nurses

women practitioners: in 1800s, 40; barriers to, 111f; Brown and, 210; as interns, 120; Reid as, 210–11; in research, 120–1; trustees and, 120

Women's Auxiliary: array of volunteer activities, 214–16; and Department of Recreation and Volunteer Services, 215; and 5Fifty5 shop, 213; founding of, 210–12; fundraising, 211, 212, 213–14; hours of unpaid work, 214–15; membership numbers, 212; membership social class, 211; and parents of hospitalized children, 189; and play spaces within hospital, 215; "quiet room," 233; supplementary hospital services, 212, 213–14; as supplementing female workforce, 217; and telethons, 296; tours on opening of University Avenue hospital, 212; training for members, 212; transporting patients during TTC strike, 214

Women's College Hospital, 121, 250, 258, 322
Women's Medical College, 111f
Workman, Joseph, 36
worthiness: charity and, 13, 29; of respectable poor, 149
Worton, Ron, 316, 331
Wright, F.H., 39

X-ray services/equipment, 70f, 77, 78, 94, 151

York University, medical school proposed for, 261, 265
Young, Judith, 187–8
Young, T. Kue, 350
Young Women's Christian Association, 25–6
Yuz, Steven, 269–70

Zeidler, Eb, 299
Zeidler Roberts Partnership, 300
Zipursky, Alvin, 354
Zlotkin, Stanley, 357